DIAGNOSTIC RADIOLOGY

of the

Dog and Cat

J. KEVIN KEALY, M.V.M., M.R.C.V.S., D.V.R.

Professor and Head,
Department of Veterinary Surgery,
  Obstetrics and Radiology,
University College Dublin,
Veterinary College of Ireland,
Dublin, Ireland

Former Head of Radiology,
Iowa State University,
Ames, Iowa

1979

W. B. SAUNDERS COMPANY   Philadelphia · London · Toronto

W. B. Saunders Company: West Washington Square
Philadelphia, PA   19105

1 St. Anne's Road
Eastbourne, East Sussex BN21 3UN, England

1 Goldthorne Avenue
Toronto, Ontario M8Z 5T9, Canada

Library of Congress Cataloging in Publication Data

Main entry under title:

Diagnostic radiology of the dog and cat.

1. Veterinary radiography.   2. Cats – Diseases – Diagnosis.
   3. Dogs – Diseases – Diagnosis.   I. Kealy, J. Kevin.

SF757.8.D5   636.7′08′960757   78–54517

ISBN 0–7216–5306–5

Diagnostic Radiology
of the Dog and Cat   ISBN   0-7216-5306-5

Last digit is the print number: 9   8   7   6   5   4   3   2   1

FOR

JOAN

and

JOHN, STEPHANIE, PAUL,
MICHAEL, COLETTE, and JANE

PREFACE

This book has been written for students and small animal practitioners. The basic concept was to provide a simple, introductory guide to the interpretation of radiographs, illustrating normal anatomy and the more commonly encountered abnormalities and anomalies. While it is true that different disease entities may cause similar radiographic changes, nonetheless the recognition of certain radiologic signs as indicators of specific disease processes is important, especially for the novice. The development of an orderly, logical, and consistent approach to the viewing of radiographs is a prerequisite for advancement in the art and science of interpretation.

In attempting to keep the book to a reasonable size and at the same time to provide an adequate introduction to the subject, many decisions had to be made as to what to include and what to exclude. Such decisions are necessarily arbitrary and subjective. It is understandable, therefore, that the finished product may not please everybody. If, however, this offering proves acceptable and useful to those for whom it is intended, the effort expended in its production will have been adequately rewarded.

KEVIN KEALY
Dublin. April, 1979.

v

ACKNOWLEDGMENTS

I am happy to express my sincere gratitude to the many colleagues who were so generous with their time and patience in assisting me with various aspects of this work.

I am particularly indebted to Dr. Russell Mitten, Radiologist at Iowa State University, who, at considerable inconvenience to himself, allowed me repeated access to his files, read the manuscript, and made many useful suggestions, virtually all of which were adopted. I received continued support and encouragement from Dr. W. M. Wass, Professor and Head, Department of Veterinary Clinical Sciences, and from Dean Phillip Pearson at Iowa State. I am sincerely grateful to them both. I would also like to acknowledge assistance received from Mr. Tom Hall and Mrs. Jolene Jacob, x-ray technicians.

Dr. Harker Rhodes of the University of Pennsylvania advised me on many aspects of the project and Dr. Darryl Biery helped with several illustrations.

Mr. Ian Hughes of Merseyside, England, read much of the manuscript and advised on the particular problems of the practitioner. Valued assistance was also received from Dr. Myron Bernstein and Dr. Jack Dinsmore of Chicago.

In Dublin, Mr. Michael Lucey was most helpful, reading the manuscript and assisting with the illustrations. Dr. Terence Grimes provided a number of illustrations for Chapter 5. Miss Hester McAllister, Radiologist at the Dublin school, gave much useful assistance as did Mrs. Phyl Smith and Miss Colette Crosbie, our radiographers.

It is certain that the book would never have been completed were it not for the unwavering support, encouragement, and patience of Mr. Carroll Cann of the W. B. Saunders Company. I also wish to acknowledge the help and courtesy received from Mr. Sandy Reinhardt, Mrs. Laura Tarves, Mr. Ray Kersey, Mr. Bill Lamsback and Miss Karen O'Keefe.

About half the material used originated in the school at Dublin, the rest at Iowa State University. I am grateful to my clinical colleagues and friends in both schools who put their case records at my disposal.

Finally, while I have had the assistance of many people, the errors are peculiarly my own and I would appreciate having my attention drawn to them.

CONTENTS

Chapter 6

THE RADIOGRAPH

Competent radiologic practice presupposes the availability of good quality radiographs. Familiarity with the basic principles underlying the production of radiographs is a prerequisite for the radiologist. Accurate positioning of the animal under investigation, correct exposure factors, the use of grids and other ancillary aids, and good darkroom technique all influence the quality of the radiograph. The use of a technique chart is essential for consistent results. Consistency is important, particularly when studies have to be repeated over a period of time to assess the progress of a case. If the radiographs in such studies are not comparable, errors of interpretation are liable to occur. Radiographs may be of poor quality because of improper positioning, improper exposure technique, or poor darkroom technique. It is hazardous to attempt to interpret such radiographs.

Radiographic technique is discussed in this book only in so far as is necessary for a proper understanding of points of interpretation. The necessary detailed information on technique can be found in any of the several works devoted to this topic.

A radiograph is a composite shadow of structures and objects in the path of an x-ray beam recorded on film. Because a radiograph is, in essence, a shadowgraph, the geometric rules applicable to the formation of shadows are

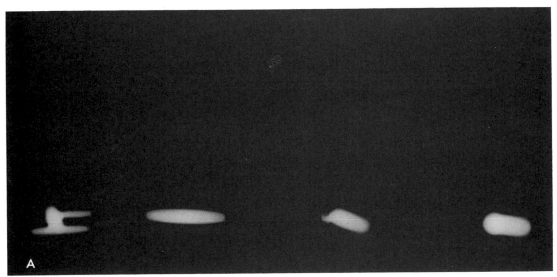

FIGURE 1–1. The necessity for two views. *A,* Four objects have been radiographed in an end-on position. On this view alone, insufficient information is available to enable a comprehensive description to be given of any item.
(Illustration continued on following page.)

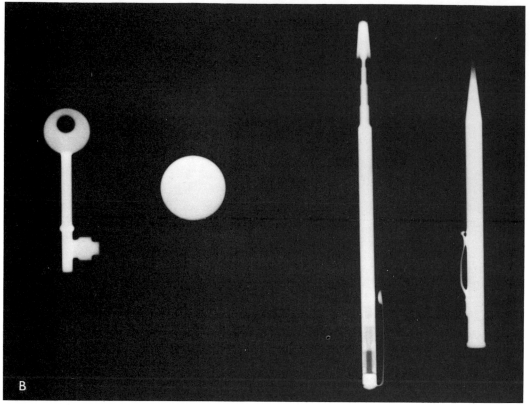

FIGURE 1–1. *Continued. B.* A second view, made at right angles to the first one, shows the items, from left to right, to be a key, a coin, a teacher's pointer, and a propelling pencil.

also valid for radiographs. Thus, the nearer the object under examination is to the film, the sharper will be its outline. Distance of an object from the film causes magnification of the resulting shadow and some distortion and blurring. The nearer an object is to the source of radiation, the greater the degree of magnification. The area being studied should, therefore, be placed as near to the film as possible. Because the radiograph is a shadowgraph and so outlines an object in only two planes, at least two views made at different angles are required in order to demonstrate the object in a three dimensional representation. The standard views are usually made at right angles to one another. (Fig. 1–1).

The radiograph is not a simple shadowgraph. The x-ray beam, or some of it, passes through the body that is under examination. Some of the incident radiation is absorbed and some is scattered. Shadows are cast not only of the outline of the body but also of structures within it. Not all substances allow x-rays to pass through them in the same way. Dense substances, like bone, inhibit the passage of radiation, while those that are less dense, such as gases, allow the rays to pass through them virtually unchanged. In between, there are substances, such as the soft tissues, that permit more radiation to reach the film than is permitted by bone but not as much as is permitted by gases. It is this differential absorption of x-rays that enables one structure to be distinguished from another.

DENSITY

A radiograph is an image made up of shadows of different densities. A distinction must be made between *subject density* and *radiographic density*.

SUBJECT DENSITY. Subject density is the weight per given volume of different body structures or other objects. Bone is more dense than muscle and muscle is more dense than fat. The denser an object the more it inhibits the passage of radiation.

RADIOGRAPHIC DENSITY. Radiographic density is a measure of the blackening of a film caused by x-rays. Where x-rays readily reach the film, the film appears black after processing. If the rays are prevented from reaching part of a film, the unaffected area will appear translucent (white) on the processed film. Between these extremes various combinations of light and dark areas are produced. Radiographic density is, therefore, dependent on subject density, for the greater the subject density the less radiation reaches the film.

Five radiographic densities can be recognized:

1. Mineral
2. Bone
3. Fluid (soft tissue)
4. Fat
5. Gas (air)

Mineral substances are very dense and inhibit the passage of virtually all incident radiation. Areas of film covered by such materials appear white on a radiograph.

Bone is not as dense as are mineral substances but it allows only little radiation to pass through it, as compared with other body tissues. Areas of film that have been covered by bone appear almost white on a radiograph.

Fluid inhibits the passage of more of the incident radiation than does gas but not as much as does bone. A fluid density lies between the whiteness of a bone density and the blackness of a gas density. Fluid densities appear grey on a radiograph. As soft tissues consist for the most part of fluid, soft tissue density and fluid density appear similar. All fluid densities appear the same. It is not possible, consequently, to distinguish radiologically between blood, chyle, transudates, and exudates.

Fat density falls between fluid and gas densities. Fat may help to outline structures that would not otherwise be seen. Perirenal fat may outline the kidneys by providing a contrasting density to the denser soft tissues.

Gases, including air, allow x-rays to pass freely through them. Areas of film covered by gas-containing organs, such as the lungs, appear dark on a radiograph.

Bone, fluid, fat, and gas occur normally within the body and are said to have biologic densities. Mineral densities are introduced into the body as contrast media or as foreign bodies. (Fig. 1–2).

A *fluid level* is the term given to the interface between fluid and gas. The fluid line is always horizontal.

The term *increased density* is used to denote a whiter shadow on the radiograph than would normally be expected. It thus refers to increased subject density as reflected on the radiograph. The increased subject density allows less radiation to reach the film. *Decreased density* denotes a darker shadow on the radiograph than would normally be anticipated. The decreased subject density allows more radiation to reach the film.

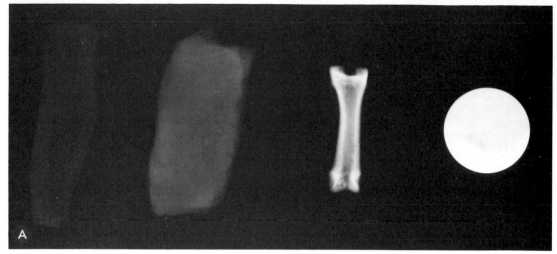

FIGURE 1–2. The five radiographic densities. *A.* A gas (air) shadow surrounds, from left to right, fat, soft tissue, bone, and mineral densities.

(*Illustration continued on opposite page.*)

All objects inhibit, to some extent, the passage of radiation. Structures that absorb little of the incident radiation are said to be *radiolucent*. They appear dark on a radiograph. Structures that inhibit the passage of most of the incident radiation are said to be *radiopaque*. *Increased radiolucency* represents decreased subject density; *increased* (radio-) *opacity* represents increased subject density. A *radiolucent defect* is an area of decreased density within a structure.

CONTRAST

Contrast means difference. Structures can be distinguished from one another on a radiograph only if they contrast with their surroundings. That is to say, they are seen when they have a different radiographic density from that which surrounds them. Structures lying in contact with one another cannot be distinguished as separate entities if they have the same density. If a structure is surrounded by a radiopaque material it will appear relatively radiolucent, while if it is surrounded by a radiolucent material it will appear relatively radiopaque.

Artifacts are markings seen on a film due to some technical fault, for example dirt in a cassette. They must be distinguished from anatomic changes.

RADIOGRAPHIC CHANGES

As well as demonstrating the varying densities of bodies under examination, the x-ray beam also demonstrates their outlines. The edges of a bone permit determination of its size and shape, and the varying densities of the cortex and medulla will also be visible. A radiograph, then, is an image consisting of the outlines of structures and their varying densities. It can be said, therefore, that as far as abnormalities are concerned, only two observations of

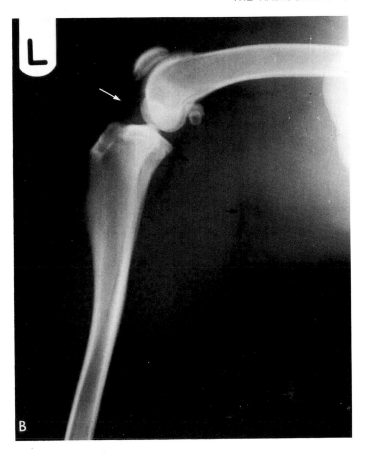

FIGURE 1-2. *Continued B.* A lateral view of a stifle joint demonstrates the five radiographic densities. A mineral density surrounds the L marker. The femur, patella, fabellae, and tibia have bone density. The muscles have soft tissue density. Fat density (arrows) is seen between the muscle planes and caudal to the straight patellar ligament. A gas (air) density surrounds the limb.

significance can be made from the study of a radiograph. One can detect the following:

(a) changes in outline, and

(b) changes in density.

Changes in outline include changes in position and contour. Pathology in an organ may be deduced from the fact that it displaces an adjacent organ. Changes in density include changes in radiographic detail; for example, changes in trabecular pattern within a bone may be the first evidence of a disease process.

STANDARD VIEWS

In order that changes in outline and changes in density be appreciated it is essential that the radiologist be familiar with the appearance of normal structures as they appear on radiographs, that is, radiologic anatomy. Since almost any structure can be rotated through 360°, it would be virtually impossible to become familiar with all the possible projections that could be produced by any given organ. Consequently, standard views of each part of the body are used. These usually consist of two views made at right angles to one another.

Agreed terms are used to describe the standard views. If a compound word is used in the description of a particular view, the first word of the compound indicates where the x-ray beam enters the body and the second word indicates where it emerges. The x-ray plate is positioned where the beam emerges. The standard views are craniocaudal, lateral, ventrodorsal, dorsoventral, and oblique.

CRANIOCAUDAL.   This term is used to describe views of the limbs made when the x-ray beam strikes the cranial aspect of a limb and emerges caudally. From the carpus and tarsus distally the term dorsopalmar is used to describe the same view. This was formerly referred to as an anteroposterior view.

LATERAL.   On the lateral view the x-ray beam is directed at right angles to its direction on the craniocaudal view. The beam is directed on to the lateral aspect of the limb and it emerges on the medial aspect. An almost similar view is produced if the beam enters the limb on the medial aspect and emerges laterally. The terms *lateromedial* and *mediolateral* are occasionally used to distinguish between views made from the lateral or medial aspects of the limbs.

VENTRODORSAL.   This term describes radiographs of the trunk, neck, or head made with the animal in dorsal recumbency. The beam enters the body on the ventral aspect and emerges dorsally. This was formerly called an anteroposterior view.

DORSOVENTRAL.   For this view the x-ray beam enters the body on its dorsal aspect and emerges on the ventral aspect. It is made with the animal in sternal recumbency. This view may be used to study the trunk, neck, or head. Its use is usually confined to the thorax and skull. It was formerly called a posteroanterior view.

OBLIQUE.   This term indicates that the view is made somewhere between the standard views made at right angles to one another.

CONTRAST MEDIA

Contrast media are frequently used as diagnostic aids. A contrast medium is a substance introduced into the body to outline a structure or structures not normally visualized or poorly visualized on plain radiographs. *Positive contrast media* are materials that are radiopaque. When introduced into the body they outline the structures that contain them. They may also outline objects within these structures that would not otherwise be seen, such as radiolucent foreign bodies. *Negative contrast media* are gases that are introduced into the body to provide contrast. Air is commonly used to outline the bladder. Carbon dioxide may be used in pneumoperitoneum to outline abdominal organs.

A *filling defect* is a space-occupying mass within a hollow organ. Contrast medium fails to fill the organ fully at the site of the defect.

VIEWING THE RADIOGRAPH

Radiographs should be viewed under optimal conditions. A room with subdued lighting is best. The radiograph is placed on a viewing box, or illuminator, which has fluorescent lighting. This gives an even light intensity over the entire film. Any other method of viewing is unsatisfactory. For anatomic reasons the entire radiograph is not evenly illuminated in most cases. Thin parts of the body will appear darker than thicker parts. It is useful to have a bright light

available to give added illumination to the darker parts. The standard illuminator is designed to illuminate the largest radiograph in common use. When viewing smaller films, light coming from the viewing screen around the film may
cause troublesome glare. Masks are available to adapt illuminators to different
sizes of films. Masks can be homemade from dark cardboard or other suitable
material. Direct light falling on the illuminator may make viewing difficult. The
use of a magnifying glass is sometimes helpful in detecting fine radiographic
detail. It is particularly helpful in the study of bone structure.

Radiographs, by convention, are placed on the illuminator with the left
side of the animal to the radiologist's right. They are so displayed throughout
this book. There is no general agreement as to whether lateral views should be
displayed with the animal's head facing toward the left or the right. The prefer-
ence appears to be for the head to point toward the left and it is so presented
here. Radiographs should always be placed on the illuminator in the same way,
to facilitate ready recognition of anatomic structures.

SYSTEMATIC APPROACH

The radiologist should train himself from the beginning to adopt a systematic approach to the viewing of radiographs. This will ensure that all of the film
is examined and not just the area in which a lesion is believed to exist. Frequently, significant changes are demonstrated away from the area of immediate
interest.

It is good radiographic practice to have the area of interest located at the
center of the film. Here there is least distortion of the image, and structures on
either side can be seen. Since the center of the radiograph tends to attract the
eye first, it is probably good practice to examine the periphery of the radiograph first and systematically progress to the center. Each structure encountered should be noted for position, normality, or abnormality. The center of the
radiograph is examined last. If an obvious lesion at the center of a radiograph
is examined first, there is a tendency to only glance over the rest of the film,
particularly if the lesion that is seen fits in with a tentative diagnosis. Any method
of viewing that ensures a systematic examination of the entire radiograph is
acceptable.

Some radiologists prefer to examine radiographs "cold," that is, without
any knowledge of the clinical picture. They then evaluate their observations in
the light of the clinical and other findings. Preconceived notions about a case
may militate against an objective assessment of the radiograph.

Beginners are prone to two kinds of error. Either they miss something that
should have been seen or they overread the radiograph. Overreading a radiograph means drawing conclusions from it that are not warranted on the objective evidence. This is most likely to happen if one has been involved in the
clinical assessment of the case and has already reached a tentative diagnosis.
There is a definite tendency to see what one wishes to see.

The ability to read radiographs thoroughly and accurately comes only with
practice and attention to detail. The interpretation of radiographs involves a
careful examination of the film coupled with a sound knowledge of radiologic
anatomy and an appreciation of the changes in structure and function caused
by disease processes. While it is essential that one be aware of the radiologic
signs commonly associated with different disease processes, it must be remem-

bered that the same disease does not always manifest itself in the same way. One disease process may be superimposed on another. Different diseases may produce similar radiologic changes. The formulation of a list of differential diagnoses is an important part of the work of the radiologist, who must be prepared to reconcile his observations with the clinical findings and with the results of ancillary diagnostic studies other than radiology.

REFERENCES

Carlson, W. (1977). Veterinary Radiology. Lea and Febiger. Philadelphia.

Douglas, S. W. and Williamson, H. D. (1970). Veterinary Radiological Interpretation. Lea and Febiger. Philadelphia.

Douglas, S. W. and Williamson, H. D. (1972). Principles of Veterinary Radiography. 2nd. ed. Williams and Wilkins Co. Baltimore.

Meschan, I. (1957). Roentgen Signs in Clinical Diagnosis. W. B. Saunders Co. Philadelphia.

Meyer, Wendy. (1977). Radiography Review. Radiographic Density. J.A.V.R.S. XVIII. 5. 138.

Morgan, J. P., Silverman, S. and Zontine, W. J. (1975). Techniques of Veterinary Radiography. The Printer, Davis, California.

Ticer, J. W. (1975). Radiographic Technique in Small Animal Practice. W. B. Saunders Co. Philadelphia.

THE ABDOMEN 2

Visualization of the abdominal organs depends on a number of factors taken singly or in combination:

1. Differences in density between one organ and another.

2. The amount of fat present within the abdomen. Emaciated or very young animals with little abdominal fat show poor contrast.

3. The contents of abdominal organs vary in density. Air or gas in the stomach may outline that organ as feces may outline the colon.

In order to demonstrate detail within the abdomen special contrast procedures are frequently necessary.

RADIOGRAPHY

The standard views used to study the abdomen are the right and left lateral recumbent and the ventrodorsal. The ventrodorsal is to be preferred to the dorsoventral, which tends to compress the viscera and cause irregular displacement of them. A standing lateral view may sometimes be employed, especially if peritoneal fluid is suspected. It should be remembered, however, that no fluid line will be seen unless there is a concomitant pneumoperitoneum.

For lateral projections the sternum should be supported by foam rubber pads to maintain it on the same level as the lumbar spine. The limbs should be held at right angles to the vertebral column. The x-ray beam should be collimated to include the diaphragm and the pelvic inlet. In ventrodorsal views in which the inguinal flank folds may cast marked shadows, the "frog-leg" position may be preferred to having the limbs drawn out behind.

Because the degree of contrast between the various abdominal organs is small, it is essential that good quality films be produced to get the maximum information. Adequate patient preparation and good radiographic technique are both important.

Except in emergency cases, the patient should be fasted for at least 12 hours prior to investigation and for at least 18 hours if contrast radiography is contemplated. Water may be allowed. The use of a mild cathartic administered the day before the examination is helpful. If feces are present in the colon an enema should be administered. Isotonic saline enemas or pure water enemas are recommended. The temperature of the enema fluid should be less than body temperature. This helps to cause expulsion of much of the gas that would remain in the colon if a warm enema were given.

A low kilovoltage, high milliamperage technique will enhance contrast. A grid should be used in animals that have a thickness of 10 cms or more. When determining the thickness of the abdomen the measurement should be made at the point of its greatest depth, usually over the caudal rib cage. The actual exposure should be made during the expiratory pause. (Fig. 2–1).

9

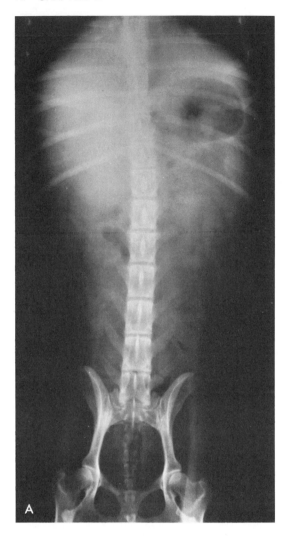

FIGURE 2–1. *A, B.* A normal canine abdomen. (*Illustration continued on opposite page.*)

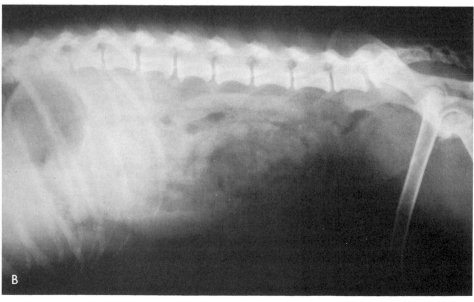

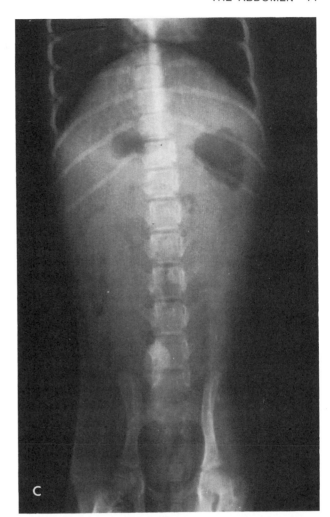

FIGURE 2–1. *Continued.* *C, D.* The abdomen of a puppy. The contrast is not as good as in the adult animal.

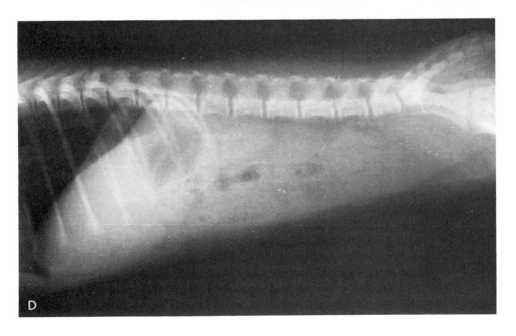

Pneumoperitonography is a useful aid in the study of the abdomen. Air, oxygen, carbon dioxide, or nitrous oxide is introduced into the peritoneal cavity by means of a syringe or a gas cylinder and a needle and three-way valve. The needle is inserted through the abdominal wall a little caudal and to the right of the umbilicus to avoid the danger of introducing gas into the spleen. Sufficient gas is introduced to distend the abdomen moderately. If abdominal fluid is present it should first be withdrawn. The procedure is not very disturbing to the patient and it can be done under deep sedation. Carbon dioxide and nitrous oxide have the advantage of being rapidly absorbed from the peritoneal cavity. If using a gas cylinder care should be taken to not overdistend the abdomen. Gas rises to the highest point within the abdomen, and thus different organs can be outlined by varying the animal's posture.

Retropneumoperitoneal visualization of abdominal organs has been described. The technique involves the insertion of a needle between the root of the tail and the anus into the retroperitoneal space. It would appear to be of limited value.

NORMAL APPEARANCE

On survey radiographs of the abdomen one can usually recognize the stomach, the small and large intestines, the liver, the spleen, the bladder, and the diaphragm. The kidneys are seen in about 50 per cent of studies. The os penis and the prepuce are seen in the male dog and teats are often seen in the female. The position and appearance of the normal viscera vary somewhat with the posture of the animal, the amount of food material present in the alimentary tract, and the respiratory movements.

ABNORMALITIES

ABDOMINAL MASSES. Masses within the abdominal cavity are due to abnormal enlargements of one or more of the intra-abdominal structures. A mass can usually be identified on plain radiographs. Some estimation of its origin may be gained from its position and the manner and degree of displacement of other organs. Sublumbar masses can be seen on lateral views. They may be due to enlarged lymph nodes, abscesses, adrenomegaly, or neoplasia of vertebrae or sublumbar structures. They displace the abdominal organs in their neighborhood ventrally. Other enlarged lymph nodes may present as intra-abdominal masses in other locations. (Fig. 2–2).

ASCITES. Ascites is the term given to a collection of extracellular fluid within the abdominal cavity. It is commonly used to describe the presence of any fluid in the abdominal cavity.

Fluid within the abdominal cavity causes the abdomen to appear more radiopaque than usual. The film may appear to be underexposed. The increased density is widely distributed throughout the abdomen causing a loss of detail in structures normally seen. This appearance is sometimes referred to as a ''ground glass'' appearance. Gas within the bowel may be seen through the fluid. Usually, the abdomen will be seen to be distended because of the fluid contained within it. Standing lateral films show an increased density in the ventral part of the abdomen, where fluid accumulates, and a more normal density dorsally. A gas-fluid interface will not be seen unless there is free gas within

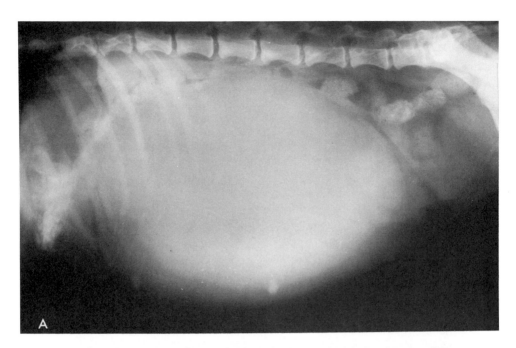

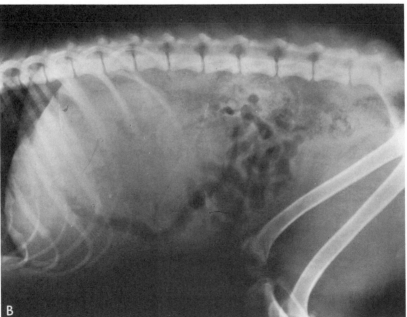

FIGURE 2–2. Intra-abdominal mass. *A.* A large mass arising in the spleen. *B, C.* This mass in the right upper quadrant of the abdomen is displacing the intestines caudally and the duodenum ventro-medially. The mass was a hydronephrotic right kidney. *D.* Masses (arrows) associated with enlarged sublumbar lymph nodes.

(Illustration continued on following page.)

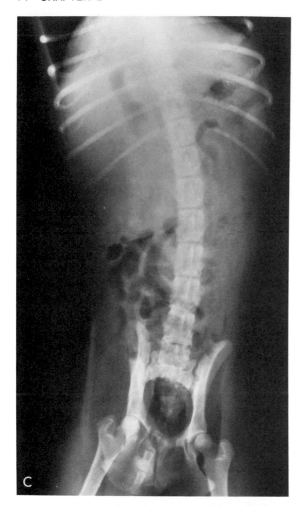

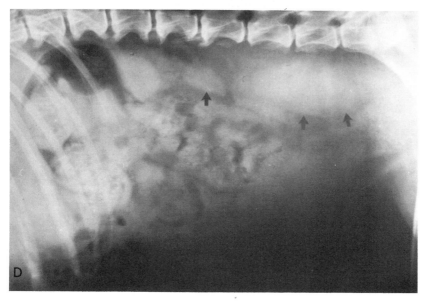

FIGURE 2-2. *Continued.*

the peritoneal cavity. Loops of intestine that contain gas tend to rise into the dorsal abdomen and "float" on the fluid. Occasionally, the faint outline of an abdominal mass may be identified through the fluid.

The fluid may be exudative or transudative in origin or it may be blood, chyle, urine, or bile. The causes of ascites are manifold and include neoplasia, congestive heart failure, hepatic disease, renal disease, hypoproteinemia, warfarin poisoning, trauma, and peritonitis. (Fig. 2–3).

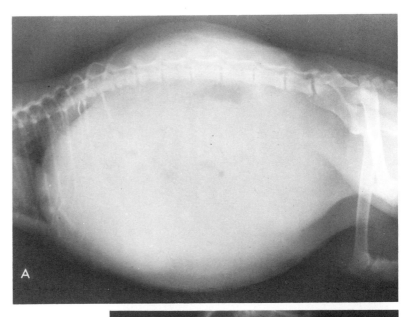

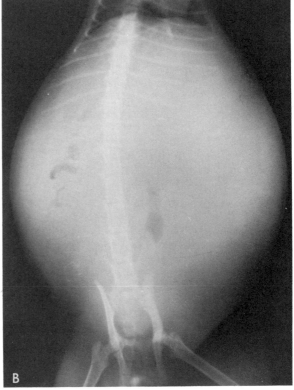

FIGURE 2–3. *A, B.* Ascites in a cat. The abdomen is grossly distended and there is loss of intra-abdominal detail. There is rotation of the abdomen on both views. The distention made accurate positioning difficult.

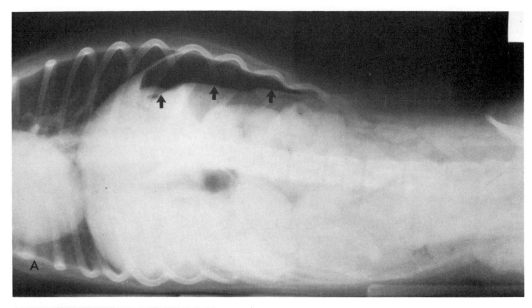

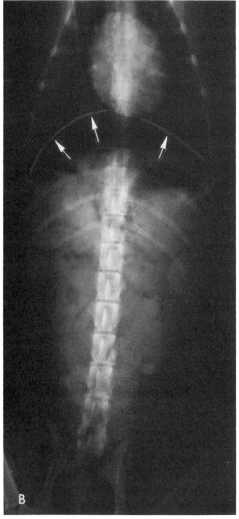

FIGURE 2–4. *A, B.* Free air within the abdomen following a laparotomy. The left lateral recumbent view (*A*) shows air (arrows) under the ribs. *B* was made with the animal supported by the forelegs. Air can be seen caudal to the diaphragm (arrows). The diaphragm lines are outlined with pencil for greater clarity.

Other conditions may give a somewhat similar appearance. Peritonitis causes a loss of detail within the abdominal shadow but the abdomen is not distended. Emaciation causes loss of abdominal detail because of fat depletion. Young animals lack intra-abdominal fat and so show poor abdominal detail. Care should be taken not to mistake a fluid-filled viscus for ascites. A grossly distended bladder can extend very far cranially into the abdomen. Perirenal cysts may be quite extensive and may simulate ascites.

Reradiographing the animal following paracentesis is often helpful in furthering a diagnosis. It can be difficult to detect small amounts of fluid radiographically.

FREE GAS IN THE ABDOMEN.   Free gas in the abdomen may be seen for several days following laparotomy. It may also be the result of a penetrating wound through the abdominal wall or of rupture of an abdominal viscus. The gas usually has an irregular shape and will be seen not to conform to the shape of any of the abdominal organs. Its position will change with changes in posture of the animal.

Free gas in the abdomen may be demonstrated on a ventrodorsal view with the animal in left lateral recumbency. The gas will be seen in the uppermost part of the abdomen under the abdominal wall. On ventrodorsal views made in right lateral recumbency there may be difficulty in distinguishing free gas from gas within the stomach. Alternatively, the animal may be supported on its hind limbs and a ventrodorsal radiograph made. The free gas will then be seen accumulated under the diaphragm. On a standing lateral view gas will be seen in the sublumbar area. (Fig. 2–4).

If gas is present in considerable amounts the various abdominal organs will be outlined by it and the film may appear to have been overexposed.

PERITONITIS.   Peritonitis causes loss of the sharp outline of the abdominal organs so that the abdomen in the affected area appears hazy or blurred. Small, irregular areas of increased density (mottling) are often evident. Fluid, if present, causes a further loss of detail. Free gas can be seen if there has been perforation of the intestine. (Fig. 2–5).

In steatitis in cats detail is diminished owing to increased density in the falciform, inguinal, and perirenal fat. It may be confused with peritonitis.

HERNIAS.   Radiography is sometimes of value in the diagnosis of a hernia.

Umbilical and Scrotal Hernias.   These are usually diagnosed on clinical examination. Displaced loops of intestine may be seen on radiographs.

Inguinal Hernia.   Radiography can help to determine the contents of an inguinal hernia. Gas shadows within the hernial outline indicate the presence of a portion of the intestine. The uterus casts a homogeneous fluid-type density as does the bladder. Fetal skeletons may be seen if the animal is in late pregnancy. A barium study can be used to determine the position of the intestine.

Ventral Hernia.   There may occasionally be doubt as to the nature of a swelling on the abdominal wall. In ventral hernia, radiographs will show gas-containing loops of intestine outside the abdomen and under the skin. The point of herniation may be seen as a discontinuity in the shadow of the abdominal wall. If necessary, intraperitoneal or subcutaneous injection of water-soluble contrast material will coat the abdominal contents and show their position.

Perineal Hernia.   Radiographs can help to determine the contents of a perineal hernia. Contrast cystography will show whether or not the bladder is in the hernia. If there is retroflexion of the bladder some difficulty may be experienced in introducing a catheter.

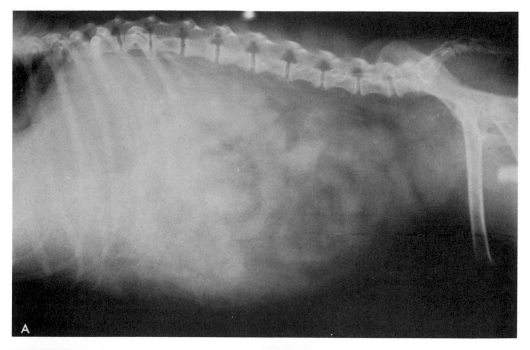

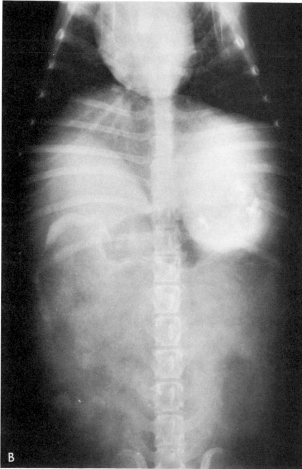

FIGURE 2–5. *A, B.* Loss of intra-abdominal detail due to peritonitis. The abdomen has a granular appearance as distinct from the homogeneous appearance of ascites. Some barium is present in the stomach and duodenum. This was a nine year old female rat terrier with chronic pancreatic necrosis.

Hiatal Hernia. This is a very rare hernia in which there is protrusion of a structure through the esophageal hiatus of the diaphragm. The cardiac area of the stomach is most likely to be involved. A barium study will show the position of the stomach. To demonstrate this hernia it is usually necessary to have the animal tilted with the head down, since the stomach may slide in and out of the thorax.

Peritoneopericardial Hernia. Abdominal organs may reach the pericardial sac through an abnormal communication between the pericardial sac and the peritoneal cavity. The cardiac outline is increased in size on radiographs and intestinal gas shadows may be seen within the cardiac shadow. Diagnosis may be difficult, particularly if the pericardial sac contains only omentum. A barium study may help.

Diaphragmatic Hernia. This hernia is dealt with in Chapter 3.

If a hernia becomes strangulated, dilated loops of bowel will be seen proximal to the herniated portion of intestine and perhaps within the herniated intestine. (Fig. 2–6).

The Liver

ANATOMY

Cranially, the liver is convex in outline and it lies mainly in contact with the diaphragm. The caudal surface is irregularly concave and lies in contact with the stomach, duodenum, pancreas, and right kidney. Of the four liver lobes, the left hepatic lobe is the largest. It may be contained within the costal arch or protrude a short, but variable, distance caudal to the ventral portion of the arch. The right medial lobe may also protrude beyond the level of the costal arch.

RADIOGRAPHY

An impression of liver size can usually be gained from a study of plain radiographs of the abdomen. It can be clearly visualized using pneumoperitonography. Lateral and ventrodorsal radiographs are made with the animal supported on its hind limbs. Cholecystography will outline the gall bladder and bile ducts but gives little information about the shape of the liver. It may assist in showing its position, for example in diaphragmatic hernia.

NORMAL APPEARANCE

The exact outline of the liver is not discernible on plain radiographs of the abdomen. On lateral radiographs it occupies a triangular area between the diaphragm and the ventral abdominal wall. Its caudal border is sharp in outline and may project a short distance caudal to the ventral portion of the costal arch. Sometimes its shadow merges with that of the spleen. This obscures its caudal limit.

On the ventrodorsal view the liver appears as a homogeneous density behind the diaphragm. Its outline is not well marked. In this view the caudal and

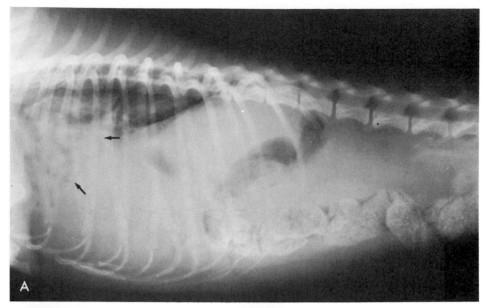

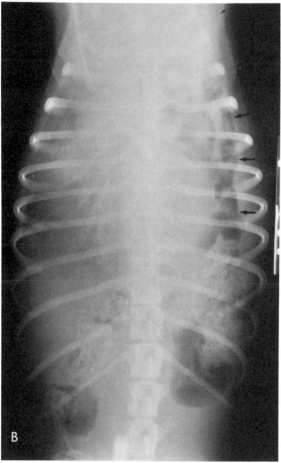

FIGURE 2–6. Hernias. *A, B.* Diaphragmatic hernia. Small intestine gas shadows can be seen within the thorax (arrows). The abdomen appears empty except for the large intestine. The diaphragm lines are obscured.
(*Illustration continued on opposite page.*)

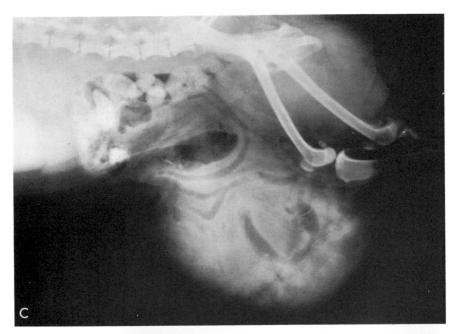

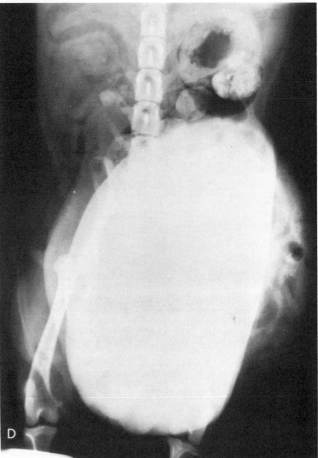

FIGURE 2–6. *Continued C, D.* A large inguinal hernia. Small intestine gas shadows can be seen within the hernial swelling on the lateral view. The hernia appears as a dense mass on the ventrodorsal view. (*Illustration continued on following page.*)

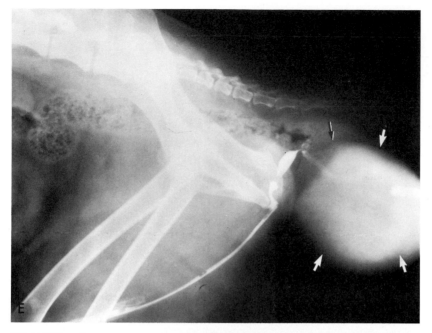

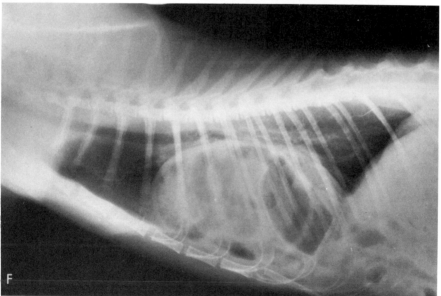

FIGURE 2-6. *Continued. E.* A perineal hernia containing the bladder. The bladder is outlined by contrast medium (*arrows*). *F.* Peritoneopericardial hernia. The cardiac shadow is enlarged and distorted Small and large intestinal gas shadows can be seen within the cardiac outline.

intermediate lobes of the lungs are superimposed on it and pulmonary vessels are frequently seen through the liver shadow. The position and shape of the liver vary with changes in position of the animal. Right lateral recumbency allows the left hepatic lobe to move caudally, causing it to cast a larger shadow than it does in left lateral recumbency. Oblique views may produce an apparent rounding of the caudoventral edge. (Fig. 2–7).

The falciform ligament appears larger on expiration than on inspiration.

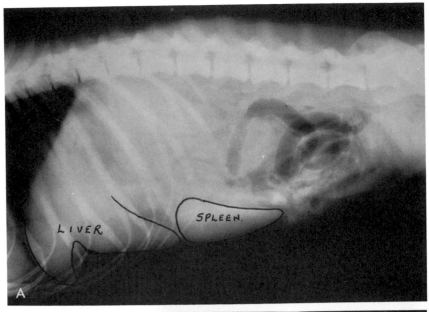

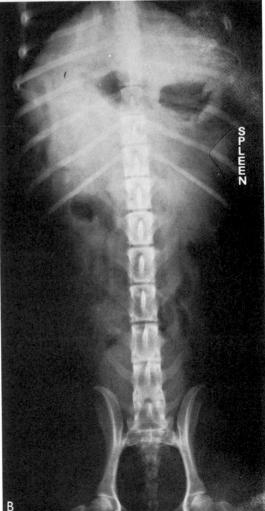

FIGURE 2-7. *A, B.* The positions of the normal liver and spleen.
(*Illustration continued on following page.*)

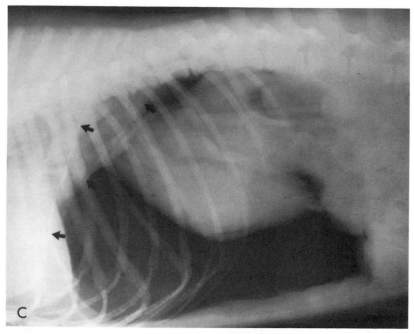

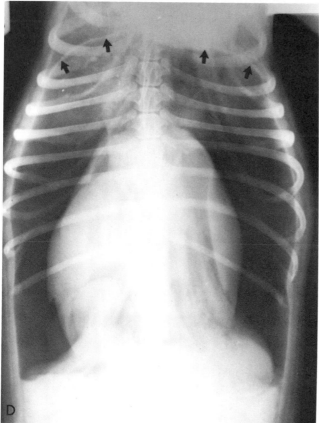

FIGURE 2–7. *Continued. C, D.* Lateral and ventrodorsal views of a normal liver outlined by pneumoperitoneum. These radiographs were made with the animal in an erect posture, that is, supported standing on the hind legs. Arrows indicate the position of the diaphragm.

ABNORMALITIES

ENLARGEMENT (Hepatomegaly). Enlargement of the liver may be the result of cardiac incompetence, primary or secondary neoplasia, inflammation, hyperplasia, infiltrative diseases such as lipidosis or amyloidosis, and engorgement with bile. Generalized enlargement is associated with rounding of the caudoventral edge, which extends further into the abdomen than it normally does. There is also displacement of those structures related to the liver. The stomach is displaced caudally, dorsally, and to the left. The duodenum is displaced to the left. The small intestine may be displaced caudally, as may the right kidney.

Localized masses within the liver may cause a variety of displacements, depending on their size and location. Thus, for example, cranial or caudal displacement of the stomach may occur with either right- or left-sided masses, because the liver is placed more to the right side than to the left. In general, however, masses in the right side of the liver tend to displace the stomach and duodenum to the left, while left-sided masses tend to displace those organs toward the right side. A mass originating in the right side of the liver may displace the tail of the spleen caudally. (Fig. 2–8).

REDUCED SIZE (Microliver). The liver may be reduced in size in cirrhosis because of scar contraction. Reduction in size may also be associated with vascular anomalies such as portocaval shunts. Reduced size of the liver is diffi-

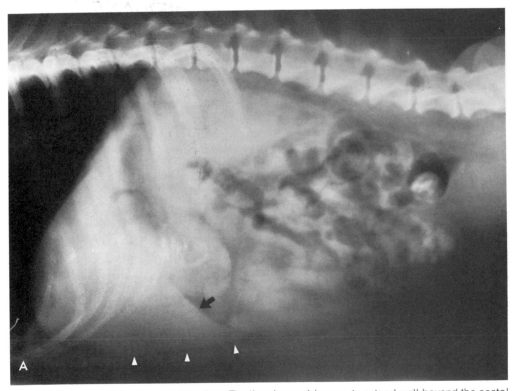

FIGURE 2–8. *A.* Enlargement of the liver. The liver (arrows) is seen to extend well beyond the costal arch.

(*Illustration continued on following page.*)

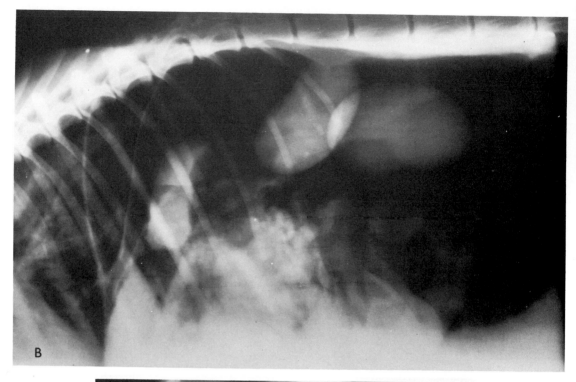

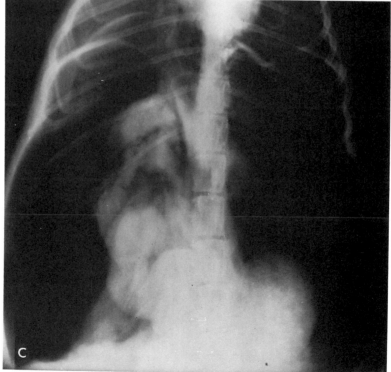

FIGURE 2–8. *Continued.   B C.*   Nodular densities in the liver demonstrated by pneumoperitoneum. The lateral view was made with the dog in ventral recumbency and fluid can be seen in the dependent part of the abdomen.

(*Illustration continued on opposite page.*)

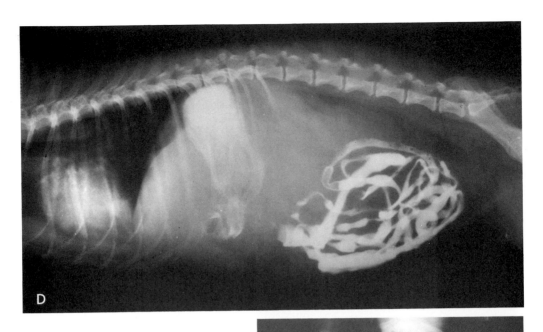

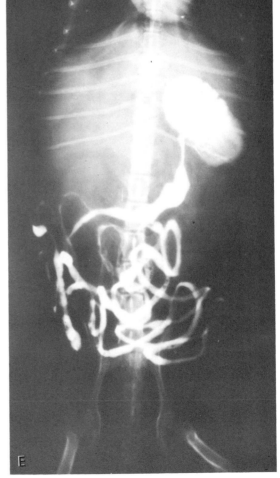

FIGURE 2–8. *Continued. D, E.* Displacement of the stomach and duodenum by an enlarged liver. The full extent of the displacement is not obvious on the lateral view. A carcinoma of the bile duct was found at autopsy. The kidneys are displaced caudally.

cult to appreciate on plain radiographs and is best seen following pneumoperitoneum. (Fig. 2–9).

CHOLECYSTITIS.   Inflammation of the gall bladder is rare in dogs and cats. Cholelithiasis (gall stones) may or may not be present.

The gall bladder and bile ducts may be demonstrated using an intravenous injection of Meglumine Iodipamide (Cholografin Meglumine. Squibb & Sons) at a dosage rate of 0.2 ml/kg body weight. The injection is given slowly and radiographs are made every 20 minutes until the gall bladder is well visualized. If a postemptying study is required a small fatty meal can be given and further radiographs made after 15 minutes. Cholecystography is not widely used, as the information likely to be gained from it is limited.

EMPHYSEMA OF THE GALL BLADDER.   Emphysema of the gall bladder has been described in the dog associated with diabetes mellitus. The radiographic findings comprised hepatomegaly and irregularly marginated radiolucent areas over the right side of the liver cranial to the pylorus.

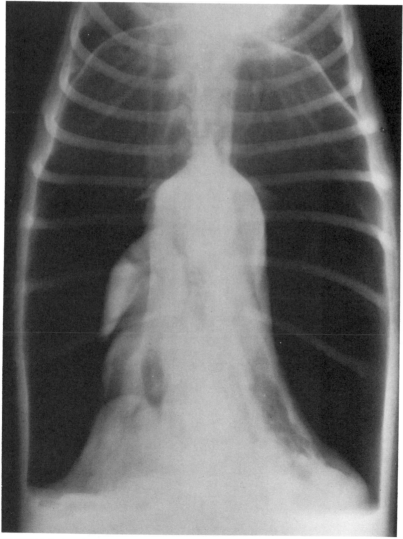

FIGURE 2–9. A small liver outlined by pneumoperitoneum. The liver was cirrhotic.

The Spleen

ANATOMY

The spleen is situated in the left cranial abdomen approximately parallel to the greater curvature of the stomach. Its head is attached to the stomach by the gastrosplenic ligament, while the rest of the organ is freely moveable. The spleen is triangular in cross section. It is related to the greater curvature of the stomach and the left kidney proximally; at its middle it is related to the colon and distally it is related to the small intestine.

RADIOGRAPHY

The spleen is usually seen on plain radiographs of the abdomen. It can be demonstrated more clearly using pneumoperitonography. It may be well visualized following intravascular injection of contrast medium.

NORMAL APPEARANCE

On the ventrodorsal view of the abdomen the spleen appears as a triangular-shaped density on the left side caudal to the stomach and cranial to the left kidney. In right lateral recumbency it is seen as a rounded oval or triangular-shaped mass in the ventral abdomen just caudal to the liver, from which occasionally it cannot be clearly distinguished. In left lateral recumbency the spleen may or may not be seen, since, because of its mobility, it may be obscured by the small intestine. It may greatly increase in size during anesthesia (Fig. 2–7A,B).

ABNORMALITIES

ENLARGEMENT. (Splenomegaly). Enlargement of the spleen may result from a variety of causes. Primary or secondary neoplasia, hyperplasia, circulatory problems, septicemia or toxemia, barbiturate or chloroform anesthesia, anemia, and torsion may all cause enlargement. Feline mastocytosis results in gross splenic enlargement. The commonest primary neoplasms are lymphosarcoma, hemangioma, and hemangiosarcoma. Nodular hypoplasia is seen occasionally in old dogs but it is difficult to demonstrate radiographically without the use of pneumoperitoneum.

An enlarged spleen displaces the stomach cranially and the small intestine dorsally and to the right. Large splenic masses may displace the colon and cecum dorsally. The direction of displacement of other organs depends on the degree of enlargement of the spleen and whether or not the entire organ is involved.

Enlargement of the spleen is the commonest cause of intra-abdominal masses. (Fig. 2–10).

ATROPHY. Atrophy of the spleen is sometimes seen in old animals. It is difficult to evaluate radiographically.

TORSION. Torsion of the spleen is seen in association with gastric dilatation and torsion.

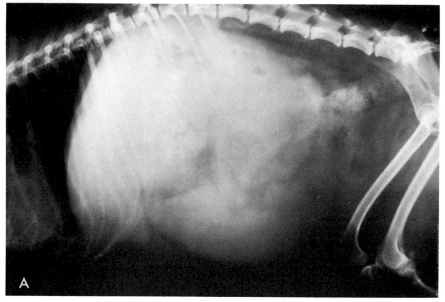

FIGURE 2-10. *A.* Enlargement of the spleen due to lymphosarcoma.
(Illustration continued on opposite page)

The Pancreas

ANATOMY

The pancreas is a V-shaped gland consisting of right and left lobes. The right lobe lies in the mesoduodenum along the right flank. It extends caudally as far as the fourth lumbar vertebra. The left lobe lies within the greater omentum. It extends caudally as far as the cranial pole of the left kidney.

RADIOGRAPHY

The normal pancreas is not demonstrable radiographically.

NORMAL APPEARANCE

The pancreas is not seen radiographically.

Abnormalities

INFLAMMATION. (Pancreatitis). Pancreatitis may be acute or chronic. It is seen most commonly in obese, middle-aged bitches. It may result in an increased density in the cranial abdomen particularly toward the right side. Swelling of the pancreas causes the duodenum to be displaced dorsally and sometimes laterally. The duodenum shows reduced peristalsis with slow passage of barium through it. If the left lobe of the pancreas is involved, there

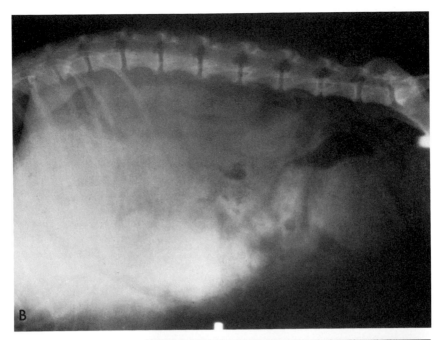

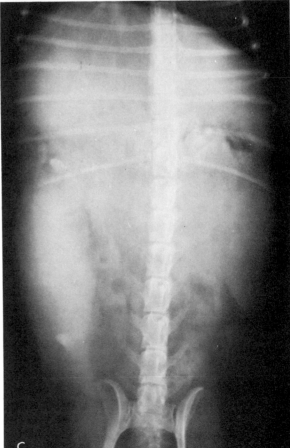

FIGURE 2–10. *Continued B, C.* Irregular enlargement of the spleen due to metastatic adenocarcinoma. The enlarged spleen is seen on both sides of the abdomen. The liver is enlarged. It also had metastatic lesions. The primary site was not determined.

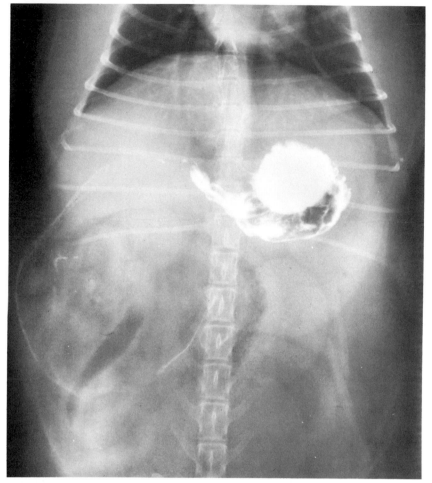

FIGURE 2–11. Displacement of the pylorus and duodenum by an inflamed pancreas. There is poor filling of the duodenum by the barium.

may be caudal displacement of the transverse colon. Granular mottling in the region of the pancreas has been reported, as has corrugation and spasticity of the duodenal wall. (Fig. 2–11).

NEOPLASIA. Neoplasia of the pancreas may cause it to increase in size and displace adjacent organs. Occasionally, the stomach is invaded by the spreading neoplasm with destruction of its wall in the affected area. (Fig. 2–12).

THE ALIMENTARY TRACT

The Esophagus

ANATOMY

The esophagus begins about the level of the middle of the first cervical vertebra and ends at the entrance to the stomach. During its course in the neck

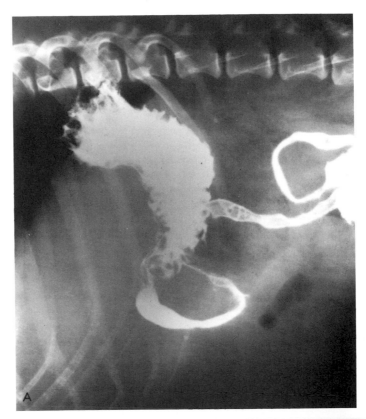

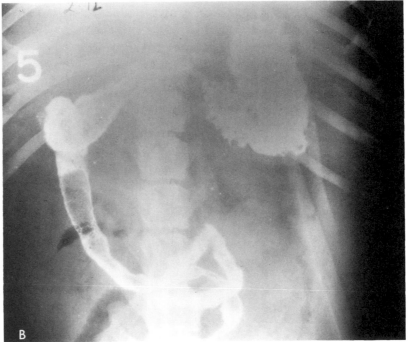

FIGURE 2–12.   *A, B.*   Displacement and invasion of the pylorus by a carcinoma of the pancreas.

it inclines toward the left side and at the entrance to the thorax it lies to the left of the trachea. Within the thorax, the esophagus lies to the left of the trachea initially but it then crosses the trachea to reach its dorsal aspect at the carina. It then courses caudally, almost in the midline, to pass through the esophageal hiatus of the diaphragm and enter the stomach dorsally.

RADIOGRAPHY

The administration of contrast material is necessary for detailed study of the esophagus. The most useful material is commercial micropulverized barium sulphate suspension. (Micropaque, Damancy & Co.; redi-FLOW, Flow Pharmaceuticals, Inc.; redi-PAQUE, Burns Biotec Laboratories; Novopaque, Picker X-ray Corporation). A barium paste (Esophotrast, Barnes-Hind Diagnostics) is useful if a special study of the mucosa is required, since it adheres better to the esophageal folds than does the more watery suspension. If the esophagus is being studied as part of a study of the gastrointestinal tract, then esophageal paste should not be used, since it is not satisfactory for outlining the stomach or intestines. If rupture of the esophagus is suspected it is preferable to use a water-soluble contrast agent instead of barium. (Gastrografin, Meglumine Diatrizoate Oral Solution, Squibb & Sons; Oral Hypaque, Sodium Diatrizoate Liquid, Winthrop Laboratories). Water-soluble agents do not give as good visualization of the esophagus as barium does.

The barium suspension is given at a dosage rate of 3 to 5 ml/kg body weight through the buccal pouch. Radiographs are made as the last of the barium is being swallowed. If the esophagus is grossly dilated, then much larger amounts of barium will be required to outline its lumen fully. Additional amounts may be given if the first study is unsatisfactory.

The esophagus should be investigated in cases of persistent regurgitation or vomiting. If there is difficulty in swallowing, contrast studies should be performed with care because of the danger of aspiration. However, small amounts of barium suspension are well tolerated in healthy lungs.

NORMAL APPEARANCE

The esophagus is not usually seen on plain films of the neck or thorax. Air or food material within the lumen will partly outline it. Normally, the esophagus contains no air or very little air. Anything more than a very small amount warrants further investigation. Air in the esophagus is frequently associated with esophageal abnormalities. It is also sometimes seen in vomiting, coughing, or dyspneic animals and in animals under general anesthesia.

Following a barium swallow some barium lodges in the longitudinal crypts between folds of the esophageal mucosa and appears as a series of regular parallel lines of almost equal width. The mucosal pattern is often irregular in appearance at the thoracic inlet. (Fig. 2–13).

The lateral projection gives most information, since in the ventrodorsal position there is considerable superimposition of other structures, especially the spine. A right ventrodorsal oblique position will help to separate the esophageal outline from the spine.

Fluoroscopically, one sees boluses of contrast material being propelled rather rapidly along the esophagus and into the stomach. The rate of travel of a

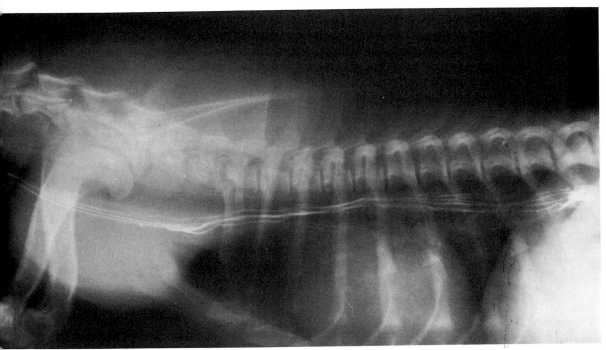

FIGURE 2–13. Normal esophagogram of a dog showing the longitudinal esophageal folds.

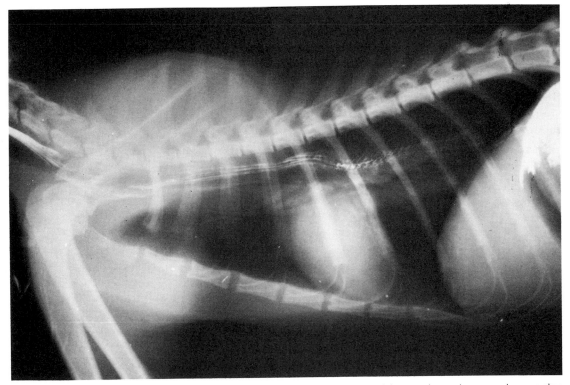

FIGURE 2–14. Normal esophagogram of a cat. The "herringbone" pattern of the esophageal mucosa is seen dorsal and caudal to the heart.

bolus may be somewhat slowed at the entrance to the chest and over the base of the heart.

In cats, the caudal third of the esophagus has transverse striations in addition to longitudinal folds. This gives it a "herringbone" appearance on barium examination. (Fig. 2–14).

ABNORMALITIES

DILATATION.   Dilatation of the esophagus may affect a portion of the organ or its entire length. A history of regurgitation of food material is a positive indication that the esophagus should be studied. Dilatation of the esophagus often results in some degree of aspiration pneumonia. Pneumonic changes in the lung fields, therefore, may accompany dilatation.

Megaesophagus.   This condition is also referred to as esophageal achalasia. The entire length of the esophagus is dilated. In the dog the disease is neuromuscular in origin, there being no anatomic cardiac sphincter. The disease is seen in young and old animals but its exact etiology remains obscure.

Radiographically, plain films of the thorax often show the dilated esophagus filled with radiopaque food material or with large amounts of air. Sometimes, food and air are present together. A barium study will reveal the full extent of the dilatation, which extends as far caudally as the diaphragm. A large amount of barium suspension may be required to demonstrate fully the extent of the dilatation. (Fig. 2–15).

Fluoroscopic examination shows absence of peristalsis or the presence of weak, inefficient peristaltic waves. The esophageal contents are seen to move with each heart beat. Standing lateral studies often show a fluid level within the

Text continued on page 40

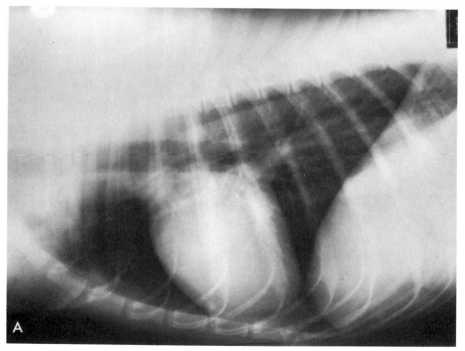

FIGURE 2–15. The esophagus. *A.* A normal thorax. The esophagus is not visualized.
(*Illustration continued on opposite page.*)

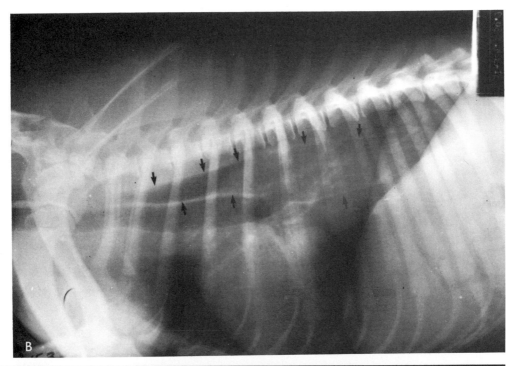

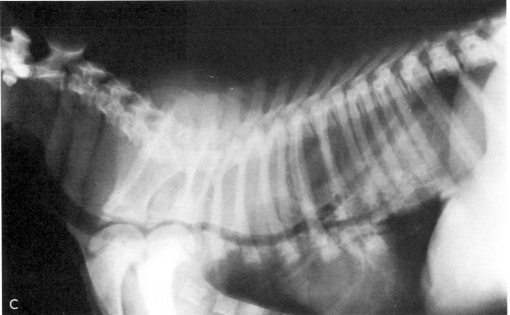

FIGURE 2–15. *Continued.* *B.* Air (arrows) can be seen within the esophagus dorsal to the trachea and in the caudal thorax. Air in the esophagus, except in very small quantities, is unusual and is often indicative of an abnormality. When air is seen, contrast studies should be performed. This was a mega-esophagus. *C, D.* The trachea is depressed by a grossly dilated esophagus. Food material within the esophagus can be seen in the caudal thorax. A barium study shows the extent of the dilatation. Mega-esophagus.

(Illustration continued on following page.)

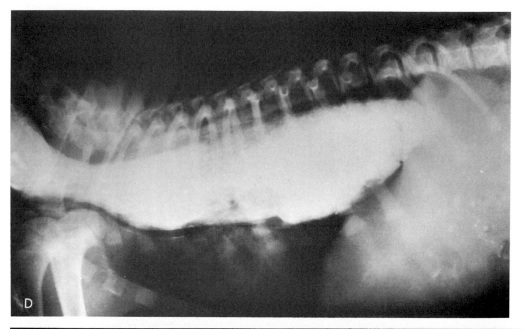

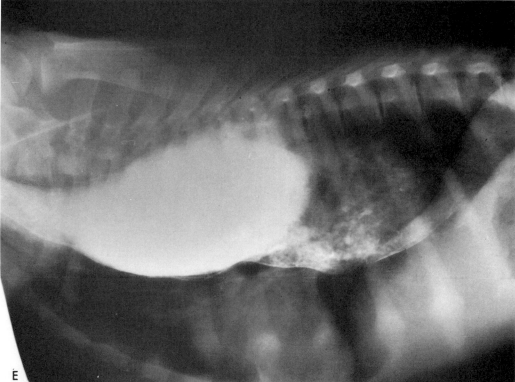

FIGURE 2–15. *Continued.* *E.* Esophageal dilatation may be so extensive that large quantities of barium are required to delineate it completely. An incomplete study may lead to an incorrect diagnosis. If insufficient barium is given, megaesophagus may simulate a vascular ring anomaly.

(*Illustration continued on opposite page.*)

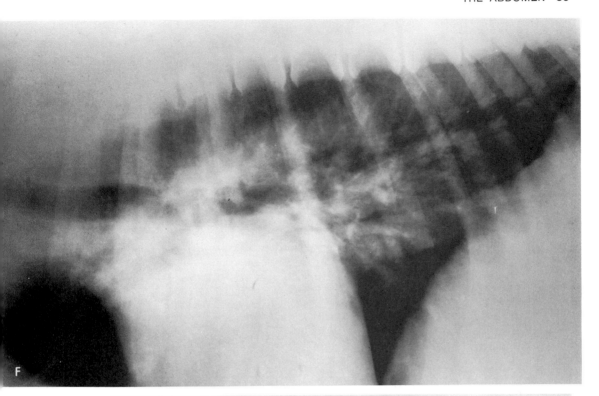

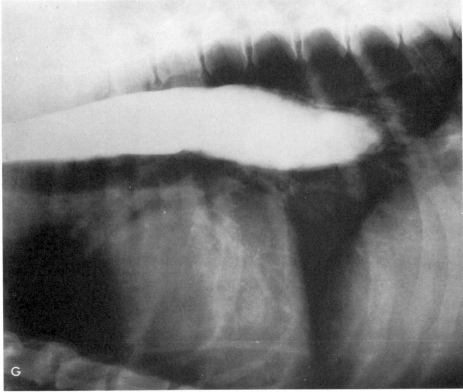

FIGURE 2–15. *Continued. F, G.* Megaesophagus. The plain chest radiograph shows widespread infiltration of the lungs due to aspiration pneumonia. The barium study shows the esophageal dilatation.

(Illustration continued on following page.)

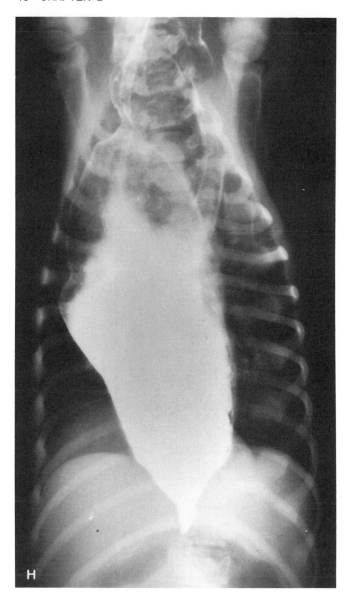

FIGURE 2–15. *Continued. H.* In mega-esophagus, the esophagus narrows sharply at the hiatus.

esophagus caused by an accumulation of liquid material ventrally and air dorsally.

Vascular Ring Anomalies. Congenital anomalies of the aortic arch system may result in vessels or vessel remnants forming bands that constrict the esophagus near the base of the heart. These are referred to as "vascular rings." Persistent Right Aortic Arch is the commonest anomaly seen, though double aortic arch, aberrant subclavian, and intercostal vessels are encountered. The anomalous vessel acts as a constricting band inhibiting proper expansion of the esophagus as food material passes along it. In time the esophagus dilates cranial to the constriction as food material continues to accumulate in it.

Persistent Right Aortic Arch. This is the commonest vascular ring anomaly. The aorta, instead of developing normally on the left side of the thorax, develops from the right primitive arch. The ductus arteriosus (ligamentum arteriosum), in its course between the aorta and the pulmonary artery, must then cross the esophagus. This results in the esophagus being trapped between the aorta on the right, the base of the heart and the pulmonary artery ventrally, and the ductus arteriosus (ligamentum arteriosum) dorsally and to the left. The ductus arteriosus, and later the ligamentum arteriosum, then acts as a constricting band that prevents normal expansion of the esophagus. As a result food material accumulates cranial to the point of constriction and this, in turn, results in a dilatation of the esophagus cranial to the base of the heart. Behind the heart the esophagus is usually normal, though persistent right aortic arch may coexist with some degree of megaesophagus.

The dilated esophagus, filled with food material, is often seen on plain radiographs, or the dilatation may be outlined by esophageal air. The trachea may be deviated ventrally. A barium study will show the dilatation of the esophagus cranial to the base of the heart and to the left of the trachea with a normal, or relatively normal, esophageal lumen caudally. The dilatation may extend well up into the neck. (Fig. 2–16).

FOREIGN BODY. Foreign bodies may be radiolucent or radiopaque. They are most commonly seen within the thoracic esophagus in the area between the base of the heart and the diaphragm. They are also seen at the entrance to the chest and less commonly at other sites. Irregularly shaped pieces of bone, such as pieces of vertebrae, are the usual offending objects. (Fig. 2–17).

Contrast material may be needed to outline a radiolucent foreign body. Barium is usually used. If rupture of the esophagus is suspected, air given by the stomach tube may be used as a contrast agent, or a water-soluble material may be used. Swallowed air occasionally outlines a foreign body.

Increased density within the thorax in the area of a foreign body indicates penetration of the esophageal wall with a resulting inflammatory reaction in the adjacent mediastinum or in the lungs, or in both. If the foreign body has been present for some time, thickening of the esophageal wall may be visible. Over a period of time a diverticulum may develop at the site of obstruction.

DIVERTICULUM. This is not a common condition. Some diverticula are occasionally seen at the entrance to the thorax. Large diverticula may form around foreign bodies, particularly in the caudal thoracic region. Barium is used to demonstrate diverticula.

Bilateral symmetric outpouching of the esophagus cranial to the diaphragm has been described.

STENOSIS. This is usually the result of damage to the wall of the esophagus either as a result of the passage of a foreign body or following surgery. The esophagus may be distended cranial to the site of the stenosis. On plain radiographs abnormal amounts of air may be seen within the esophageal lumen. A barium study will outline the area of constriction and the associated dilatation, if present. Stenosis may be missed on radiographs and is best demonstrated fluoroscopically.

SPIROCERCA LUPI INFESTATION. This parasite, which is found in the southeastern United States, southern Europe, Africa, and South America, invades the esophageal wall during its larval stage. It provokes a granulomatous reaction that appears on radiographs as an area of increased density between the base of the heart and the diaphragm. Affected animals may have difficulty swallowing. New bone formation (spondylosis) is frequently seen on the ventral aspects of the thoracic vertebrae in the neighborhood, that is, from about the

Text continued on page 45

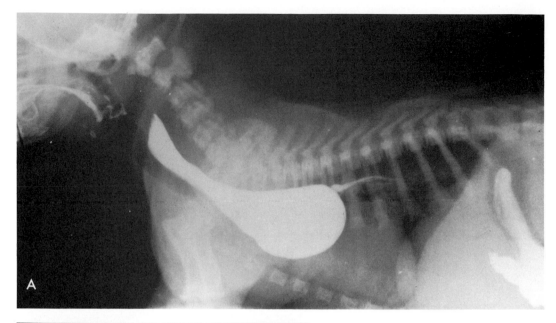

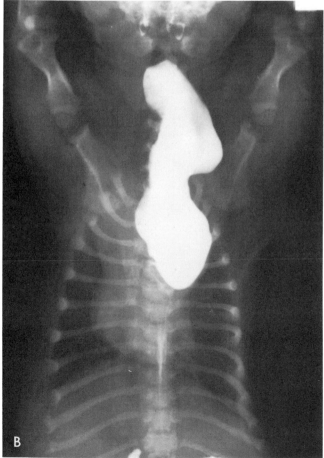

FIGURE 2–16. *A, B.* A vascular ring anomaly — in this case a persistent right aortic arch. There is marked dilatation of the esophagus cranial to the base of the heart and a normal configuration caudally.

(*Illustration continued on opposite page.*)

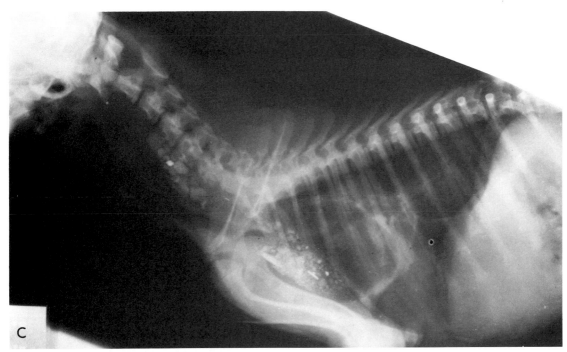

FIGURE 2–16. *Continued. C.* A vascular ring anomaly outlined by air and food material within the esophagus. The diagnosis should be confirmed by a barium study.

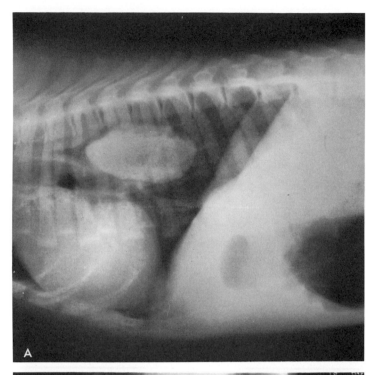

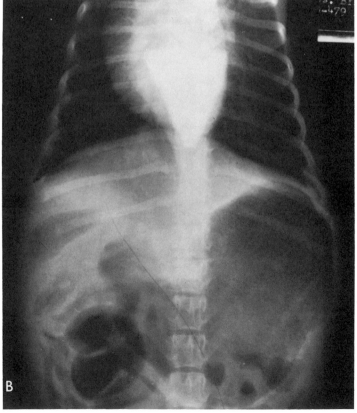

FIGURE 2–17. *A, B.* A bone in the caudal third of the thoracic esophagus. Abnormalities of the esophagus often provoke the swallowing of air. The stomach is distended and there is an excessive amount of gas in the small intestine.
(Illustration continued on opposite page.)

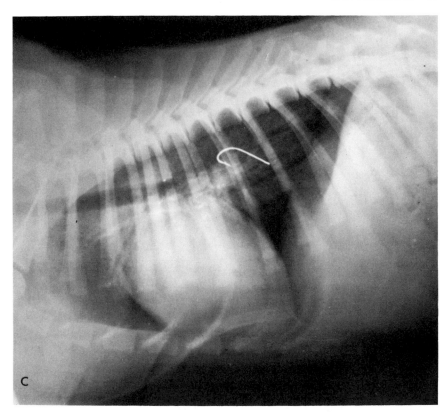

FIGURE 2–17. *Continued. C.* A fishhook in the esophagus.

seventh to the tenth thoracic vertebrae. Fibrosarcoma or osteosarcoma may develop from the esophageal lesion. A barium study will help to determine the degree of occlusion of the esophagus.

GASTROESOPHAGEAL INTUSSUSCEPTION. This is a rare condition seen in young dogs in which a portion of the stomach invaginates into the esophagus through the esophageal hiatus. The normal gastric bubble of air is not seen on plain radiographs and there may be an increased density in the caudal thorax. Gastric rugal folds are seen within the esophagus on barium examination. It may be associated with dilatation of the esophagus. If much of the stomach has passed into the esophagus it may not be possible to get barium into the stomach. The radiographic appearance will then be that of an intraesophageal mass. (Fig. 2–18).

NEOPLASIA. Neoplasia of the esophagus is rare in the dog, but squamous cell carcinoma is occasionally seen in the cat with vomiting as a common presenting sign. A barium study will show irregularity of outline of the esophagus at the site of the tumor.

ESOPHAGITIS. It is very difficult to make a definite diagnosis of esophagitis radiographically. Some irregularity in outline of the mucosal folds may be noted following a barium swallow. Air is often present within the esophageal lumen. Long-standing cases may show some thickening of the esophageal wall.

EXTRINSIC COMPRESSION. Masses within the neck or thorax not associated with the esophagus may nevertheless cause pressure on it. The increased

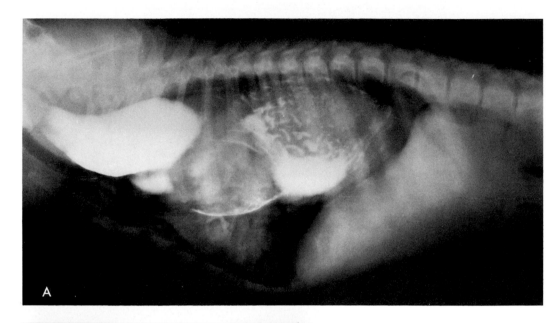

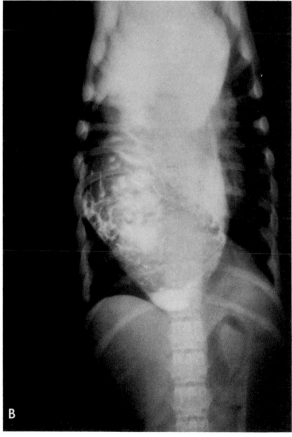

FIGURE 2–18. Gastroesophageal intussusception. *A, B.* A nine week old German Shepherd with a history of vomition and respiratory distress for two days. There is an associated megaesophagus. Gastric rugal folds can be seen within the thorax. The usual stomach shadow is not seen in the abdomen.

(Illustration continued on opposite page.)

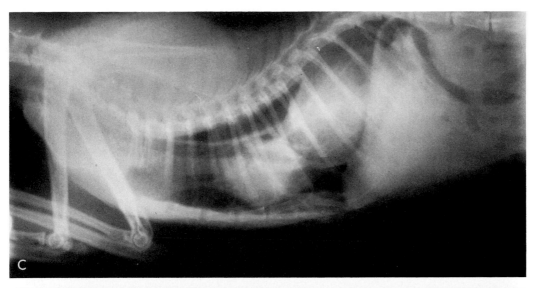

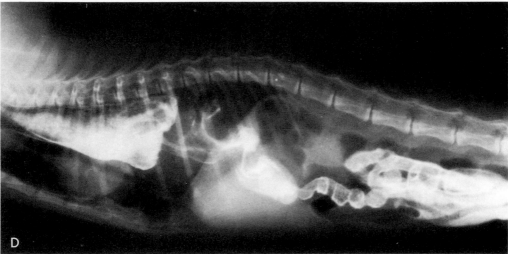

FIGURE 2–18. *Continued. C, D.* A seven month old Siamese cat with a history of intermittent vomition a variable time after feeding. The plain lateral film shows a mass in the caudal thorax. The contrast study shows a protrusion of the stomach into a dilated esophagus.

densities associated with such masses are commonly seen on plain radiographs. Air is often present within the esophagus. A barium swallow will show the site and degree of compression. The esophageal lumen, though compressed, remains regular in outline, there being no filling defect. Dilatation may occur cranial to the point of compression.

CRICOPHARYNGEAL ACHALASIA.   This condition is caused by failure of the cricopharyngeal region to relax during swallowing. If a barium swallow is given, the barium is seen to remain in the pharynx despite swallowing movements. Small amounts of barium get into the esophagus, which is dilated with air. Aspiration of barium into the larynx is often observed and barium may be forced into the nasal passages and trickle from the nose. On plain radiographs accumulations of barium are seen in the pharynx with little or no barium reaching the stomach. Fluoroscopy is required to make a diagnosis.

Cricopharyngeal achalasia should be considered in the differential diagnosis in the examination of young dogs that have difficulty in swallowing.

ESOPHAGEAL FISTULA AND ESOPHAGOBRONCHIAL FISTULA. These conditions are rarely seen. If suspected, a water-soluble contrast medium given by the mouth may confirm the diagnosis.

The Stomach

ANATOMY

The stomach lies in the central abdomen caudal to the diaphragm and the liver. For purposes of description it is divided into four regions:

1. The cardia — the portion that blends with the esophagus.

2. The fundus — the large blind pouch that lies dorsal and to the left of the cardia.

3. The body — the principal portion, extending from the fundus to the pylorus.

4. The pylorus — forms approximately the distal third. Its proximal portion, the pyloric antrum, is a thin-walled saccule that is continuous distally with the pyloric canal. The canal is surrounded by a thick double sphincter.

The body and the fundus are, for the most part, to the left of the midline, while the pyloric antrum and the pyloric canal lie to the right side. The body and the fundus are in contact with the left hemidiaphragm, while the liver lies between the pylorus and the right hemidiaphragm. The pancreas is in the angle formed between the stomach and the duodenum. When empty, the stomach is almost entirely within the rib cage and its ventral border is about one-third the depth of the abdomen from the abdominal floor. When full, the stomach reaches the floor of the abdomen and extends a variable distance caudally. In puppies, a full stomach may reach the umbilicus or beyond.

RADIOGRAPHY

Plain and contrast radiographs are necessary for a full evaluation of the stomach. Functional studies require the use of the fluoroscope.

Contrast studies may be positive, negative, or double contrast.

POSITIVE. Barium or a water-soluble iodide preparation may be used. The best positive contrast material is commercial micropulverized barium sulphate in suspension. (Micropaque, Barium Sulphate Suspension, Damancy & Co.; redi-FLOW, Flow Pharmaceuticals, Inc.; redi-PAQUE, Burns Biotec Laboratories; Novopaque, Picker X-ray Corporation). Commercial preparations may be given undiluted. Suspensions of pure barium sulphate are not satisfactory, since their performance within the alimentary tract is not always predictable, because of their tendency to flocculate. The dose of the micropulverized barium suspension is 2 to 5 ml/kg body weight given slowly into the buccal pouch. Alternatively, it may be given by a stomach tube using a mouth gag. If a double contrast study is to be performed, air through a stomach tube or a carbonated beverage (30 to 60 ml) may be given before or after the barium.

Negative contrast alone is not very satisfactory for outlining detail within the stomach.

If perforation of the esophagus, stomach, or intestine is suspected a water-soluble iodide compound should be used instead of barium. (Oral Hypaque, Sodium Diatrizoate Liquid, Winthrop Laboratories; Gastrografin, Meglumine Diatrizoate Oral Solution, Squibb & Sons). These preparations should be given at a dosage rate of 7 ml/kg body weight. They may be given by a stomach tube, as they are very bitter. The water-soluble agents will be absorbed from the mediastinum or peritoneal cavity, whereas barium will not. Organic iodides are contraindicated in dehydrated subjects. It should be remembered that such agents pass through the alimentary tract faster than does barium and they usually do not give the same clarity of outline. In the distal parts of the intestine they become diluted, due to their hypertonicity, and detail is lost. They should be employed, therefore, only when there are specific indications for their use.

NEGATIVE. Room air given by a stomach tube at a dosage rate of 6 to 12 ml/kg body weight, or a carbonated beverage (30 to 60 ml) may be used. Negative contrast alone is not a satisfactory method of studying the stomach but it may be useful in the demonstration of a radiolucent foreign body.

DOUBLE CONTRAST. A combination of positive and negative contrast agents is used. As the stomach almost always contains some gas or swallowed air, virtually all contrast studies of the stomach are, to some extent, double contrast studies. Double contrast studies are particularly valuable in studying the gastric mucosa.

It is most important that the animal be properly prepared prior to the barium examination. The animal should be fasted for 18 to 24 hours and water should be withheld for at least three to four hours prior to the examination. Anticholinergic drugs should be withheld for the previous 24 hours. An enema may be required to clear the colon. The use of a mild cathartic agent 24 hours before the examination is also helpful. Little or no information can be gained from a contrast study if large amounts of food material are present within the stomach. Barium should be used sparingly. Indeed it is preferable to administer too little rather than too much, since more can be given if required. Too much barium obscures all detail.

Anesthetic agents and tranquilizers may considerably affect gastric emptying time and the transit time of barium through the intestines. Acetylpromazine maleate (Acepromazine, Ayerst Laboratories) at a dosage rate of up to 1 mg per pound body weight has been shown to have little effect in this regard. Triflupromazine hydrochloride (Vetame. E. R., Squibb & Sons) is said to slow barium passage time in a predictable manner and so facilitates detailed study of segments of the gastrointestinal tract.

Plain radiographs should be made immediately before the barium is administered to exclude the possibility of the barium masking a foreign body or a lesion that might otherwise have been seen. Following barium administration right and left lateral, ventrodorsal, dorsoventral, and oblique views should be made. Occasionally a standing lateral view may be helpful. One must ensure that barium is seen to fill all parts of the stomach. Following the initial studies further radiographs are made at 20 minute intervals up to one hour and thereafter hourly until a diagnosis is made or until all the barium has left the stomach. If a full gastrointestinal series is required, then further radiographs are made hourly until most of the contrast material has reached the colon. A 24 hour film is sometimes useful if there has been delayed gastric emptying.

NORMAL APPEARANCE

The stomach usually contains fluid and some gas or air. The gas is often referred to as the "stomach bubble." The fluid and gas change position with changes in position of the animal. Thus, if an animal is radiographed in right lateral recumbency, the gas will be seen in the fundus and in the body. Conversely, in left lateral recumbency gas will be seen, for the most part, in the pyloric antrum. Gas in a viscus tends to rise to the highest point possible. In lateral views the pylorus is seen end-on and often casts quite a dense circular shadow that may be mistaken for a foreign body within the stomach. In lateral views a line drawn through the fundus, body, and pylorus may be perpendicular to the vertebral column, may be parallel to the ribs or may lie somewhere between these two extremes. In the ventrodorsal view a line drawn through the fundus and pylorus will be perpendicular to the vertebral column. Lateral and ventrodorsal views are usually adequate as survey radiographs.

Following a barium meal the position of the barium within the stomach will depend on the position of the animal and will be the opposite of the position occupied by gas. In right lateral recumbency barium will be seen in the pyloric antrum, while in left lateral recumbency it will be seen in the body and the fundus. In the ventrodorsal position, barium will accumulate in the fundus and cardia, while in the dorsoventral position it will gravitate to the body and the pyloric antrum. Right dorsoventral oblique views show the pylorus best.

An adequate study of the stomach entails visualization of all regions. In the normal stomach rugal folds are clearly seen. They should be regular in outline, parallel to one another, and smooth. They may appear linear or tortuous depending on the degree of distention of the stomach. The spaces between the folds should be about as wide as the folds themselves. In a normal animal, properly prepared, barium will appear in the duodenum within a few minutes of giving it. It is frequently seen there on the first radiograph made after its administration. Varying times have been given for complete emptying of the stomach. It is probable that the average emptying time in the fasting animal is about three and one-half hours, but it may vary considerably. In nervous animals the passage of barium into the duodenum at the beginning of the study may be delayed for up to 30 minutes or more. In such cases it is often helpful to return the animal to its cage after the barium has been given and then to continue with the study after about 30 minutes. Delayed emptying due to nervousness must not be confused with that seen in pyloric malfunction.

Fluoroscopy will show contractions of the stomach. Peristaltic waves will be seen to pass across the body, through the pyloric antrum up to the pyloric canal. At the end of each contraction the pylorus relaxes and allows a stream of contrast material to pass into the duodenum. During fluoroscopic examination the animal should be rolled over to ensure that barium reaches all parts of the mucosal surface and that all parts of the stomach are seen. (Fig. 2–19).

ABNORMALITIES

FOREIGN BODY. Many foreign bodies are radiopaque and are, therefore, readily seen on plain films of the abdomen. Occasionally, radiolucent objects are encountered. These may be demonstrated using barium or air contrast. Small amounts of barium should be used as too much may obscure the outline of a foreign body. The use of a double contrast technique may be helpful. Frequently

Text continued on page 55

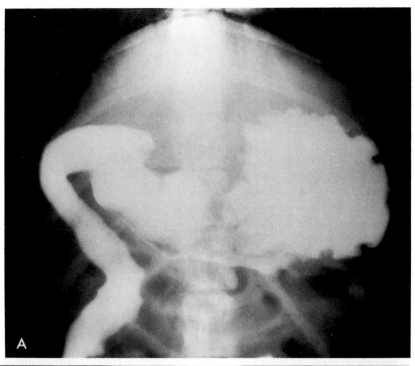

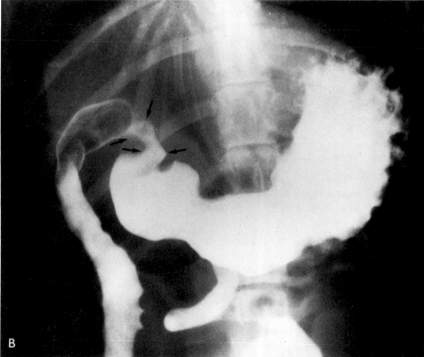

FIGURE 2–19. *A.* A ventrodorsal view of the stomach shows that in this position most of the barium has collected in the fundus. Some barium and gas are seen in the body and pyloric antrum. *B.* In the dorsoventral view barium fills the body and the pyloric antrum. The pylorus (arrows) is seen as a narrow passage between the pyloric antrum and the duodenum. The indentations in the wall in the fundic region are due to mucosal folds.

(Illustration continued on following page.)

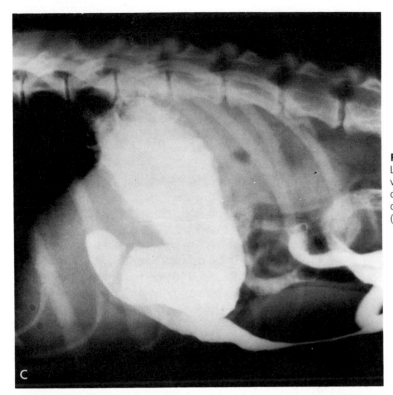

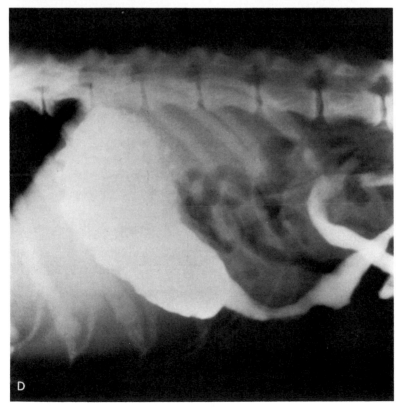

FIGURE 2–19. *Continued. C, D.* Left and right lateral recumbent views show the changes in outline of the stomach and duodenum with changes in the animal's posture. (*Illustration continued on opposite page.*)

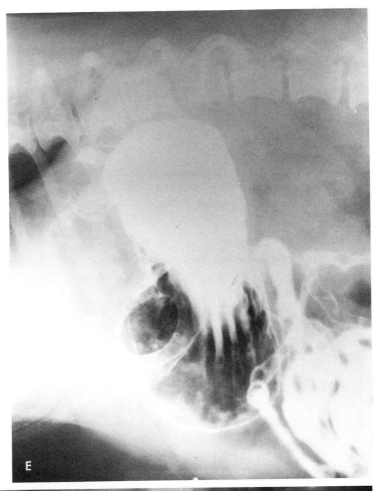

FIGURE 2–19. *Continued. E, F.* These are double contrast studies of the stomach. Double contrast gives good visualization of the rugal folds. (*Illustration continued on following page.*)

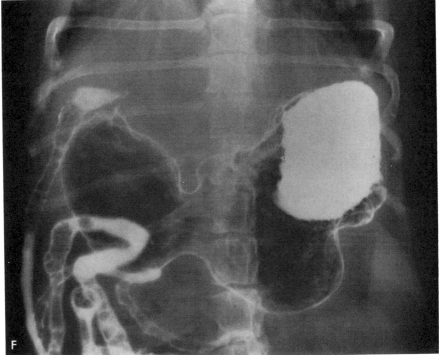

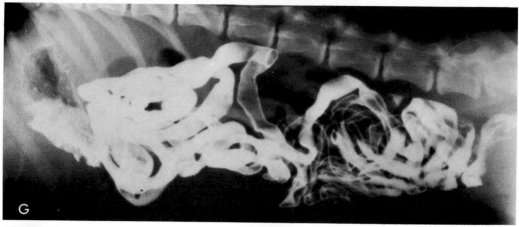

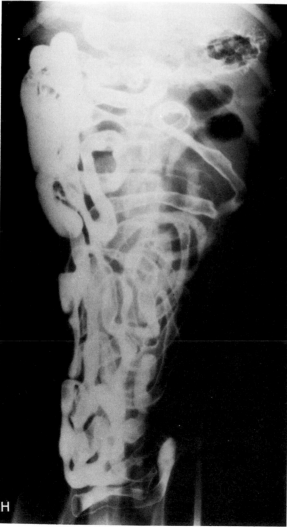

FIGURE 2–19. *Continued.* *G, H.* These show the stomach and small intestine two and one-half hours after the administration of barium.

the foreign body is most clearly seen when most of the barium has left the stomach. It is then outlined by the residual barium adhering to it. A foreign body may occasionally obstruct the pylorus, provoking persistent vomiting. (Fig. 2–20).

GASTRITIS.　Gastritis is not easy to diagnose with certainty radiographically. A thickened gastric wall or thickened rugal folds may be seen. An inflamed stomach often empties more rapidly than a normal one.

GASTRIC DILATATION AND TORSION.　Dilatation of the stomach may result from obstruction of the pylorus or from atony of the stomach wall. Acute gastric dilatation may occur with or without torsion. Torsion is most frequently seen in large breeds of dogs. The etiology is uncertain, but it may be associated with over-eating prior to exercise or with excessive drinking of water. There may be a hereditary predisposition. In acute gastric dilatation, the stomach is grossly distended with gas and the intestines are displaced caudally.

Torsion is a common complicating factor in gastric dilatation. Viewed ventrodorsally, the torsion is usually clockwise, the stomach rotating about its longitudinal axis. The stomach may be so dilated as to appear to fill almost the entire abdomen. Frequently, a fold of the stomach wall can be seen. The spleen may undergo torsion also. It will be engorged and displaced dorsocaudally. It is often difficult to see. The pylorus is displaced toward the left side. The duodenum and intestines may contain large amounts of gas. Usually, the degree of dilatation is much greater with torsion than with simple dilatation.

Swallowed air, often associated with esophageal pathology, may cause a mild degree of gastric dilatation (Fig. 2–21).

PYLORIC OBSTRUCTION.　The pylorus may be obstructed for a number of reasons: foreign body, pyloric stenosis, pylorospasm, gastric neoplasia. Hepatic, splenic, or pancreatic masses may cause pressure on the pylorus and inhibit passage of food material through it. The common presenting sign is persistent vomiting.

The usual radiographic signs of pyloric obstruction are delayed emptying of the stomach and, in long-standing cases, gastric dilatation. Large quantities of semiradiopaque food material may be seen within the stomach even after fasting. A large amount of fluid is often present within the stomach. Fluoroscopic examination is often very helpful.

Following the administration of barium, peristaltic waves can be seen pushing the barium into the pyloric antrum but little or no barium reaches the duodenum. Occasionally, a very thin stream of barium is seen to pass through the narrowed canal, the so-called "string sign." It is important that the animal be properly fasted before the radiographic examination. In a properly fasted animal barium should be seen in the duodenum within a few minutes of its administration. In cases of pyloric obstruction it may be retained within the stomach for several hours.

Pyloric stenosis (hypertrophy) may be congenital or acquired. Thus pyloric obstruction may be seen at any age. It is important to differentiate between true pyloric obstruction and pylorospasm. Some nervous animals may retain barium in the stomach for long periods of time because of the stress of the examination and the upsetting effects of unfamiliar surroundings. It is often helpful to return the animal to its cage for 30 minutes if delayed emptying is present. The examination is continued after that time. On reexamination, if barium has passed freely into the duodenum then a diagnosis of pyloric obstruction is not warranted. Pylorospasm

Text continued on page 61

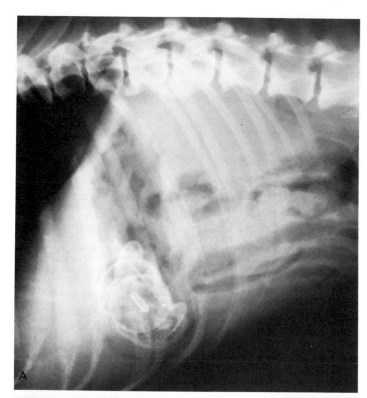

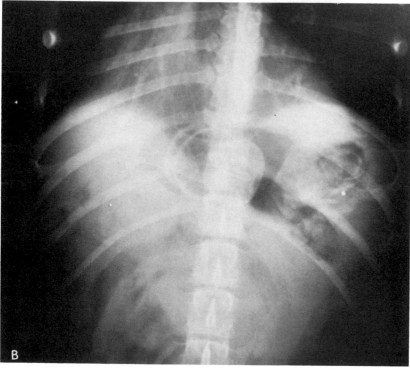

FIGURE 2–20. *A, B.* A radiopaque foreign body in the stomach.
(*Illustration continued on opposite page.*)

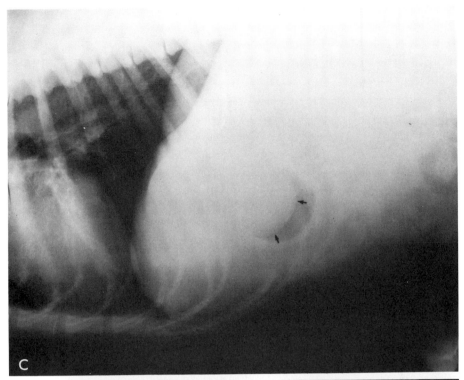

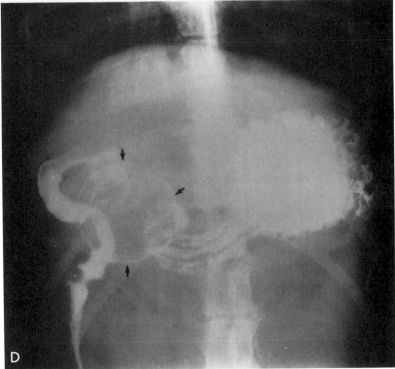

FIGURE 2–20 *Continued. C, D.* On the lateral view (C), gas within the stomach partly outlines a foreign body (arrows). Following administration of barium, the object is more clearly seen on the ventrodorsal view (D) (arrows). It was a rubber ball.

(Illustration continued on following page.)

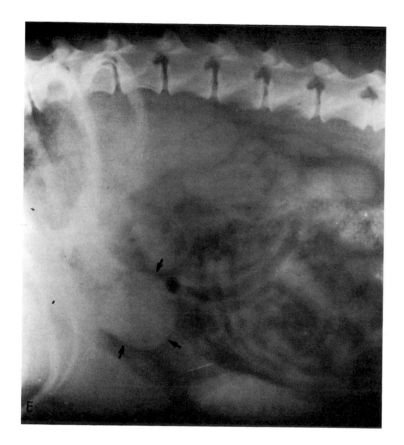

FIGURE 2–20 *Continued. E* The pylorus seen end-on (arrows) should not be mistaken for a foreign body. (The liver appears enlarged).

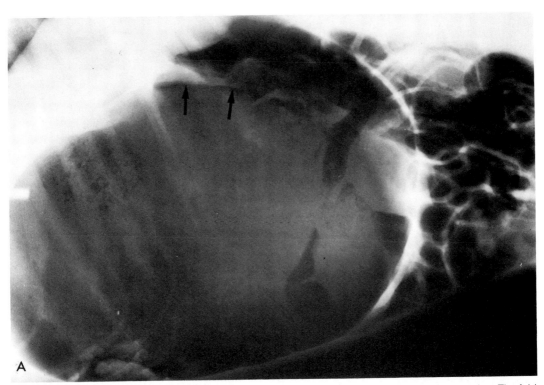

FIGURE 2–21. *A.* Gastric dilatation. Dilatation of such a severe nature is usually associated with torsion. The fold in the stomach wall (arrows) indicates that this is a case of gastric torsion. The dog presented with persistent retching, abdominal pain, and a very tense abdomen.

(*Illustration continued on following page.*)

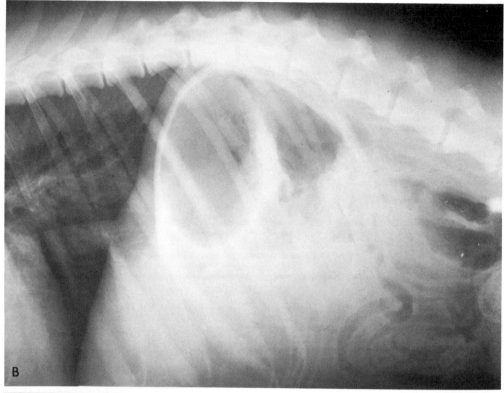

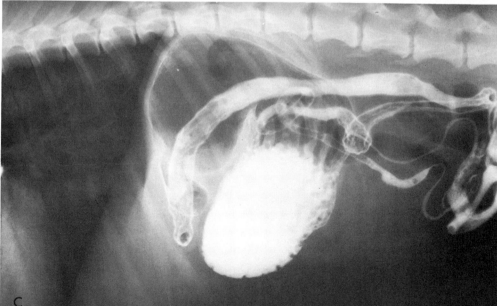

FIGURE 2–21 *Continued. B–D.* A partial rotation of the stomach. On the plain radiograph (B) the stomach appears folded on itself. The contrast studies confirm the diagnosis. The pylorus is displaced toward the left side (arrow).

(*Illustration continued on opposite page.*)

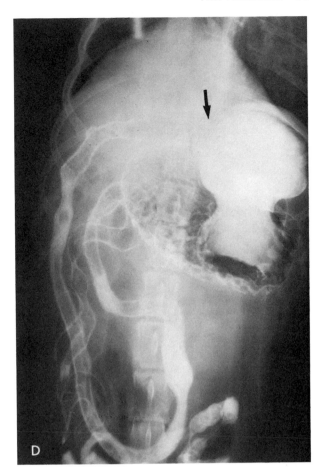

FIGURE 2–21. *D.* See legend on opposite page.

may also be overcome by administering a spasmolytic drug. If, despite cage rest and the use of spasmolytics, barium does not pass into the duodenum for an abnormally long time, for example for an hour or more, then a diagnosis of pyloric obstruction should be made. Distention of the stomach may sometimes be appreciated because of radiopaque food material within it. (Fig. 2–22).

NEOPLASIA. Neoplasia of the stomach is relatively rare in dogs and cats. The diagnosis may be difficult. Neoplasms of the pancreas may invade the stomach. The radiographic signs of gastric neoplasia include the following:

(1) Absence or gross distortion of the normal pattern of rugal folds and thickening of the stomach wall.

(2) The presence of an intraluminal mass, sometimes outlined by the gastric gas bubble.

(3) Failure to outline the stomach fully on barium examination — a so-called "filling defect."

(4) Ulceration of the stomach wall. Barium may fill the ulcer crater and persist there unchanged in outline over a series of radiographs. In profile it will appear as an outpouching of the gastric lumen. A radiolucent halo may be seen around the ulcer crater.

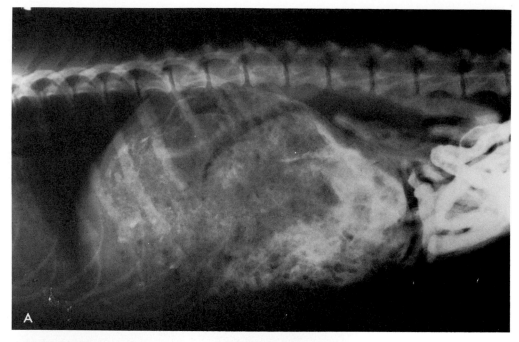

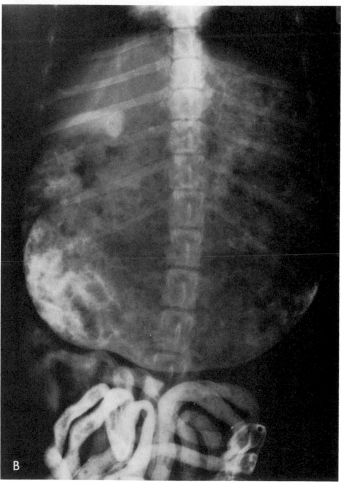

FIGURE 2-22. *A, B* Gross distention of the stomach. This results from prolonged interference with gastric emptying.

(5) Rigidity of the stomach wall. This is failure to transmit peristaltic waves. It may be noted on serial radiographs as an unchanging outline of part of the stomach wall or it may be observed fluoroscopically. Observed changes should be demonstrated on several films to preclude the possibility of mistaking normal features associated with contractions of the stomach for abnormalities.

A negative radiographic examination of the stomach does not mean that no neoplasm is present. Benign ulceration is very rare. (Fig. 2–23).

DISPLACEMENT.   The stomach may be displaced by masses within the abdomen. Enlargement of the liver will cause the stomach to be displaced. The stomach may be displaced into the thorax in cases of diaphragmatic hernia. (Fig. 2–9).

GASTROESOPHAGEAL INTUSSUSCEPTION.   This is dealt with in the section on the esophagus. (See page 45).

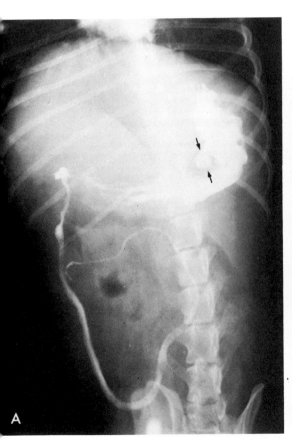
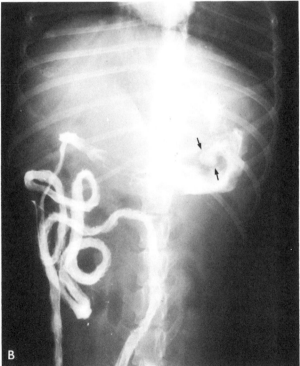

FIGURE 2–23. *A–D.*   Gastric ulceration in a case of reticulum cell sarcoma. The dog presented with a history of losing weight and anorexia for six weeks. Barium is seen to be retained in an ulcer crater in several radiographs made over a period of about 90 minutes. The ulcer remains fixed in position and shape (arrows). The radiolucent area about the ulcer, sometimes called the ulcer "halo" represents swelling and edema of the surrounding gastric mucosa.

(*Illustration continued on following page.*)

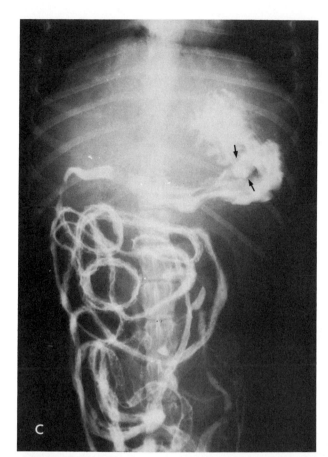

FIGURE 2–23. *Continued. C, D.* See legend on preceding page.

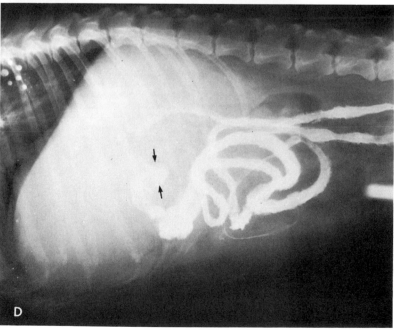

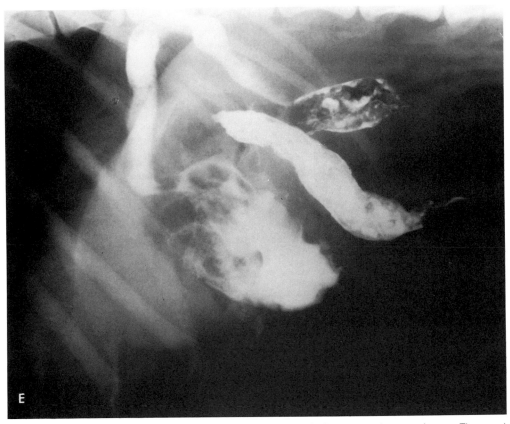

FIGURE 2–23. *Continued. E.* Gross distortion of the stomach due to an adenocarcinoma. The rugal folds are widened, irregular, and absent in places. Fluoroscopically, the lesser curvature appeared rigid.

The Small Intestine

ANATOMY

The small intestine extends from the pylorus to the ileocolic junction. It occupies the ventral portion of the abdomen caudal to the stomach and the liver. It measures about 3.5 times the length of the body in the living animal.

THE DUODENUM. The duodenum is the first part of the small intestine. Its cranial portion is continuous with the pylorus and forms the cranial duodenal flexure from which it courses dorsolaterally and caudally. The cranial part is known as the duodenal cap or bulb. Dorsally and laterally it is in contact with the liver and medially it is in contact with the pancreas. The descending portion of the duodenum runs caudally to about the level of the sixth lumbar vertebra, where it turns medially to form the caudal flexure. It then runs obliquely forward and to the left as the ascending portion and becomes continuous with the jejunum at the duodenojejunal flexure. The duodenum has a short mesentery and it is relatively fixed in position.

THE JEJUNUM AND ILEUM. The jejunum and ileum form most of the small intestine. They are suspended by a long mesentery and so are freely moveable within the abdomen. There is no clear division between the jejunum and the ileum. The term ileum is applied to the short, usually contracted, terminal part of the small intestine. It ends at the ileocolic valve, which is within the duodenal loop, or ventral to the ascending portion of the duodenum. The jejunum and ileum form numerous coils in the midventral abdomen.

RADIOGRAPHY

On plain lateral and ventrodorsal radiographs the small intestine can be recognized because of the mixture of gas and food material within it. The small intestine of the cat contains less gas than does that of the dog.

Detailed studies of the small intestine require the use of contrast material. Preparation of the animal and the administration of barium are carried out as described for the examination of the stomach. A somewhat larger quantity of barium suspension than that recommended for gastric studies gives better filling of the small intestine. Up to 12 ml/kg body weight of a 30 per cent weight per volume suspension has been recommended. After giving the barium meal, lateral and ventrodorsal radiographs should be made immediately and thereafter every 20 minutes for the first hour and then hourly until a diagnosis is made or until most of the barium has reached the colon. Fluoroscopy is used to study function and determine if normal peristalsis is present. Pneumoperitoneum is sometimes helpful. The use of a compression band assists in reducing the effect of respiratory movements on the abdomen.

NORMAL APPEARANCE

The duodenum is fairly fixed in position. The jejunum and ileum have a wide range of movement and are readily displaced by other organs or by masses within the abdomen. Gas and food material are seen within the lumen of the small intestine. The duodenal loop is easily recognized on contrast studies, but it is very difficult to distinguish individual coils of the jejunum and ileum because of their tortuous course.

The mucosal pattern of the small intestine is not as well marked as in man. Barium studies show a smooth or finely villous pattern. Frequently, sharply defined barium-filled outpouchings are seen along the course of the duodenum. These are normal and they have been called "pseudoulcers." They are the result of mucosal thinning over submucosal lymphoid follicles. They should not be confused with true ulcers, which are very rare. (Fig. 2–24).

In a normal study the contrast material remains homogeneous in appearance and maintains a continuous column as it passes along the intestine. The caliber of the bowel should be uniform, though a full duodenum may be slightly wider than the jejunum and ileum. Peristaltic waves are seen as areas of contraction on radiographs. Serial studies should be made to ensure that such contractions do change in size and position. The usual transit time of barium through the small intestine of the dog varies from about one to four hours. Transit time is faster in cats. (Fig. 2–19).

Fluoroscopically, peristaltic waves are seen to pass along segments of the intestine, pushing the barium ahead of them. Secondary waves cause some of the contrast material to flow in a retrograde direction, thus imparting a churning motion to the intestinal contents.

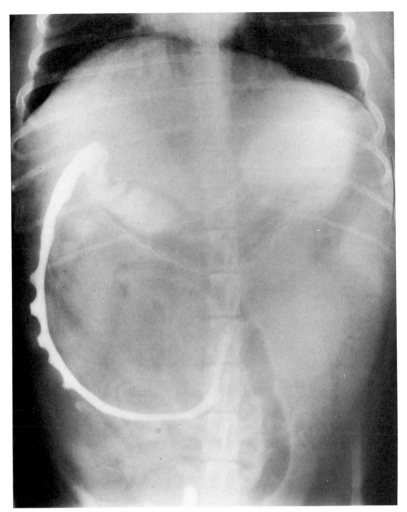

FIGURE 2–24. Pseudoulceration of the duodenum.

ABNORMALITIES

In studies of the small intestine plain radiographs often give some indication of abnormality and they should be studied routinely before proceeding to contrast radiography.

OBSTRUCTION (Ileus). Obstruction of the small intestine may result from several causes. Vomition, depression, and abdominal tenderness are common presenting signs. Mechanical obstruction may be due to foreign bodies, intussusception, incarcerated hernias, volvulus, neoplasia, and mesenteric infarction. Obstruction may also be due to functional failure of peristalsis. Pressure from extrinsic masses rarely causes obstruction of the small intestine, because of the mobility of the jejunum and ileum.

Radiographically, acute obstruction is characterized by the presence of gross distention of a loop or loops of bowel with gas, or fluid, or a combination of both. Standard lateral and ventrodorsal views are usually adequate to demonstrate it.

As the dog's intestine normally contains some gas, the demonstration of gas-capped fluid levels on standing lateral projections is not particularly helpful in making a diagnosis. The level of obstruction can often be gauged from the length of gas-filled intestine seen proximal to the point of obstruction. Swallowed air, such as that seen sometimes with esophageal disease, may be present in the small intestine. It does not distend the bowel grossly.

On barium examination there may be delayed gastric emptying and slow passage of barium along the intestine. The fluid present in the bowel dilutes the barium. It is probably inadvisable to proceed with a barium examination when dilated loops of intestine have been demonstrated. Such cases require surgery, and any information gained by such a procedure is unlikely to affect management of the case. Furthermore, the administration of barium further distresses the animal and frequently provokes vomition. (Fig. 2–25).

FOREIGN BODY. Radiopaque foreign bodies are readily seen on plain radiographs. Radiolucent objects are occasionally outlined by gas within the intestine. Barium may be required to demonstrate a radiolucent foreign body. If obstruction is not complete, the foreign object is often most clearly seen after the main column of barium has passed, when it will be outlined by traces of barium adhering to it. If the foreign body is long and pliable, such as a piece of string, then the intestine tends to push together on itself along the foreign body. This results in a gathering

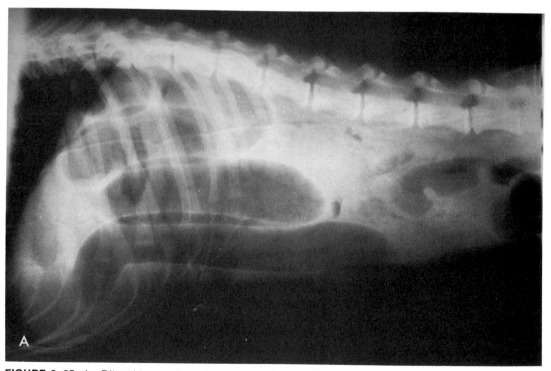

FIGURE 2–25. *A.* Dilated loops of small intestine indicative of acute obstruction. *B.* If barium is administered to an animal with an acute obstruction, the barium mixes with the fluid in the dilated intestine. It may not reach the point of obstruction. Such studies rarely yield information of significant value. *C.* Gas-capped fluid levels in the small intestine of a dog with postoperative ileus. There is some fluid and free gas within the abdominal cavity. This is a standing lateral view.

(*Illustration continued on opposite page.*)

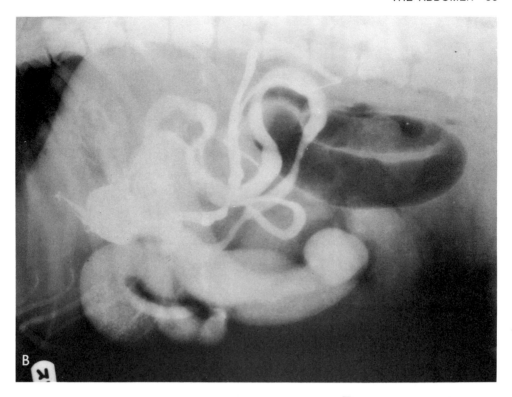

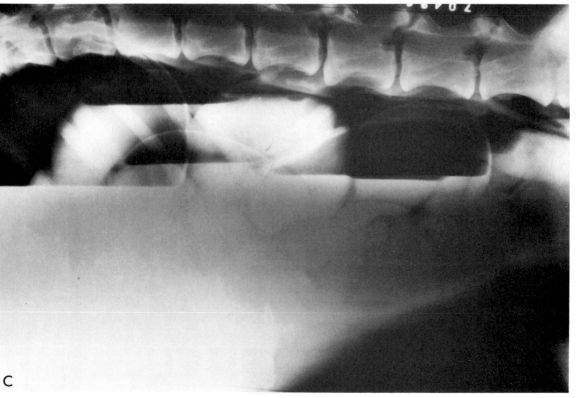

FIGURE 2-25. *Continued. B, C. (See legend on opposite page.)*

together of the coils of the intestine in the midabdomen. The resulting appearance has been likened to a gathered flounce or accordion pleats.

If a foreign body causes complete obstruction, then dilated gas and fluid-filled loops of intestine will be seen proximal to the obstruction. Most obstructing foreign bodies are found in the jejunum. Many foreign bodies pass through the intestine without causing any symptoms. (Fig. 2–26).

INTUSSUSCEPTION. This is most commonly seen in young dogs. The symptoms are vomiting, abdominal pain, the passage of mucus or blood, and frequently a palpable mass in the abdomen. Intussusception may cause a complete or an incomplete obstruction. If the obstruction is complete, dilated gas and fluid-filled loops of bowel are seen proximal to the intussusception. The colon is empty. If the obstruction is incomplete there is little, if any, distention of the bowel and feces are usually present in the colon. Occasionally, the mass of the intussusception is dense enough to cast a shadow on the radiograph. Thin lines of gas may be seen representing gas in the distal segment of intestine surrounding the intussusceptum.

If the obstruction is incomplete and there is a doubt about the diagnosis, a barium enema is probably the most satisfactory method of demonstrating an intussusception. The barium will outline the intraluminal mass. Circular mucosal folds (coil spring pattern) are often seen indicative of an intussuscepted portion of intestine. The barium enema sometimes reduces the intussusception but in such cases there is usually a recurrence within hours. If possible, barium enemas should be observed fluoroscopically. Barium given by the mouth is not as satisfactory as an enema. The time taken to demonstrate the intussusception is much longer than with an enema and the administration of barium may provoke vomiting. (Fig. 2–27).

INTESTINAL STRICTURE. The bowel may be constricted as a result of intrinsic causes or as a result of pressure from without. Stricture from extrinsic pressure is unusual, since the small intestine tends to become displaced rather than compressed by extrinsic masses. If a stricture has been present for some time the intestine proximal to it dilates and becomes filled with radiopaque impacted food material. If there is no dilatation of the bowel, strictures can be demonstrated by barium, but serial radiographs should be used to demonstrate the unchanging nature of the narrowed segment. Peristaltic contractions should not be mistaken for strictures. (Fig. 2–28).

ENTERITIS. Enteritis is often difficult to diagnose radiographically. Common radiographic signs of enteritis include the following:

(a) The presence of abnormal amounts of gas widely distributed throughout the intestine but not dilating it. Swallowed air, particularly associated with esophageal abnormalities, is sometimes present in considerable amounts in the small intestine. It should not be mistaken for endogenous gas. In enteritis the gas is present in long narrow streaks, whereas swallowed air tends to be present in sufficient quantity to cause some dilatation of the intestinal loops. Furthermore, swallowed air is usually present in the stomach as well as in the intestine.

(b) Rapid passage of barium through the intestine indicates hypermotility and may be associated with enteritis. This is best observed fluoroscopically.

(c) Barium may fail to fill the lumen of the intestine and it may appear as a thin streak along the affected lengths of the intestine.

(d) Irregularities in mucosal pattern, including ulceration and uneven distribution of barium along the mucosa, may indicate enteritis.

(e) Thickening of the intestinal wall may be a concomitant of inflammatory

Text continued on page 83

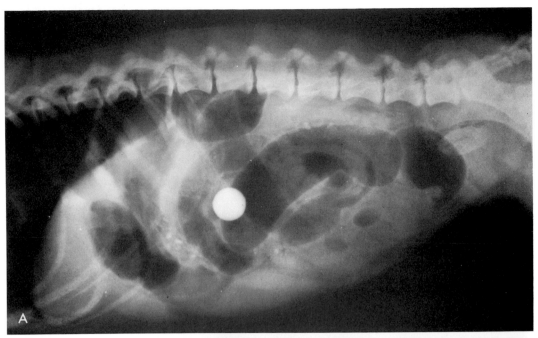

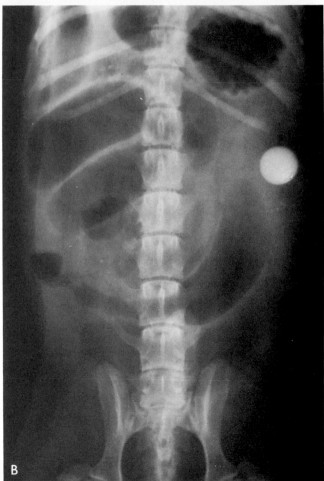

FIGURE 2–26. *A, B.* A radiopaque foreign body that is causing an acute obstruction.
(*Illustration continued on following page.*)

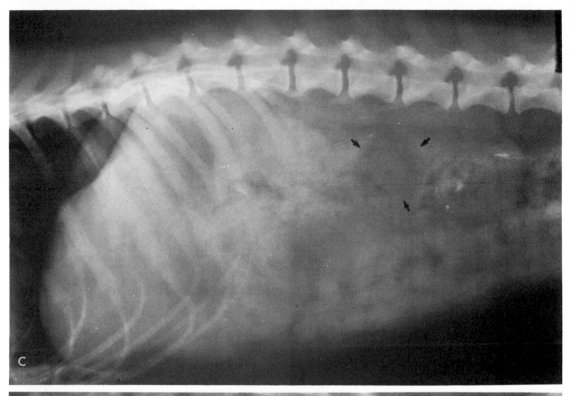

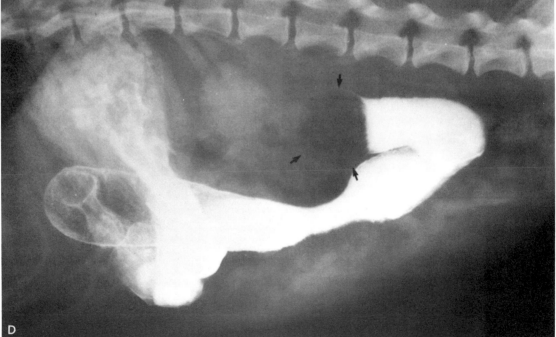

FIGURE 2–26 *Continued. C, D.* A plain radiograph of the abdomen of this dog with a history of vomiting shows an indistinct circular shadow in the dorsal abdomen (arrows) A barium study outlines a foreign body obstructing passage of the barium. The object was a rubber ball.

(*Illustration continued on opposite page.*)

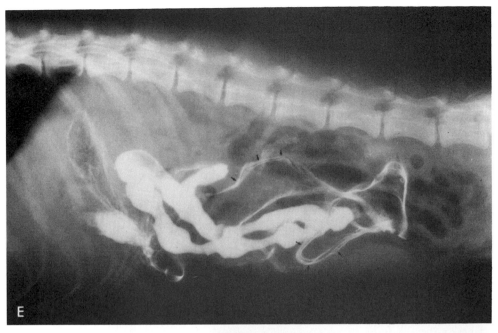

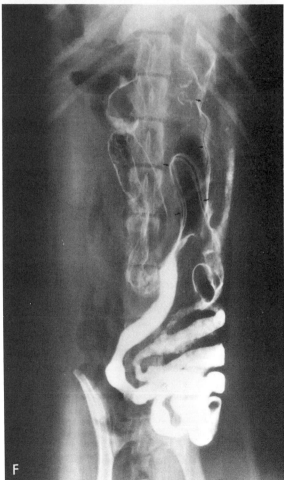

FIGURE 2–26 *Continued. E, F.* Ascarid worms (arrows) in the small intestine. (*Illustration continued on following page.*)

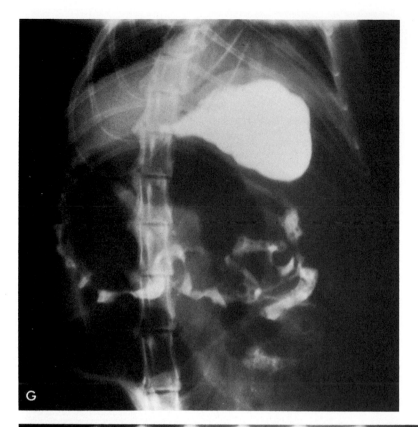

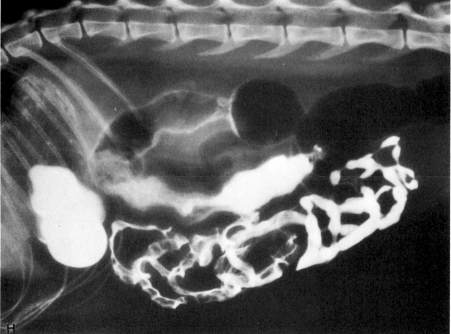

FIGURE 2–26 *Continued. G, H.*   A string foreign body. The ventrodorsal view shows puckering of the duodenum which is drawn cranially. The lateral view, made some time later, shows puckering of the small intestine distal to the duodenum. The string can be seen in places, outlined by the barium.

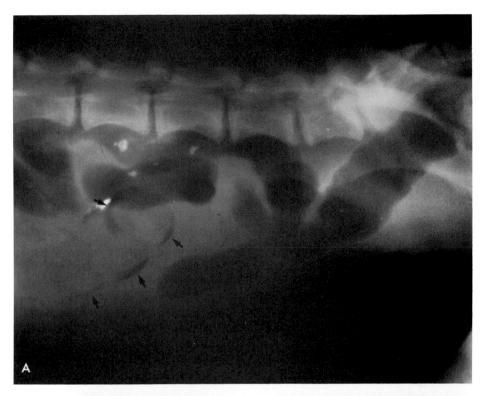

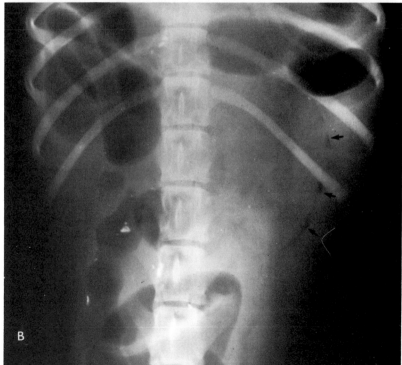

FIGURE 2–27. *A, B.* Plain radiographs of a dog with an intussusception show gas (arrows) trapped between the intussuscipiens and the intussusceptum. This is not usually seen.

(Illustration continued on following page.)

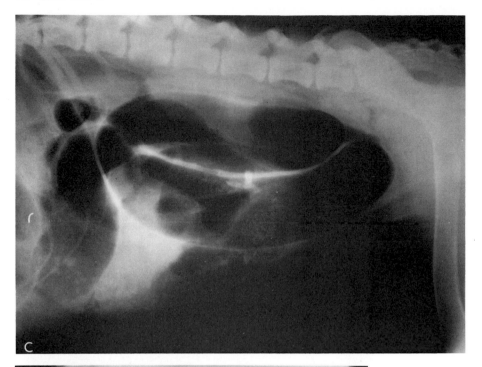

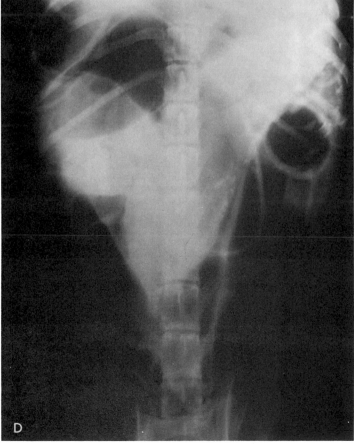

FIGURE 2–27 *Continued. C, D.* An acute intestinal obstruction with gross dilatation of loops of small intestine. This proved to be an intussusception. (*Illustration continued on opposite page.*)

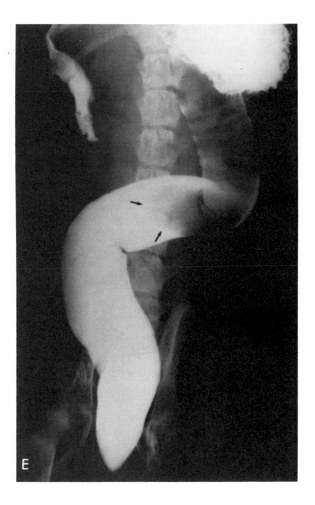

FIGURE 2–27. *Continued. E–K.* An intussusception is best demonstrated by a barium enema. *E.* An intussusception is clearly outlined by the barium. Its distal limit is indicated by the arrows. Proximally, the characteristic "coil-spring" appearance of intussusception can be seen. This is due to folding of the mucosa. Some barium is present in the stomach and duodenum.

(*Illustration continued on following page.*)

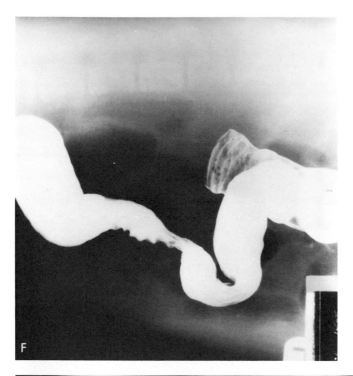

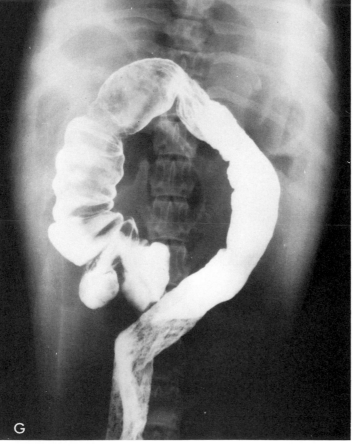

FIGURE 2-27. *Continued. F* through *K* are cases of intussusception demonstrated by barium enemas.
(*Illustration continued on following pages.*)

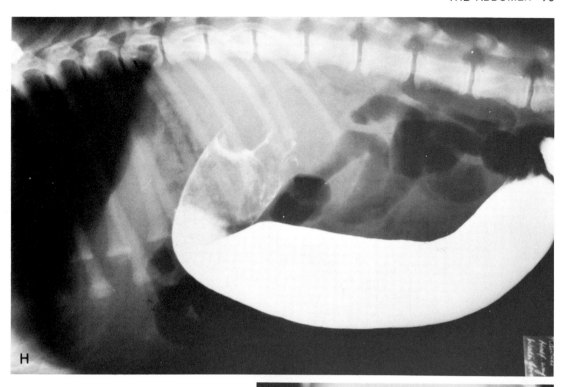

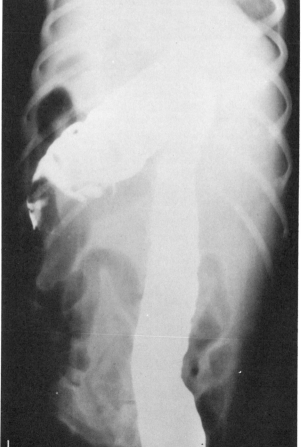

Figure 2–27. *Continued.*

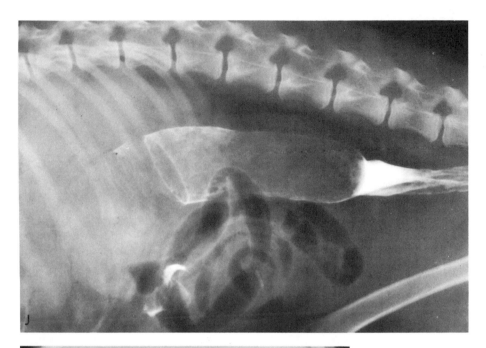

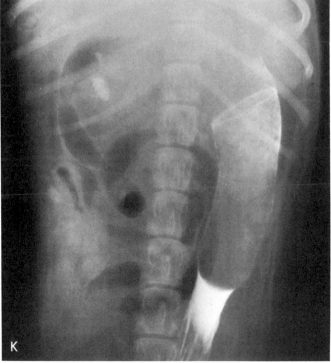

FIGURE 2–27. *Continued. J, K.* See legend on page 78.

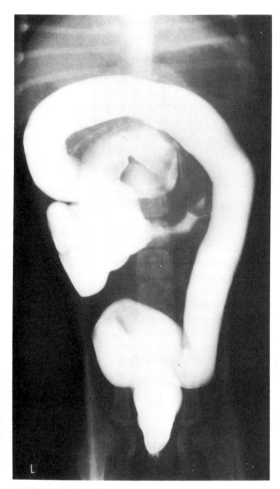
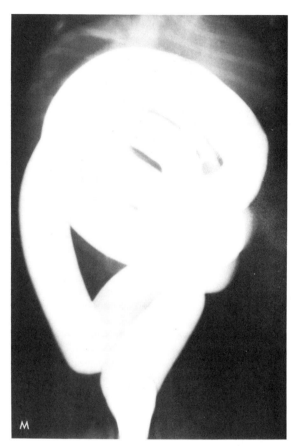

FIGURE 2–27. *Continued. L, M. L* shows an intussusception in the distal jejunum outlined by barium. *M*—The same case showing how too much barium may mask the abnormality. Unless carefully administered a barium enema may cause reduction of an early intussusception which then tends to recur within hours. Where possible barium enemas should be observed fluoroscopically.

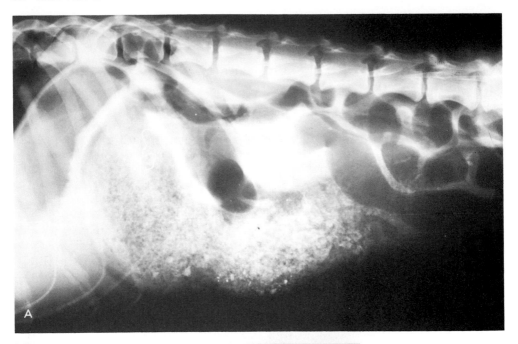

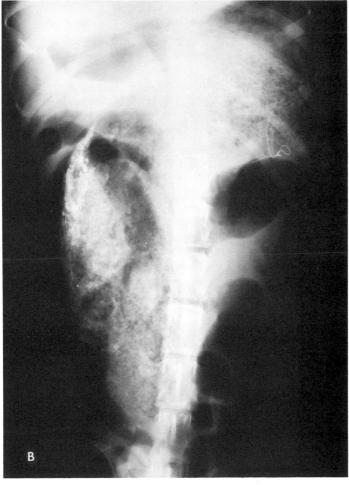

FIGURE 2–28. *A–C.* Plain radiographs of the abdomen show a large mass of impacted ingesta within the intestine. A barium enema (C) shows that the mass is not in the colon. The small intestine was grossly distended and impacted proximal to a constriction in the ileum. Distended loops of small intestine indicate that an obstruction is present. This was a five year old coonhound that had been losing weight for five months. It frequently vomited after eating. The stricture of the ileum found at surgery was thought to be due to recanulation of an intussusception.

(*Illustration continued on opposite page.*)

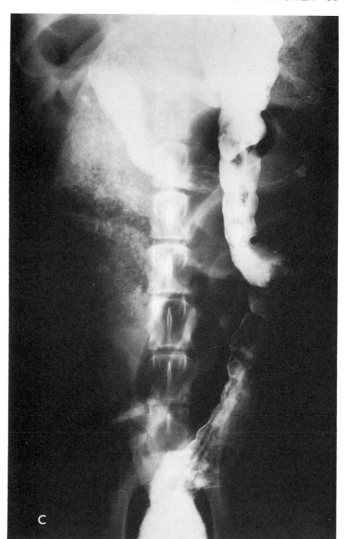

FIGURE 2–28 *Continued. C. See legend on opposite page.*

change. This can be demonstrated using barium in association with pneumoperitoneum. This sign is difficult to observe without double contrast.

(f) Small nodular filling defects have been described associated with enteritis. (Fig. 2–29).

NEOPLASIA. Intestinal neoplasia is more common than is gastric neoplasia, though both are relatively rare. A neoplasm in the wall of the intestine tends to produce an annular constricting lesion, narrowing the intestinal lumen. Intraluminal masses produce constant filling defects on barium examination. Ulceration may be present with loss of the normal smooth mucosal pattern. (Fig. 2–30).

MALABSORPTION SYNDROME. This may be the cause of persistent diarrhea in dogs. The radiographic changes are often not characteristic. They may include dilatation of the intestine, fragmentation of the barium column, and irregularity of the mucosal pattern due to excessive secretion within the intestine.

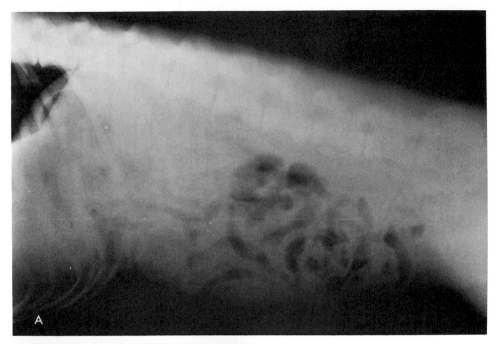

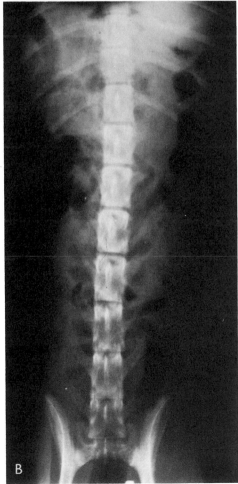

FIGURE 2-29. *A, B* Excessive amounts of gas in the small intestine suggest enteritis.

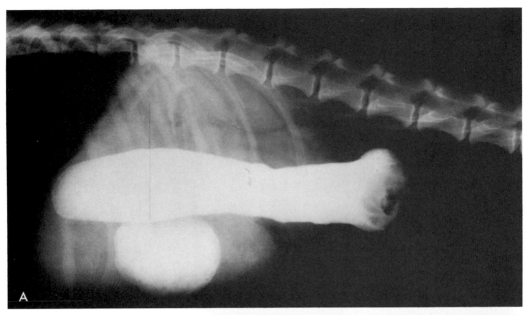

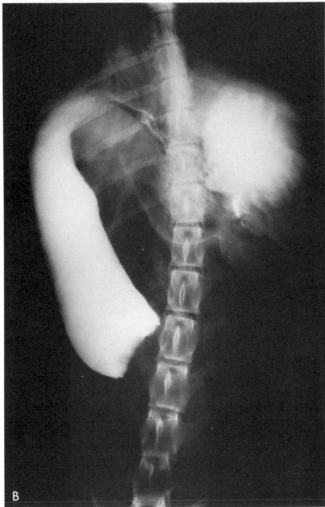

FIGURE 2–30. *A, B.* Obstruction of the duodenum due to an adenocarcinoma. The barium column shows an irregular edge and a large filling defect at the point of obstruction. The duodenum is dilated proximal to the obstruction.

(*Illustration continued on following page.*)

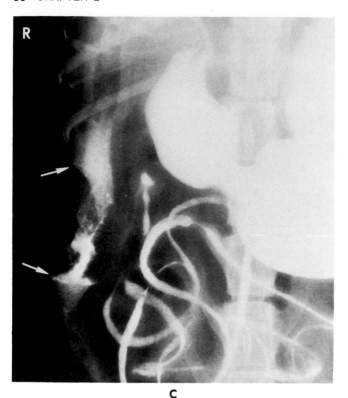

R

C

FIGURE 2–30 *Continued. C.* Oral barium contrast study on a 10 year old female cocker spaniel dog that had a history of intermittent vomiting, anorexia, and weight loss over the past month. On abdominal palpation a small moveable mass was felt in the right cranial quadrant. The contrast radiograph outlines localized, irregular luminal narrowing of the proximal duodenum with a sharply defined shelf deformity at the transition zone between normal and abnormal bowel (arrows). The mucosal surface of the lesion is nodular and ulcerated. The radiographic findings are the classic "napkin ring" or "apple-core" deformity of an annular bowel neoplasm. Surgical resection of the tumor was done and the histologic diagnosis was fibrosarcoma. (From Gomez, J. A. The gastrointestinal contrast study. Methods and Interpretation. The Veterinary Clinics of North America. Radiology. Nov., 1974. W. B. Saunders Co. Philadelphia.)

The Large Intestine

ANATOMY

The large intestine is composed of the cecum, the colon, the rectum, and the anal canal.

In the dog the cecum is a diverticulum of the proximal colon with which it communicates through the cecocolic valve. It does not communicate directly with the ileum. The cecum is twisted on itself to give it a corkscrew shape. It lies within the duodenal loop. In the cat it is a straight blind pouch.

The colon is divided into ascending, transverse, and descending parts. It is shaped like a question mark or a shepherd's crook. The right colic flexure unites the ascending and transverse portions, while the transverse and descending parts form the left or splenic flexure. The ascending colon lies ventral to the right kidney. It is related to the right limb of the pancreas dorsally and to the duodenum on the right. To the left and ventrally it contacts the small intestine and cranially it touches the stomach. The transverse colon is related to the stomach cranioventrally and to the left limb of the pancreas craniodorsally. Caudally it is in contact with the small intestine. The descending colon lies to the left of the midline and extends from the splenic flexure to the pelvic inlet. Dorsally it is in contact with the iliopsoas muscle, but cranially it is related to the left kidney and ureter. Medially it is related to the ascending duodenum and laterally to the spleen. Elsewhere it is bounded by the small intestine. Caudally it lies above the bladder and uterus. The descending colon is sometimes longer and more tortuous than usual and it is then referred to as a "redundant colon."

The rectum is the terminal portion of the colon beginning at the pelvic inlet and ending at the anal canal. Ventral to the rectum in the female is the vagina, in the male the prostate gland and the urethra.

RADIOGRAPHY

The large intestine is usually seen on plain radiographs because of the feces and gas within it. Detailed studies require a barium enema.

Before carrying out a barium enema it is useful, though not essential, to have the animal fasted for 18 to 24 hours prior to the procedure. A mild cathartic may be administered. General anesthesia is desirable to eliminate straining. The colon should be thoroughly washed out with saline or warm water to remove all feces. Tepid solutions are said to result in less gas accumulation within the colon than warm ones. A cuffed rectal catheter (Bardex Cuffed Rectal Catheters, Bard Hospital Division, C. R. Bard, Inc.) is used to introduce the barium suspension. The concentration of the suspension should be about 15 to 20 per cent (w/v) and it can be prepared from any of the commercial liquid suspensions of barium recommended for study of the upper gastrointestinal tract. Gravity flow, from a large container, is more satisfactory than using a syringe. The amount used is approximately 20 to 30 ml/kg body weight given slowly. If fluoroscopy is available it should be used. If not, then frequent radiographs are necessary during the procedure to assess the degree of filling of the colon. It should be filled completely to its physiological capacity but not overdilated. Radiographs taken in the ventrodorsal position are best for evaluating the degree of filling. When the colon has been filled lateral and ventrodorsal radiographs are made. The colon is then evacuated and post evacuation films are made. Finally, air, in equal volume to the evacuated barium suspension is injected and double contrast radiographs are made in lateral and ventrodorsal projections. (Fig. 2–31).

NORMAL APPEARANCE

On plain radiographs the colon is seen with varying degrees of clarity depending on the contents. A barium enema reveals a smooth mucosal surface.

ABNORMALITIES

FECAL RETENTION.   Fecal retention is evidenced by the presence of dense masses of fecal material in the colon and rectum. These masses may be very dense, approaching the density of bone. They may be so dense that obstipation results. (Fig. 2–32).

MEGACOLON (Hirschsprung's disease).   This is a condition in which there is gross dilatation and hypertrophy of the colon proximal to a narrowed, aganglionic segment at its distal end. Dogs and cats are affected. The condition is often first recognized in adult life. The clinical signs comprise constipation, the passage of blood-stained mucus, and occasionally diarrhea, even in the presence of hard masses of feces.

On plain radiographs, masses of dense feces are seen in a dilated colon. The terminal aganglionic segment and the rectum are usually empty. This helps to distinguish the condition from simple fecal impaction in which feces are often seen in the rectum. A barium enema will confirm the presence of a terminal aganglionic

Text continued on page 93

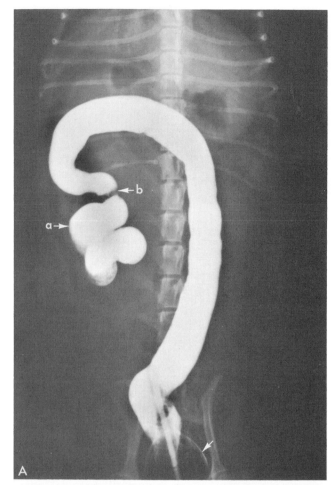

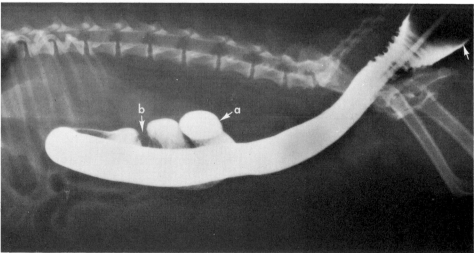

FIGURE 2–31. A, B. Positive contrast study of the colon. The wall is smooth in outline and the lumen is uniform in width. The colon assumes a "shepherd's crook" or "question mark" configuration in the VD view. In this study, the cecum (*a*) and cecocolic valve (*b*) are seen. Cecal opacification during radiography of the colon is not always satisfactory. Note the air-filled cuff of the Bardex catheter (arrows). (From Ticer, J. W., 1975, Radiographic Technique in Small Animal Practice., W. B. Saunders Co., Philadelphia)

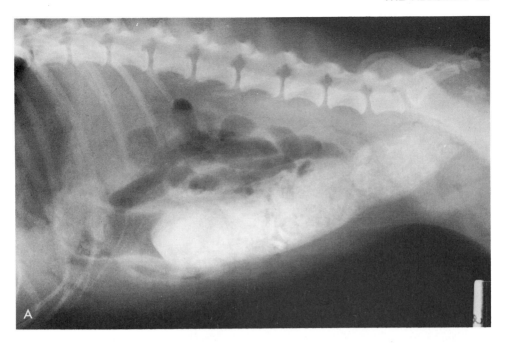

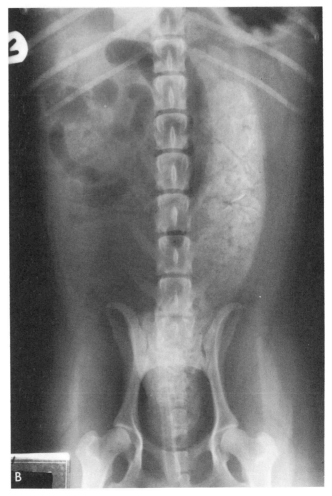

FIGURE 2-32. *A, B.* Fecal retention in a dog. Fecal material can be identified in the colon and rectum. The presence of quantities of fecal material in the colon and rectum does not necessarily imply that the animal is constipated. House trained dogs may show fecal retention on radiographs if they have not had an opportunity to defecate prior to radiography.

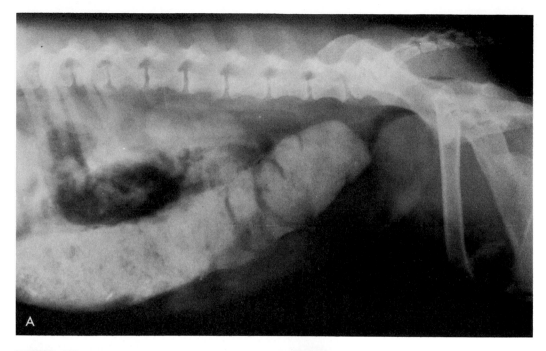

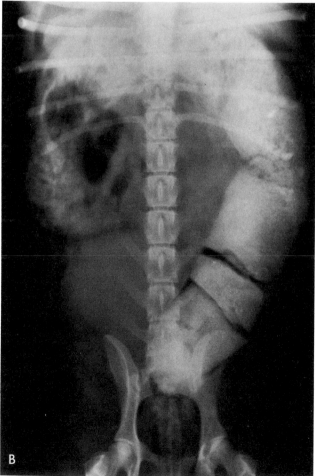

FIGURE 2–33. *A, B.* Megacolon. The colon is distended and impacted with hard, dense fecal material. The terminal aganglionic segment and the rectum are empty. The prostate gland is enlarged and is in the antepubic position. It narrows the lumen of the rectum. However, this would not account for the degree of impaction.

(*Illustration continued on opposite page.*)

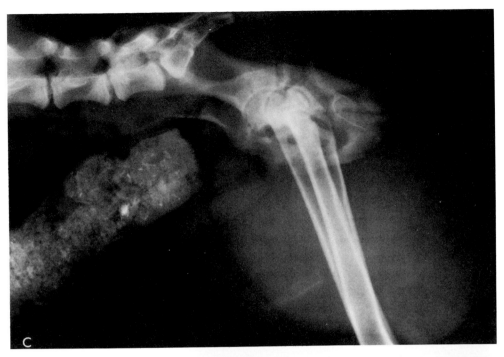

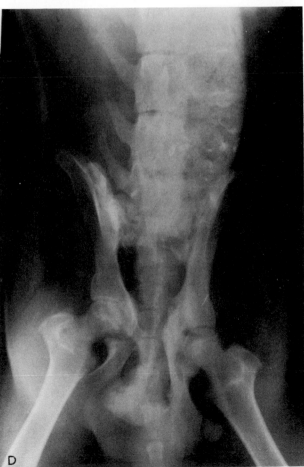

FIGURE 2–33 *Continued. C, D.* Obstipation due to old pelvic fractures.

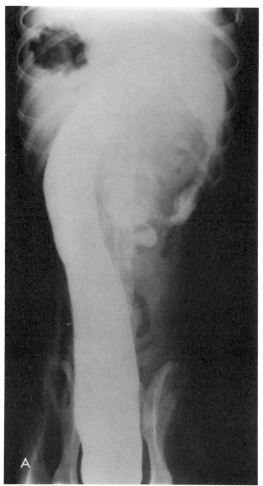

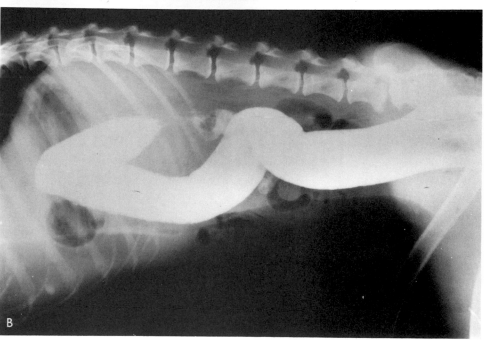

FIGURE 2–34. *A, B.* A barium enema fails to fill fully the ascending colon and cecum despite the fact that some barium has reached the ilium. The colonic mucosa is irregular in appearance. The dog was infected with Trichuris vulpis.
(*Illustration continued on opposite page.*)

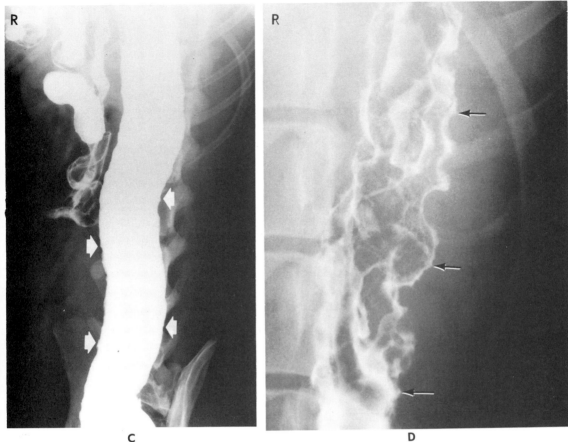

FIGURE 2–34. *Continued. C, D.* Barium enema radiographs of a two year old female boxer dog that had intermittent, bloody diarrhea for the previous six months. (*C*), The barium-filled descending colon (right ventrodorsal oblique positioning) is distensible but exhibits diffuse, superficial mucosal ulcerations (arrows). The partially filled ileum has a smooth mucosal pattern. (*D*), A close-up of the postevacuation barium enema radiograph of the descending colon reveals prominent tortuous mucosal folds that produce a rugose pattern. The folds appear finely nodular and there are numerous flecks of barium clinging to small superficial ulcers (arrows). Large intestinal biopsy disclosed canine histiocytic ulcerative colitis. (Courtesy of Gomez. Vet. Clinics of North America. Nov. 1974. Pp. 822–823.)

contracted segment. In most cases, however, the diagnosis can be made from plain radiographs. Muscular spasm may cause contraction of the intestine about the enema catheter; this should not be mistaken for permanent contraction. Such spasms are transient.

Dilatation of the colon due to chronic constipation is sometimes seen in older dogs. It is referred to as "pseudomegacolon" or "obstipation." It may be due to old healed pelvic fractures, neoplasia, strictures, or foreign bodies. No contracted distal segment is present. (Fig. 2–33).

COLITIS. The principal clinical sign of inflammation of the colon is straining (tenesmus). Diarrhea, often blood stained, and the frequent passage of small amounts of feces are also suggestive of the condition. Colitis may be acute or chronic, ulcerative, or granulomatous.

Radiographically, thickened mucosal folds, narrowing of the colonic lumen, ulceration, and spasm may be seen on barium enema examination. The changes seen are variable, and supplementary proctoscopic examination is advisable. (Fig. 2 34).

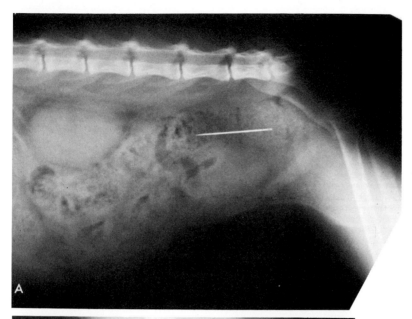

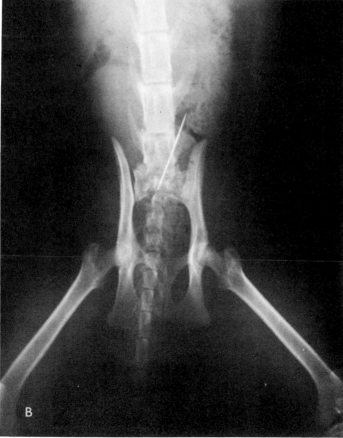

FIGURE 2–35. *A, B.* A needle in the large intestine of a cat. Two views are necessary to demonstrate its position. Needles and other sharp objects frequently pass through the alimentary tract without causing any signs.

FOREIGN BODIES. Foreign bodies in the colon and rectum are seldom of clinical significance, as they are usually passed out without difficulty. It is important to be sure of their position and at least two views at right angles to one another are necessary. Occasionally, sharp pieces of bone or pointed foreign objects may become lodged in the colon or rectum; radiography may be used to identify their position with accuracy. (Fig. 2–35).

DISPLACEMENT. The colon may be displaced by intra-abdominal masses, such as enlarged sublumbar lymph nodes, or by an enlarged prostate gland. A full bladder displaces the colon. Sometimes the colon is somewhat longer than usual and part of the descending colon may be seen on the right side (redundant colon).

INTUSSUSCEPTION. This has been discussed in connection with the small intestine. If the colon is involved the lesion is best demonstrated by barium enema, in which the mass of the intussusception will be seen protruding into the colon. (Fig. 2–27).

NEOPLASIA. This is not common. Blood in the feces and constipation may be presenting signs. Annular constrictions due to neoplasia may result in pseudo-megacolon. Barium enema examination will outline areas of constriction or ulceration. Filling defects are seen. Double contrast studies are valuable in outlining polyps. (Fig. 2–36).

IMPERFORATE ANUS, ATRESIA RECTI, ATRESIA COLI. These are rare congenital conditions. Radiography is used to determine the extent of the deficiency. In the case of imperforate anus a metallic probe is placed against the anal dimple and a radiograph is made with the animal suspended by the hind limbs. This position ensures that the gas in the intestine will rise to outline the posterior limit of the bowel. An estimate can then be made of the distance between the gas and the metallic probe. A similar technique can be used in cases of atresia of the colon, the metal probe being inserted into the rectum.

THE URINARY SYSTEM

This system comprises the kidneys, the ureters, the bladder, and the urethra.

The Kidneys and Ureters

ANATOMY

The kidneys are bean shaped in appearance. They are retroperitoneal, one on either side of the aorta and caudal vena cava. They lie in an oblique direction, tilted cranioventrally. The left kidney is less firmly attached to the dorsal wall than is the right and hence is more variable in position. Both kidneys move somewhat during respiration. The kidneys of the cat are more freely moveable than those of the dog.

The left kidney, cranially, is in contact with the spleen, the greater curvature of the stomach, the pancreas, and the left adrenal gland. Dorsally, it is related to the sublumbar muscles and caudally it is in contact with the descending colon. Medially, it is related to the descending colon and the ascending duodenum. Ventrally, it is related to the descending colon.

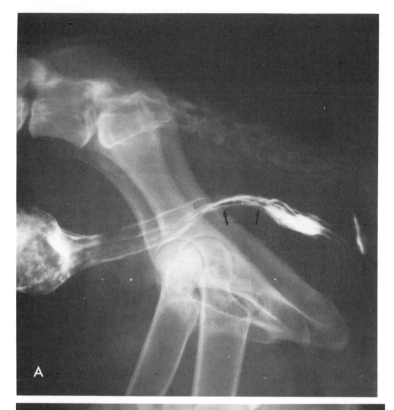

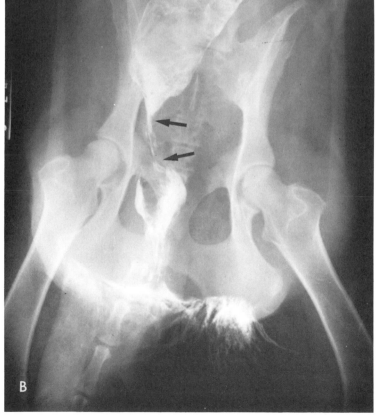

FIGURE 2–36. *A, B.* A persistent fill
ing defect in the rectum (arrows) due to
an undifferentiated carcinoma. The pa
tient was a nine year old spayed female
with a history of difficult defecation and
dribbling of urine.

The right kidney, cranially, lies in the renal fossa of the caudate lobe of the liver. It is related to the right adrenal gland. Medially, it is close to the caudal vena cava. Ventrally, it is in contact with the right limb of the pancreas and the ascending colon.

The kidneys may be displaced caudally by a full stomach or cranially by an enlarged uterus.

The ureters are tubular structures that carry urine from the kidneys to the bladder. The ureters begin at the renal pelvis and course caudoventrally to the bladder, which they enter at the trigone through oblique slit-like openings. They are extraperitoneal.

RADIOGRAPHY

The kidneys are seen clearly in about 50 per cent of plain studies of the abdomen. The clarity with which they are seen depends on the amount of perirenal fat present and on the absence of food material within the alimentary tract. They are often more clearly seen on lateral radiographs, in which they are partially superimposed on one another.

The radiographic appearance of the kidneys varies with changes in the animal's position. In lateral recumbency the uppermost kidney rotates on its long axis, profiling the hilar notch. Right and left lateral recumbent views are, therefore, recommended for optimum visualization of both kidneys. Movements of the diaphragm cause a change in position of the kidneys. In right lateral recumbency the right kidney may be displaced cranially. The superimposition of the kidneys on one another is less, therefore, in right lateral recumbency than it is in left.

Since plain films usually give poor delineation of the kidneys, contrast radiography using organic iodide contrast material is often used to study the urinary tract. This procedure is referred to as intravenous urography. General anesthesia or deep sedation is advisable. Survey radiographs should always be made prior to the use of contrast agents. A variety of contrast techniques may be employed.

Low Volume, Rapid Infusion. The dose of contrast material is given rapidly into a peripheral vein after the animal has been placed in dorsal recumbency over the cassette. The dose of contrast agent recommended is 850 mgI/kg body weight with the maximum dose not exceeding 35g. A radiograph is made immediately. Ventrodorsal and lateral radiographs are then made as quickly as possible and again at one minute, four minutes, and 15 minutes after completion of the injection. Left and right ventrodorsal oblique views are necessary to outline the terminal ureters.

Compression may be applied to the caudal abdomen to improve opacification of the ureters. If compression is to be used it should be applied before the injection is made. The dose is then reduced to 425 mgI/kg body weight. A standard compression device may be used or foam rubber pads may be bandaged tightly onto the ventral aspect of the abdomen cranial to the pubis. It has been suggested that compression may cause distortion of the ureters and so it is advisable to make further radiographs after the compression has been removed.

The low volume, rapid injection technique gives very good results.

High Volume, Drip Infusion. 1200 mgI/kg body weight is mixed with an equal volume of 5 per cent glucose solution. This is given slowly over a period of 10 minutes. Lateral and ventrodorsal radiographs are made at the end of the infusion and a compression device is applied. Further radiographs are made after 10 minutes and the compression band is then released. If kidney function is abnormal, compression is reapplied and further films are made 20 minutes later. The terminal ureters can be demonstrated on oblique views after the compression has been removed.

This method also gives good visualization but is more time-consuming than the rapid infusion method. It is recommended in cases of renal failure.

LOW VOLUME, SLOW INFUSION. Contrast material at a dosage rate of 425 mgI/kg body weight is injected slowly over two or three minutes. Radiographs are made immediately and thereafter at five minute intervals until the urinary system is outlined. Definition may be improved by the use of compression. This is the least satisfactory method.

Several preparations of contrast material are available commercially (Conray 280 or Conray 420, Meglumine Iothalamate or Sodium Iothalamate, Mallinckrodt Chemical Works and May & Baker, Ltd.; Hypaque M 75%, Sodium and Meglumine Diatrizoates, Winthrop Laboratories; Renovist II, Sodium and Meglumine Diatrizoates, Squibb & Sons). These are all satisfactory. Untoward reactions following injection are rare, though vomiting occasionally occurs after rapid injections. These agents may be given to uremic patients unless there is severe dehydration. Perivascular injection may result in sloughing. Increasing the dose beyond the levels recommended does not improve opacification.

The patient should be fasted for 24 hours prior to the study and a mild cathartic given. Water should be withheld for 12 hours, as mild dehydration improves opacification of the kidneys. Water should not be withheld if there is severe renal insufficiency. An enema may be necessary to remove fecal material. Five to 10 units of vasopressin given an hour prior to radiography will reduce intestinal gas. (Fig. 2–37).

PNEUMOPERITONOGRAPHY. The kidney outlines may be demonstrated using pneumoperitoneum.

NORMAL APPEARANCE

The left kidney lies in the area from the second to the fifth lumbar vertebrae. The right kidney is more cranial, in the area from the thirteenth thoracic to the third

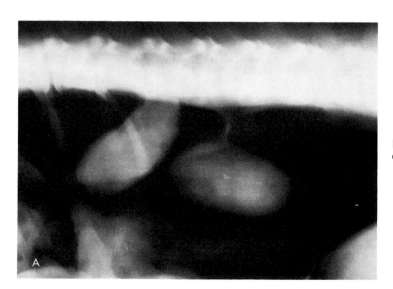

FIGURE 2–37. *A.* The kidneys outlined by pneumoperitoneum.

(Illustration continued on opposite page.)

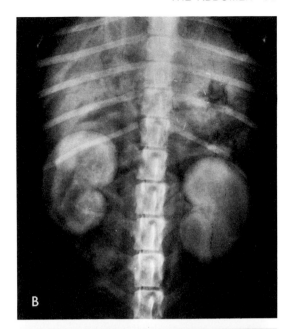

FIGURE 2–37 *Continued. B–D.* Contrast studies of normal kidneys. Nephrogram (*B*). This radiograph was made ten seconds after the injection of contrast medium. The cortex can be distinguished from the medulla because of its rich blood supply. Figures *C* and *D* are normal urograms.

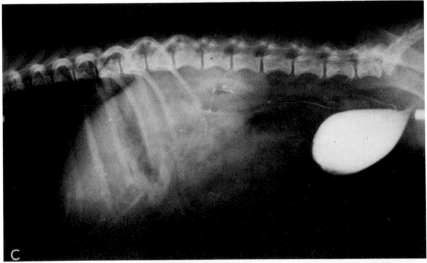

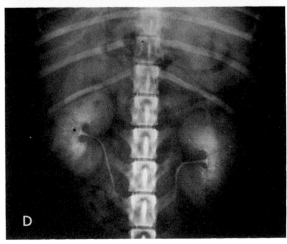

lumbar vertebra. The normal kidney is approximately 2.5 to 3.5 times the length of the second lumbar vertebra. The normal feline kidney is approximately 2.4 to 3 times the length of the second lumbar vertebra. The cranial limit of the right kidney is seldom seen on plain radiographs because of its close relationship with the liver.

The position of the kidneys varies with respiration and the degree of distention of the stomach. Position is more variable in the cat than in the dog. Measurements related to the vertebral bodies are not to be considered accurate. Normal kidneys may be larger or smaller than the lengths suggested, Abnormality should be suspected, however, if a kidney is less than 2.5 or more than 3.5 times the length of the second lumbar vertebra.

On contrast studies, both kidneys should be well visualized. Films made during the stage of opacification of the kidneys are called "nephrograms." The kidneys should be smooth in outline and the renal pelves and ureters should be clearly seen. (Fig. 2–37).

On fluoroscopy, peristaltic waves are seen in the ureters. The upper portion of the ureter is seen to fill with contrast material and then a peristaltic wave sweeps it into the bladder.

Failure of the kidneys to excrete contrast material satisfactorily may indicate loss of renal function. However, this is but a crude test of kidney function and other methods should be used to evaluate it.

ABNORMALITIES

Radiographic examination does not always reveal characteristic signs of kidney or ureteral disease. It may give information as to the number, size, position, shape, and density of the kidneys. One can then assess how the findings compare with normal studies. When variations are seen they have to be explained pathophysiologically. It would be unrealistic to attempt to correlate all the possible changes with pathologic or physiologic aberrations. The discussion will be confined, therefore, to manifestations of abnormality seen in the more common disease conditions.

CONGENITAL DEFECTS. One kidney may be absent (aplasia), congenitally deformed, misplaced (ectopia), or very small and nonfunctional. If one kidney is nonfunctional the other one may be hypertrophied. Congenital hydronephrosis has been described with hypertrophy of the opposite kidney.

These defects are best demonstrated using intravenous pyelography. Pneumoperitoneum may also be employed.

HYDRONEPHROSIS. This usually follows obstruction of a ureter. The obstruction may be caused by impingement on the ureter by an abdominal mass or by calculi, stricture of the ureter, or accidental ligation of a ureter during surgery. Following obstruction there is progressive pelvic distention with atrophy of the kidney parenchyma, resulting in the kidney becoming a large fluid-filled sac. Occasionally, obstruction of a ureter may result in atrophy without hydronephrosis.

Radiographically, the enlarged kidney is often seen as an abdominal mass with a tissue or fluid density. It must be distinguished from other possible intra-abdominal masses. Intravenous contrast radiography will outline the normal kidney but there will be no excretion of contrast medium through the affected kidney if urine flow has ceased. Hydroureter is seen proximal to the point of ureteral obstruction with a dilated kidney pelvis in cases in which urine excretion is still occurring. (Fig. 2–38).

Text continued on page 105

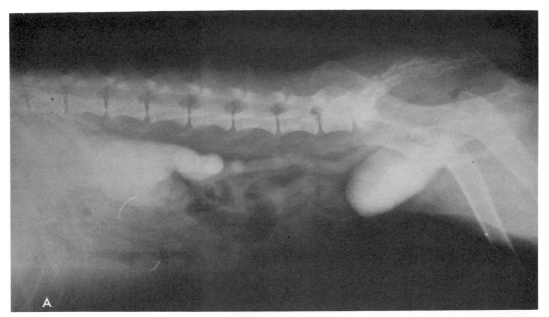

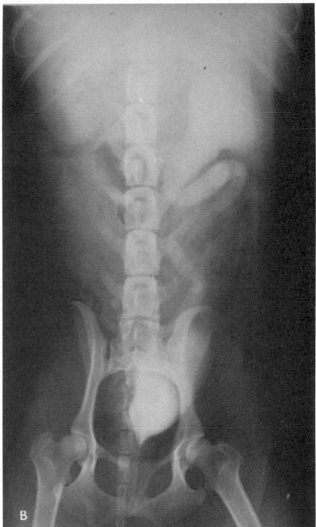

FIGURE 2–38. *A, B.* Hydronephrosis and hydroureter. The radiographs were made fifteen minutes after rapid injection of contrast medium. The left ureter is grossly dilated, as is the left renal pelvis. *(Illustration continued on following page.)*

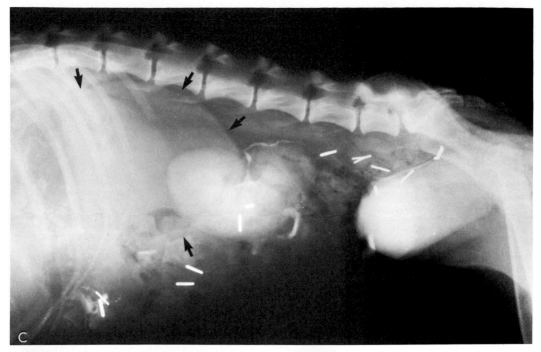

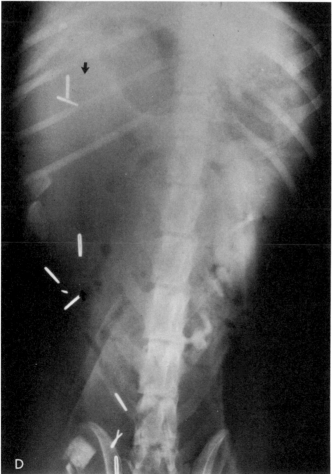

FIGURE 2–38 Continued. C, D. A large hydronephrotic right kidney (arrows). It presents radiographically as an intra-abdominal mass. The contrast studies show normal excretion on the left side and no excretion of contrast medium on the right. The cause of the hydronephrosis was clamping off the ureter with a hemostatic clip during surgery for a postspay granuloma. Numerous hemostatic clips are seen.

(Illustration continued on opposite page.)

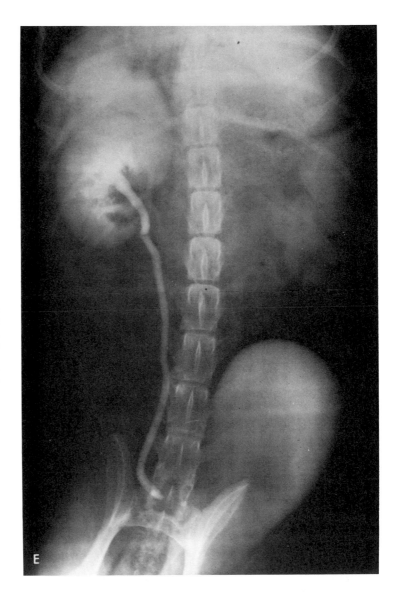

FIGURE 2–38 *Continued. E.* A non-functioning left kidney. Compression was used to improve visualization. This accounts for the right ureter appearing wider than usual.
(*Illustration continued on following page.*)

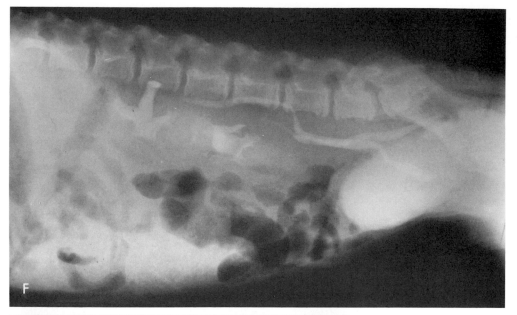

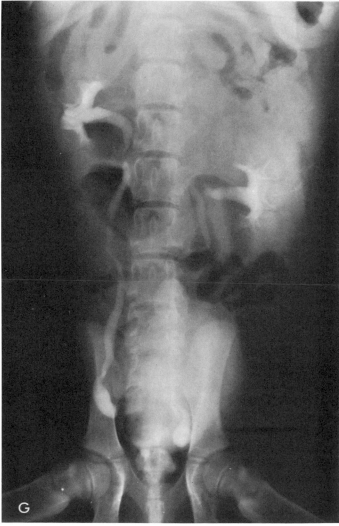

FIGURE 2–38 *Continued F, G.* Dilatation of the ureters and kidney pelves in a dog with pyelonephritis. This was a four month old puppy with a history of hematuria and vomiting for eight days.

RENAL CALCULI.   Calculi are seen as radiopaque densities within the kidney. They tend to be centrally located. Occasionally, a single large calculus is seen that occupies the kidney pelvis and extends up into the renal diverticula. Such a calculus is referred to as a "stag-horn" calculus. Calcifications within the kidney parenchyma should not be mistaken for calculi. Urate calculi are usually radiolucent and cystine calculi may or may not be radiolucent. Contrast studies are necessary to demonstrate radiolucent calculi. Good patient preparation is essential when examining for calculi, as small calculi may be obscured by intestinal contents. (Fig. 2-39).

RUPTURE OF THE KIDNEY.   Rupture of a kidney may occur as the result of trauma. On plain radiographs one may detect a retroperitoneal density that obliterates the psoas shadow. On intravenous pyelography, contrast material will be seen in the retroperitoneal area. A high-dose contrast technique is advised to overcome the reduced excretion that results from nephron damage. (Fig. 2-40).

Intracapsular hemorrhage, if severe, will cause an increase in kidney size.

NEOPLASIA.   Neoplasia of the kidney is not common. Carcinoma arising from the tubular epithelium is the most common malignant neoplasm in the dog. Malignant lymphoma is the commonest renal neoplasm in cats. Bilateral involvement is usual.

The radiographic demonstration of neoplasia, whether primary or secondary, depends on whether or not demonstrable changes in size and function are present. Frequently, the findings are not specific. Neoplasia should be considered in the differential diagnosis if kidney enlargement is present or if the kidney is irregular in outline. Carcinomas often involve one pole of the kidney only. Pneumoperitoneum is useful in demonstrating kidney shape. Intravenous pyelography will show changes in shape and function. The presence of pulmonary metastases may confirm a diagnosis of renal neoplasia.

RENAL CYSTS.   Cysts may be single or multiple. Cysts usually cause a distortion of the outline of the kidney, which may be seen on plain radiographs. Contrast studies will outline changes in shape and function of the kidney. Radiographic examination alone seldom yields sufficient specific information to make a diagnosis of renal cysts. Polycystic disease, in which parts of the renal parenchyma are replaced by cysts, is sometimes seen in young dogs and cats.

Perirenal cysts may surround a normal or a nonfunctional kidney. On plain radiographs they appear as intra-abdominal masses that cannot be distinguished from enlarged kidneys. (Fig. 2-41).

NEPHRITIS.   Nephritis is not usually diagnosed on radiographs. Small nodular kidneys may indicate chronic interstitial nephritis. Kidney size may be reduced in some cases of nephrosis. End-stage kidneys are small.

INFARCTION.   Areas of infarction can be demonstrated as nonfunctional areas using contrast radiography.

The Ureters

CONGENITAL ANOMALIES.   Ectopic ureters may occasionally be the cause of urinary incontinence in young female dogs. The ectopic ureter may open into the vagina, the body of the uterus or into a uterine horn. Incontinence is not a feature of the condition in the male, where the ectopic ureter may open into the urethra. Ectopic ureter may be bilateral. It is frequently associated with some degree of dilatation.

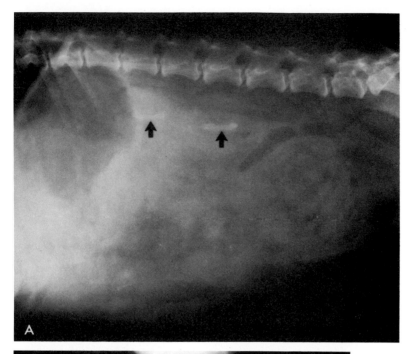

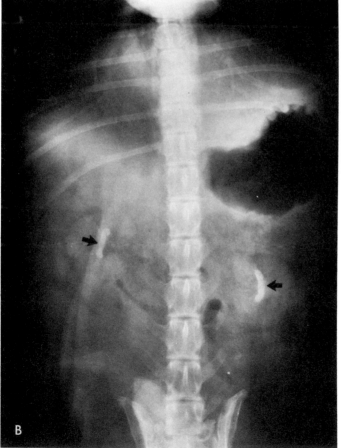

FIGURE 2–39. *A B.* Calculi (arrows) are seen in both kidneys.

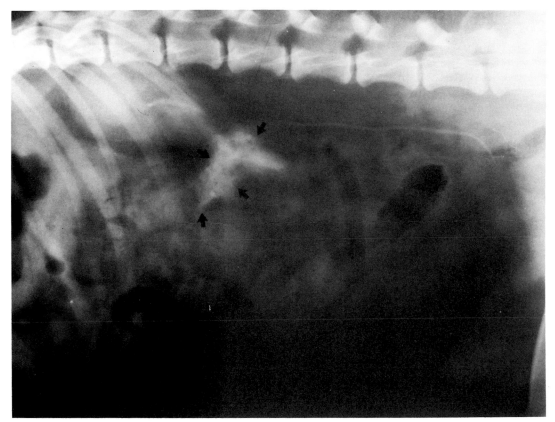

FIGURE 2-40. Rupture of a kidney. On this intravenous urogram contrast medium (arrows) is seen to leak out into the retroperitoneal space from a ruptured kidney. Contrast material is seen in the ureter of the normal kidney.

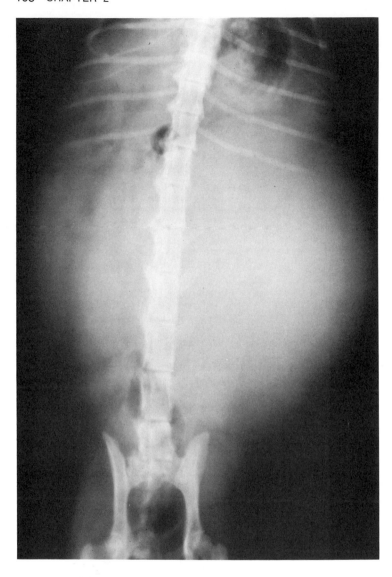

FIGURE 2–41. This abdominal mass in a cat was due to a large perirenal cyst An excretory urogram showed function in both kidneys.

An ectopic ureter may be demonstrated either by intravenous pyelography or by retrograde urography if the opening of the ectopic ureter is accessible. The abnormal ureter will be seen to bypass the bladder. (Fig. 2–42).

URETERAL CALCULI.   These are very rare, but occasionally a small calculus passing down from the kidney to the bladder may obstruct the ureter. A very careful search is necessary to detect the presence of such a calculus on a radiograph. Adequate preparation of the patient is vital to eliminate the possibility of food material in the intestine being mistaken for a calculus.

RUPTURE OF THE URETER.   This is usually the result of trauma. On intravenous pyelography contrast material will be seen to leak out from the affected ureter at the site of rupture. Rupture usually occurs near the kidney. It may be followed by stenosis.

HYDROURETER.   Hydroureter may result from blockage of a ureter due to the presence of a calculus. It may also result from damage to the ureter, resulting in stenosis. Contrast studies will show a dilated ureter proximal to the point of

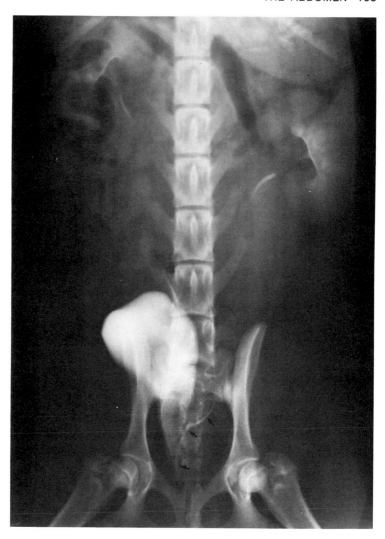

FIGURE 2–42. This nine month old bitch had a history of urinary incontinence. An ectopic ureter (arrows) can be seen bypassing the bladder.

obstruction. If the condition persists, hydronephrosis will follow. Blockage of the ureter may also result from a bladder abnormality, such as a neoplasm, inhibiting ureteral emptying. (Fig. 2–38).

The Bladder

ANATOMY

The urinary bladder is a hollow organ that varies in size and position depending on the amount of urine it contains. When empty, it lies entirely, or almost entirely, within the pelvis. The bladder of the cat lies more cranial than that of the dog.

Dorsally the bladder is related to the small intestine and the descending colon. In the female the cervix and body of the uterus are in contact with it. Ventrally, when distended, it is related to the abdominal wall.

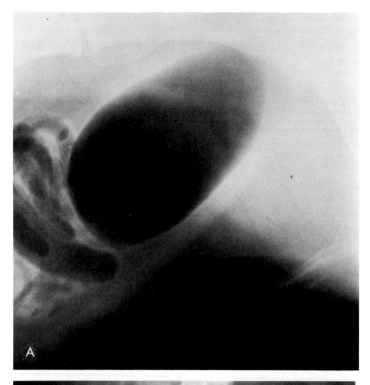

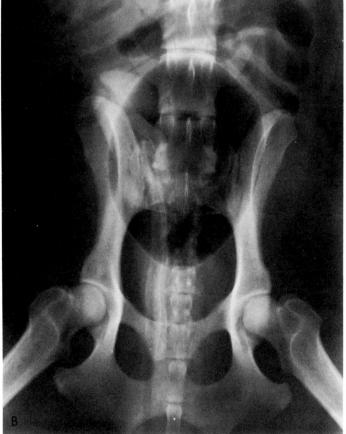

FIGURE 2–43. *A. B.* A normal pneumocystogram in a dog. The bladder wall is smooth and thin.
(Illustration continued on opposite page.)

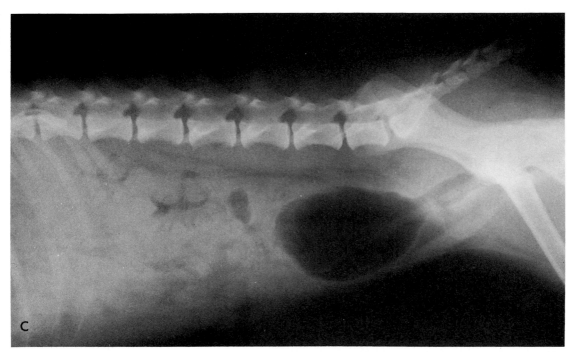

FIGURE 2–43 *Continued. C.* In this study air has passed from the bladder into the ureters and renal pelves. The bladder is displaced cranially by an enlarged prostate gland.

RADIOGRAPHY

When the bladder contains some urine it is seen on plain radiographs. Detailed study requires the use of a contrast medium. The patient should be fasted for 18 to 24 hours, if possible, and a cleansing enema given about an hour before the study is to be performed. Various methods are used to outline the bladder.

PNEUMOCYSTOGRAPHY. Air, at a dosage rate of 6 to 12 ml/kg body weight is injected into the bladder through a flexible catheter using a three-way stopcock and a large syringe. The bladder should be moderately distended. Recoil pressure on the plunger of the syringe or an escape of air about the catheter are indications that sufficient air has been injected. Carbon dioxide or nitrous oxide may be used instead of air. Flexible male catheters are suitable for both males and females. Sedation or general anesthesia will facilitate the procedure. (Fig. 2–43).

POSITIVE CONTRAST CYSTOGRAPHY. Any aqueous organic iodinated medium recommended for urography is suitable. The contrast agent should be diluted with sterilized water or saline to a concentration of 5 per cent w/v of iodine. The contrast material is injected until the bladder is moderately distended. This usually requires about 6 to 12 ml/kg body weight of diluted contrast agent. Intravenous injection of contrast material will also outline the bladder. (Fig. 2–44).

DOUBLE CONTRAST CYSTOGRAPHY. Air may be used with positive contrast material to give a double contrast radiograph. Sterile barium sulphate in a 15 to 20 per cent suspension has also been used to provide double contrast radiographs. The barium is injected into the bladder by means of a catheter. It is not necessary to distend the bladder but the animal is rolled over several times to disperse the barium suspension over the bladder wall. As much of the barium as possible is then aspirated through the catheter and air is injected until the bladder is mod-

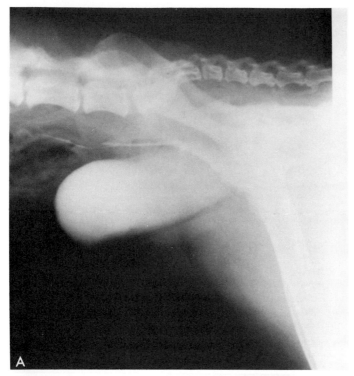

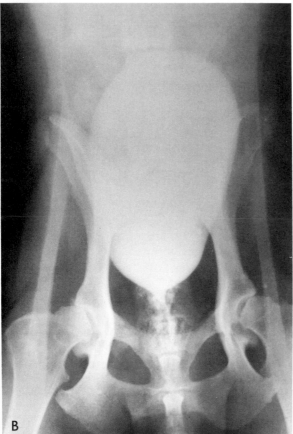

FIGURE 2–44. *A, B* A positive contrast study of the bladder.

erately distended. Barium may provoke inflammatory reaction in the bladder and is not the contrast material of choice (Fig. 2–45).

All these techniques may be combined with pneumoperitoneum if necessary. One should avoid giving an opinion on bladder contrast studies unless the bladder has been adequately distended.

NORMAL APPEARANCE

The empty bladder may not be seen on radiographs. It can be seen when it contains urine. It is seen as a pear-shaped density in the caudal abdomen with its narrow end toward the pelvis. It is best seen on lateral views. When it contains urine the bladder is intra-abdominal. When full, the bladder may displace the small intestine cranially and the ascending colon to the right. The bladder itself may be displaced cranially by an enlarged prostate gland.

Following contrast cystography the bladder should be uniformly distended and there should be no filling defects or leakage into the abdominal cavity. The wall should be thin and regular in outline. Occasionally, particularly in young animals, contrast material may be seen in the ureters. The prostate ducts will not be opacified if the prostate is normal.

ABNORMALITIES

CYSTITIS.   No radiographic changes may be seen in cases of acute cystitis. In chronic cystitis the bladder wall is often thickened. This is best shown by a combination of pneumocystography and pneumoperitoneum. Distention of the bladder may be difficult if the wall is thickened. Mucosal irregularity is frequently seen in chronic cystitis. Cystitis has been described associated with diabetes mellitus. In such cases gas may be seen within the bladder wall. Localized or diffuse thickening of the wall may also be associated with neoplasia. (Fig. 2–46).

CALCULI.   Cystic calculi are common in dogs. Most calculi in dogs are composed of phosphates, which are radiopaque and are readily seen on plain radiographs. Oxalate calculi are also radiopaque. Urate and cystine calculi are often radiolucent and may require contrast studies to demonstrate their presence. Air bubbles, introduced into the bladder with positive contrast material, may simulate calculi. In positive contrast cystography calculi appear as filling defects within the contrast medium. They may be masked if too much contrast is used or if it is too concentrated. Calculi in the female are usually large. Pneumocystography can be useful in helping to identify calculi. (Fig. 2–47).

A careful examination is often necessary to detect the presence of small calculi, as they can easily be missed or masked by feces in the colon.

Cats are not often affected with calculi. Females are more often affected than males and the calculi are usually phosphate in composition.

NEOPLASIA.   Neoplastic growths are not usually seen on plain radiographs unless there is calcification. Malignant tumors are more common than benign ones. The papilloma is the most common benign neoplasm, while the transitional cell carcinoma is the most common malignant one. Polyps are sometimes seen. Secondary invasion of the bladder by a neoplastic growth is rare. Neoplasia of the bladder occurs in older dogs. It is not often seen in cats.

Malignant tumors are usually very invasive and the ureters or urethra are frequently involved, resulting in obstructive lesions. Hematuria is a common presenting sign.

Text continued on page 118

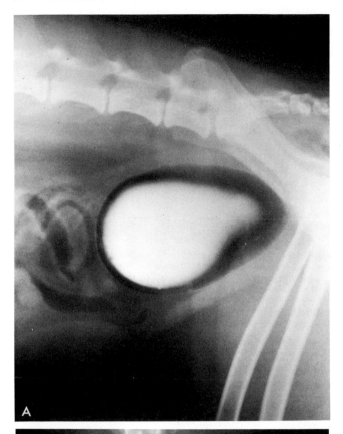

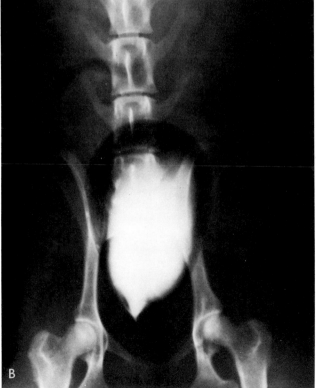

FIGURE 2–45. *A, B* A double contrast study of the bladder using a water-soluble contrast agent and air.

(*Illustration continued on opposite page.*)

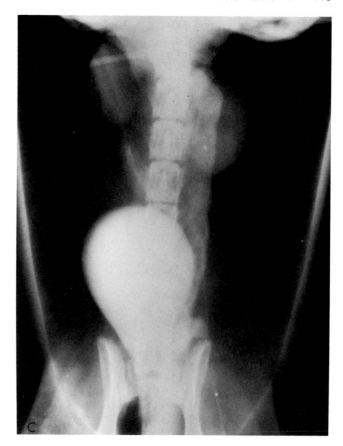

FIGURE 2–45 *Continued C.* The bladder and kidneys are demonstrated using pneumoperitoneum and a water-soluble contrast agent in the bladder. The animal was suspended by the hind limbs while the radiograph was being made.

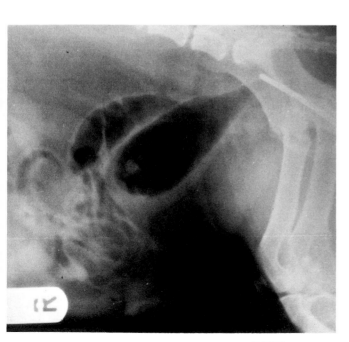

FIGURE 2–46. A thickened bladder wall due to chronic cystitis, demonstrated by pneumocystography. Calculi are seen within the bladder. (Courtesy of Dr. Robin Lee).

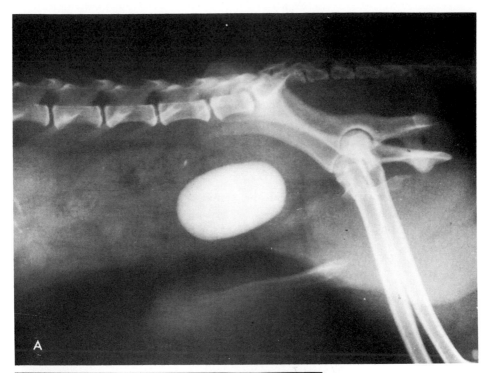

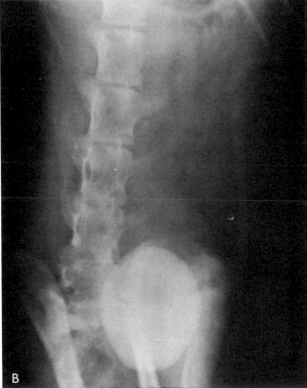

FIGURE 2–47. *A, B.* A large single calculus in the bladder of a dog. Large single calculi are more commonly seen in females. (There are fractures of the pubis and sacrum).

(Illustration continued on opposite page.)

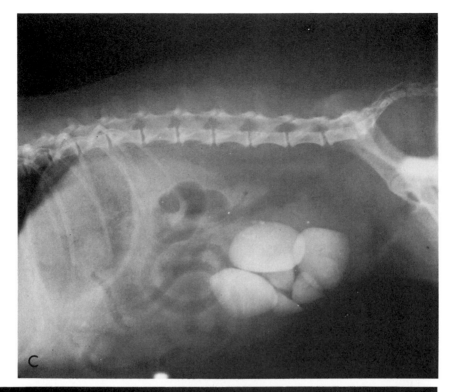

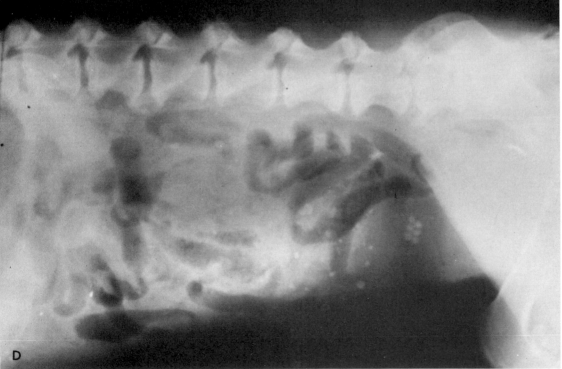

FIGURE 2–47 *Continued.* *C.* Multiple cystic calculi. *D.* Calcifications in the omentum may simulate cystic calculi. A contrast study should be performed to positively identify densities within the bladder.

Infiltrating lesions may cause thickening of the bladder wall and irregularities in the mucosa that can be difficult to differentiate from cystitis. Pneumocystography will demonstrate masses protruding into the lumen of the bladder. Irregularities in the wall are often best shown by positive contrast or double contrast studies. Blood clots within the bladder may be mistaken for tumor masses. (Fig. 2–48).

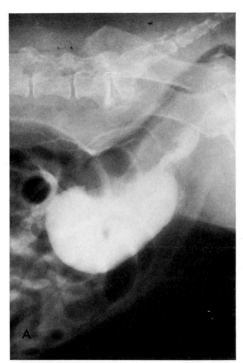

FIGURE 2–48. Neoplasia of the bladder. *A, B.* This eleven year old bitch presented with cystitis, a swollen vulva, and a full abdomen. The intravenous urogram shows a thickened bladder wall (arrows), a large filling defect around the neck of the bladder and in the dorsal bladder wall. Nodular densities project into the lumen. The ventrodorsal view shows that the defect is mostly on the left side. This was an inoperable transitional cell carcinoma.

(*Illustration continued on opposite page.*)

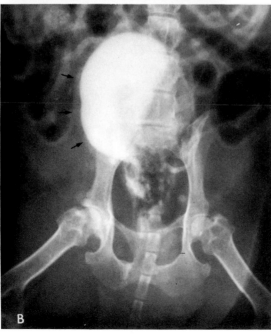

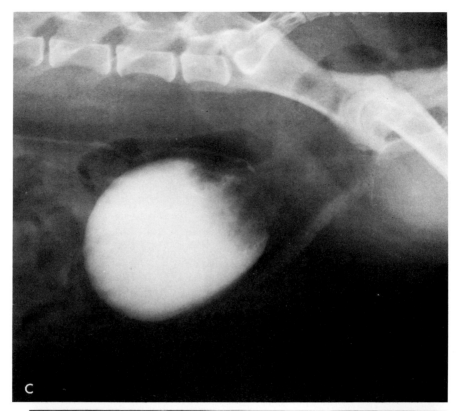

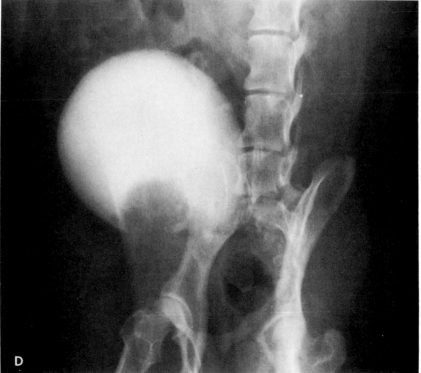

FIGURE 2–48. *Continued C, D.* A large filling defect is seen in the caudal region of the bladder. The mass was a bladder carcinoma.

(Illustration continued on following page.)

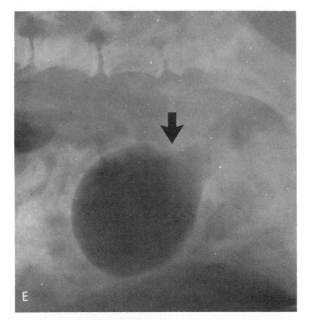

FIGURE 2–48. *Continued. E, F.* This fourteen year old male dog had a history of difficulty in defecation. The prostate was enlarged and tender. The pneumocystogram shows cranial displacement of the bladder with a very wide prostatic urethra. A filling defect can be seen at the neck of the bladder (arrow). A positive contrast study outlines the filling defect more clearly. The apparent irregularity of the wall at the floor of the bladder is due to intraluminal blood clots. The diagnosis was carcinoma of the bladder.

(*Illustration continued on opposite page.*)

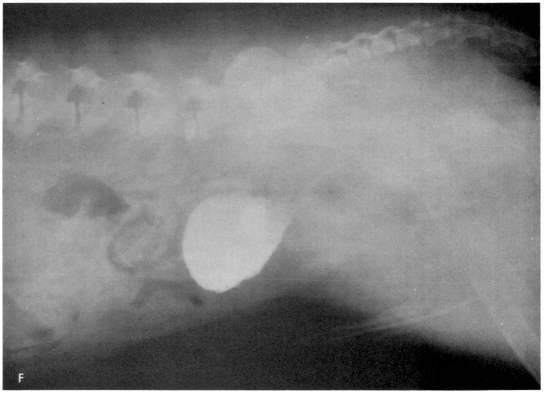

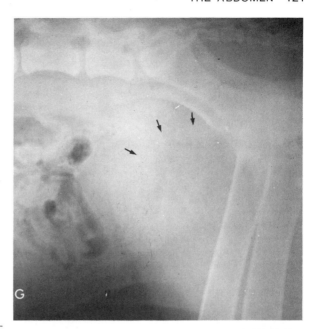

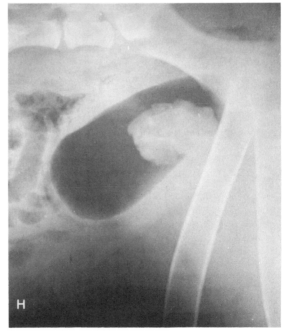

FIGURE 2–48. *Continued. G, H.* A lateral radiograph of the abdomen of this bitch with hematuria shows a faint calcific density in the caudal abdomen (arrows). A pneumocystogram shows a large intraluminal mass attached to the bladder wall. The diagnosis was fibrosarcoma.

Obstruction to the outflow of urine from the ureter may be caused by invasive lesions in the bladder, resulting in hydroureter or hydronephrosis.

RUPTURE.   Rupture of the bladder may result from trauma or rarely from a difficult parturition. The rupture cannot be demonstrated on plain radiographs. Fluid, however, may be seen within the abdominal cavity and there will be absence of the bladder shadow. Probably the easiest method of demonstrating rupture is to introduce some positive contrast medium by means of a catheter. This will leak into the peritoneal cavity where it can be readily seen. Air can also be used and leakage of it into the peritoneal cavity is conclusive evidence of rupture. A con-

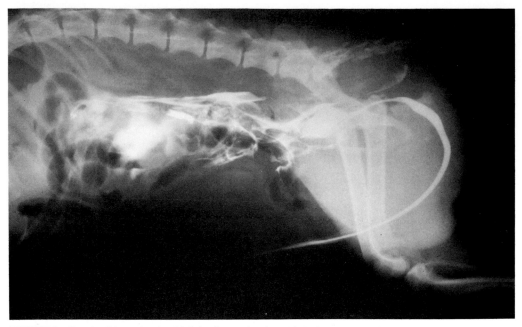

FIGURE 2–49. In this animal, which had sustained multiple fractures of the pelvis, positive contrast material introduced by a catheter has leaked from the bladder into the peritoneal cavity, indicating rupture of the bladder.

trast study should be carried out in every animal that has sustained severe injury to the pelvis, if the bladder is not seen on plain radiographs. (Fig. 2–49).

DIVERTICULUM. Occasionally, a diverticulum may be found in the bladder wall. A diverticulum is usually the result of trauma. It is best demonstrated by a positive contrast study, in which it will be seen as an outpouching from the wall. Urine is sometimes retained within a diverticulum, and in such cases the positive contrast material will be seen as a persistent density in the affected area of the bladder. Small, congenital diverticula are occasionally seen at the site of attachment of the urachus. (Fig. 2–50).

HEMORRHAGE. Cystitis is sometimes accompanied by intraluminal hemorrhage. Trauma or neoplasia may also cause bleeding. Large blood clots may form in the bladder. They may be mistaken for neoplastic growths. They are, however, moveable within the bladder and are not attached to the wall. They can be flushed out with saline. Flushing will not affect the appearance of a neoplasm. (Fig. 2–51).

RETROFLEXION. The bladder is sometimes displaced caudally in cases of perineal hernia. This can be difficult to demonstrate radiographically. The condition may be suspected if there is absence of the usual bladder shadow. The density of the overlying thigh muscles prevents visualization of the displaced bladder. Contrast studies, either positive or negative, may be helpful. There may, however, be difficulty in introducing a catheter because of the retroflexion. (Fig. 2–7).

DISPLACEMENT. Any large mass in the caudal abdomen may displace the bladder. The commonest cause of displacement is enlargement of the prostate gland. An enlarged prostate gland displaces the bladder cranially.

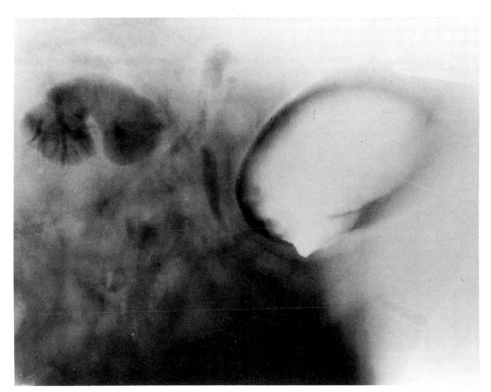

FIGURE 2–50.   A diverticulum in the wall of the bladder. The wall is markedly thickened around the defect. Air has entered a ureter and outlines a renal pelvis.

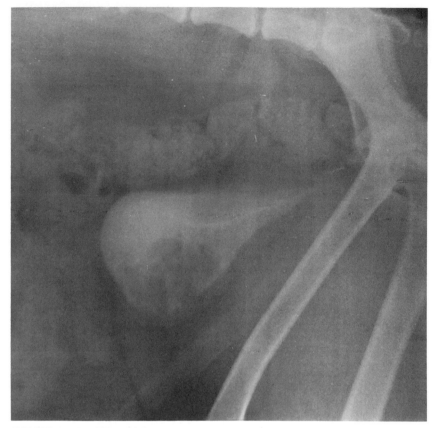

FIGURE 2–51. Filling defects are seen within the bladder on this positive contrast study. The defects were due to blood clots. The bladder wall is thickened. (Courtesy of Dr. Robin Lee).

DISTENTION. The bladder may be seen to be grossly distended in house-trained dogs and cats that have not had an opportunity to void urine prior to the radiographic examination. Distention may also be seen following damage to the spinal cord or as a result of urethral calculi. (Fig. 2–52).

PERSISTENT URACHUS. On rare occasions, persistent urachus causes dribbling of urine from the umbilicus. A positive contrast study of the bladder will show leakage into the urachus.

VESICOURETERAL REFLUX. This is often seen in young dogs. The incidence decreases after about the third month of age. It is more frequently seen in lateral recumbency. In older dogs reflux may be associated with cystitis or other abnormalities of the bladder. Persistent reflux may result in an ascending infection of the ureter and kidney.

The Urethra

ANATOMY

The urethra is the canal that carries urine from the bladder to the exterior. In the male it also transports seminal secretions.

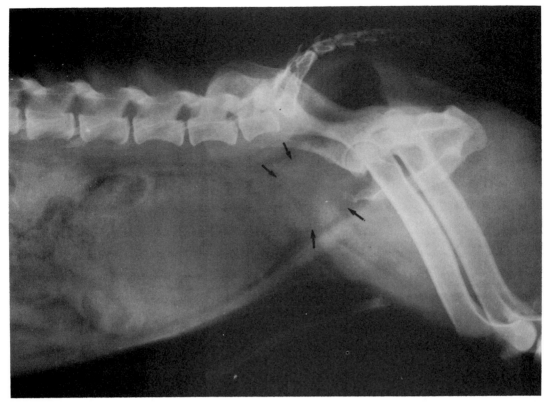

FIGURE 2-52 Distention of the bladder. There is a fracture of the pelvis and the prostate gland is enlarged (arrows)

In the male the proximal portion of the urethra passes through the prostate gland. Distally it lies along the ventral aspect of the os penis. In the female the urethra is short, extending from the bladder to the urethral orifice, which lies just caudal to the vaginovestibular junction.

RADIOGRAPHY

The urethra is not seen on plain radiographs. It can be demonstrated by the introduction of positive contrast material through a catheter. It is also seen on micturating radiographs if contrast medium is present within the bladder.

NORMAL APPEARANCE

On contrast studies the urethra is smooth in outline. The prostatic urethra is somewhat wider than the extrapelvic urethra. Normally, contrast material does not enter the prostatic ducts.

ABNORMALITIES

CONGENITAL ANOMALIES. Congenital anomalies of the urethra are extremely rare. Absence of the urethra has been reported. Abnormal openings of the

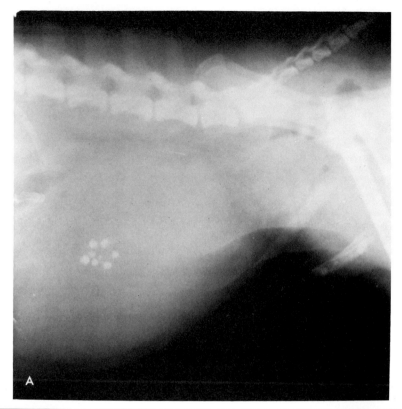

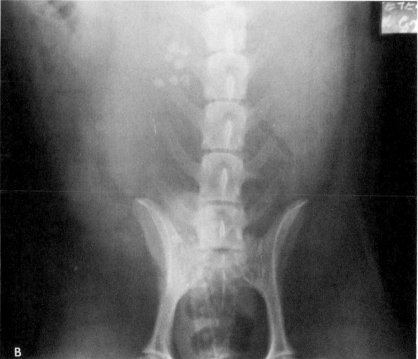

FIGURE 2–53. *A, B.* Cystic and urethral calculi. Small calculi are present in the bladder and along the course of the urethra at the os penis. The bladder is distended owing to urethral obstruction.

(Illustration continued on opposite page.)

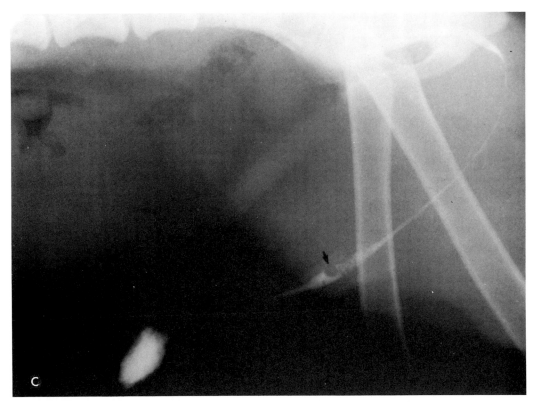

FIGURE 2–53. *Continued. C.* A radiolucent calculus outlined by positive contrast (arrow). Air bubbles should not be mistaken for calculi In this case the filling defect in the urethra was demonstrated on several radiographs. The bladder is distended and the animal had difficulty in passing urine for several days.

urethra on the ventral aspect of the penis, into the rectum, into the vagina in the female, and in the perineal region have been encountered. Anomalies require the use of contrast studies to demonstrate them radiographically. They are usually evident on clinical examination.

CALCULI. The most common abnormality associated with the urethra is the presence of urethral calculi in male dogs. These are usually radiopaque and are readily seen on plain radiographs. The best view is the lateral recumbent. Some difficulty may be encountered in identifying them within the prostatic urethra or in the area of the ischial arch unless there has been adequate penetration of the tissues. The most common sites at which calculi are seen are the proximal extremity of the os penis and in the area of the ischial arch. Positive contrast studies are required to outline radiolucent calculi. They appear as filling defects within the column of contrast material. Air bubbles should not be mistaken for calculi. Calculi are rarely demonstrable in cats, as obstructing material is often mucoid in nature. (Fig. 2–53).

RUPTURE. Severe trauma to the pelvic area may result in rupture of the urethra. It may also be ruptured during the passage of a catheter. A positive contrast study will show leakage of contrast material into the periurethral tissues. (Fig. 2–54).

STENOSIS. Stenosis of the urethra may follow fracture of the penis or surgical interference. Contrast radiography is required for its demonstration.

NEOPLASIA. Urethral neoplasia is very rare.

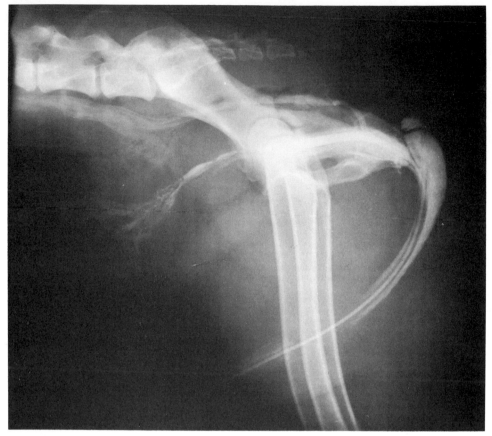

FIGURE 2–54 The urethra has been ruptured during passage of a catheter. Contrast medium has leaked into the periurethral tissues and into the venous drainage system.

THE GENITAL SYSTEM

The Male

The organs of radiographic interest are the penis, the prostate gland, and the testes.

ANATOMY

The os penis is much longer in the dog than in the cat. It tapers distally. The proximal two-thirds carries a groove ventrally in which lies the corpus cavernosum urethrae and the urethra.

The prostate gland encompasses the proximal part of the urethra and the neck of the bladder. It lies on the pelvic symphysis. Its position changes with distention of the bladder. When the bladder is full the prostate is drawn forward to lie cranial to the pubis. When the bladder is empty the prostate is intrapelvic in position.

The testes are in the scrotum, which lies between the thighs. The left testicle is placed more caudally than is the right.

NORMAL APPEARANCE

Except for the os penis, the penis is not seen on plain radiographs. The os penis is seen on the ventral aspect of the abdomen. The prepuce is also usually seen both on lateral and ventrodorsal views of the caudal abdomen. It may be mistaken for an intra-abdominal mass on the ventrodorsal view.

The scrotum casts a marked shadow at the caudal aspect of the pelvis.

ABNORMALITIES

FRACTURE OF THE OS PENIS. Fracture of the os penis is occasionally encountered. It is readily seen on plain radiographs. Fracture of the os penis may result in stenosis of the urethra. (Fig. 2–55).

TESTICULAR ENLARGEMENT. Enlarged testicles are seen radiographically on plain films but they are more readily appreciated on clinical examination. Radiography may be of value in demostrating the presence of an intra-abdominal mass in the case of a retained testicle, particularly if it is neoplastic and enlarged. (Fig. 2–56).

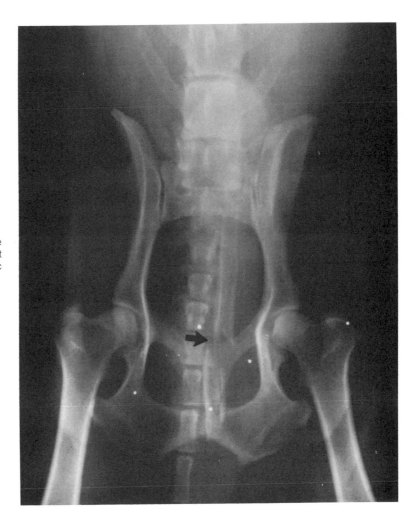

FIGURE 2–55. A fracture of the os penis (arrow). Some small shot grains can be seen in the pelvic area.

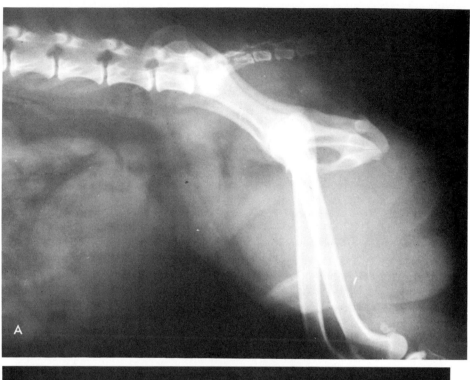

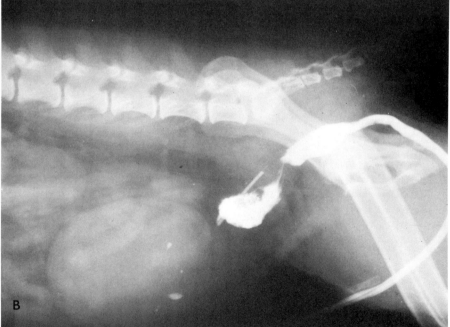

FIGURE 2–56. *A, B.* The plain radiograph shows a mass in the caudal abdomen. Contrast medium distinguishes it from the bladder. The mass was an enlarged intra-abdominal testicle that had undergone torsion.

ENLARGEMENT OF THE PROSTATE GLAND.   The prostate gland is seen on plain radiographs when it is enlarged. It is best seen on the lateral view of the caudal abdomen, in which it protrudes into the abdomen beyond the pelvic brim. An enlarged prostate gland displaces the bladder cranially. An evaluation of prostate size should be made with the bladder empty or almost empty. It can be clearly shown using pneumocystography. Some compression of the rectum above the enlarged gland may also be seen on the lateral view.

Enlargement of the prostate gland may be due to hypertrophy, cyst formation, prostatitis, or neoplasia. It is virtually impossible to distinguish between these conditions radiographically. In the case of prostatitis, air or positive contrast material will sometimes leak into the prostatic ducts following cystography. This may help to distinguish inflammatory changes from hypertrophy or neoplasia. Cysts may sometimes fill with air during pneumocystography.

Pneumoperitoneum may be used to demonstrate enlargement of the prostate gland. (Fig. 2–57 and 2–52).

The Female

ANATOMY

The uterus consists of a neck, a body, and two horns. The horns are completely within the abdomen. The body is partly in the abdomen and partly in the pelvis. The left ovary lies between the abdominal wall and the descending colon about the level of the third or fourth lumbar vertebra. The right ovary lies ventral to the right kidney and dorsal to the descending duodenum. It is a little more cranially placed than is the left ovary.

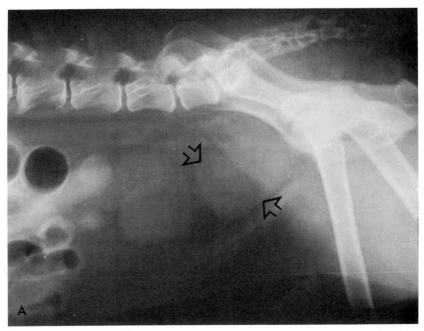

FIGURE 2–57. *A.* An enlarged prostate gland (arrows). The almost empty bladder can be seen cranial to the prostate. Either density could be interpreted as being urinary bladder. A pneumocystogram would identify the bladder.

(*Illustration continued on following page.*)

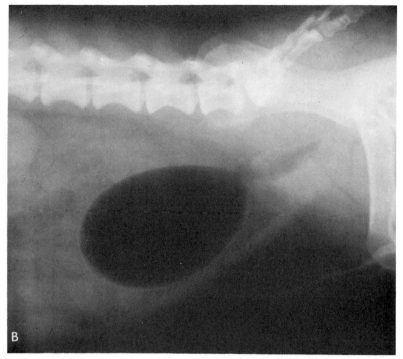

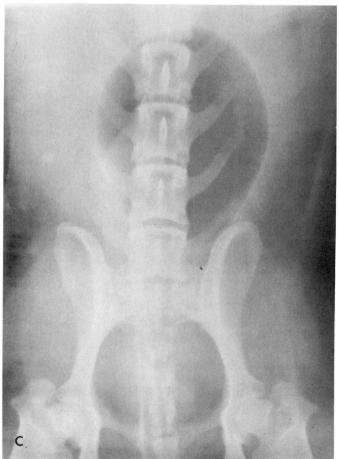

FIGURE 2–57. *Continued. B, C.* Pneumocystography shows the bladder to be displaced cranially by a mass caudal to it. The commonest cause of such displacement is an enlarged prostate gland.

(Illustration continued on opposite page.)

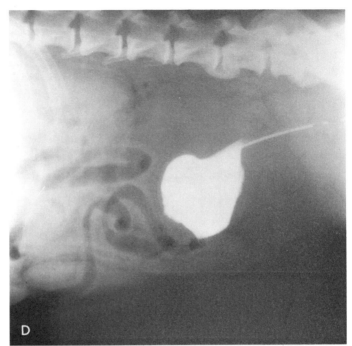

FIGURE 2–57. *Continued. D, E.* A contrast study of this bladder shows it to be displaced cranially by a large mass in the caudal abdomen. The mass is more clearly seen using pneumoperitoneum. There was a large abscess in the prostate gland.
The pneumoperitoneum study was made with the animal suspended by the hind limbs. These studies are not sufficient to evaluate the bladder, as the lumen is not completely filled.

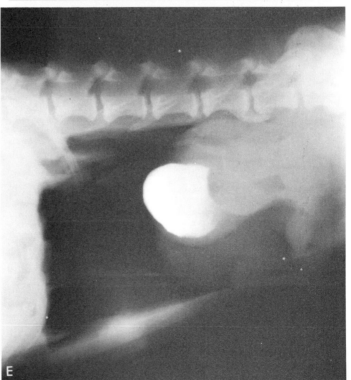

NORMAL APPEARANCE

The genital tract of the female is not seen on plain radiographs in the nongravid animal unless the uterus or ovaries are enlarged. During pregnancy the uterus gradually enlarges. It can be seen clearly on radiographs after about the fifth week of pregnancy — occasionally earlier. The only diagnosis that can be made at this time is one of uterine enlargement. Individual fetal swellings are seldom identifiable. At about the 45th day of pregnancy the fetal bones begin to ossify. It may be several days later before all the bones have become visible and an estimate made of the number of fetuses present. Counting of fetuses is best done by counting the skulls, because when several fetuses are present overlapping of one skeleton on another makes recognition of individuals difficult. The pregnant uterus lies on the floor of the abdomen during the last half of pregnancy. (Fig. 2–58).

ABNORMALITIES

DYSTOCIA. Radiography is often used to demonstrate abnormal presentations. The number of fetuses present can also be ascertained. Radiography is also useful in determining whether or not a fetus remains in the uterus after parturition has apparently been completed. (Fig. 2–59).

FETAL DEATH AND MUMMIFICATION. After the fetus dies, and provided no infection is present, resorption of soft tissues results in the bony structures of the fetus becoming very much more prominent than usual. If infection is present physometra, gas in the uterus, will be seen. Mummified fetuses show dense bones with the skeletons having a compressed appearance and occupying a relatively small area. They appear to be rolled-up. Live fetuses have a gentle curve to the spine. Unless there is evidence of mummification or of gas in the uterus it is generally not possible to tell whether or not fetuses are alive on radiographic evidence alone. Gas within the fetus itself is evidence of death. Overlapping of the cranial bones is evidence of fetal death. (Fig. 2–60).

ECTOPIC PREGNANCY. In ectopic pregnancy, the fetuses have a very dense appearance due to absence of fluid within them. The appearance is often similar to mummification. Frequently the fetuses lie in the abdomen distant from the position of the uterus.

PYOMETRA. Pyometra is evidenced radiographically by the presence of an enlarged uterus. It is seen in the caudal abdomen as a large coiled mass that displaces the small intestine cranially. The mass has a homogeneous, fluid-type density. It is usually not possible to distinguish enlargement due to pregnancy from enlargement due to pyometra unless fetal ossification has taken place. Both conditions may or may not exhibit fusiform swellings. Ossification of fetal skeletons is the best radiographic evidence of pregnancy. (Fig. 2–61).

Pressure applied to the caudal abdomen by means of a wooden spoon or other radiolucent implement may improve visualization of the uterus by displacing the small intestine and the bladder away from it. Positive contrast studies of the uterus are unlikely to yield any valuable information.

METRITIS. Metritis is not a radiographic diagnosis. If it causes enlargement of the uterus then the enlarged uterus may be seen.

NEOPLASIA. Uterine neoplasia is extremely rare. The associated mass may be seen on plain radiographs or may be outlined by pneumoperitoneum. (Fig. 2–62).

Text continued on page 143

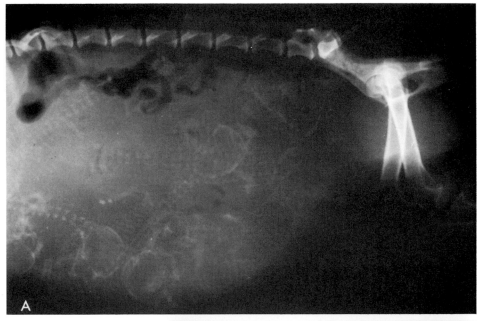

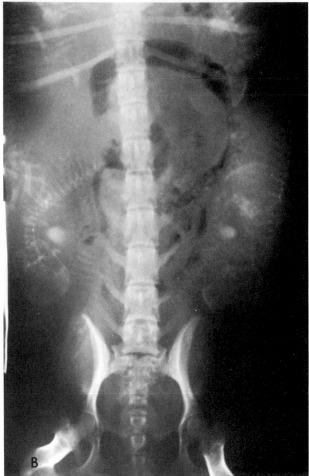

FIGURE 2–58. *A, B.* A normal pregnancy in a bitch.

(Illustration continued on following page.)

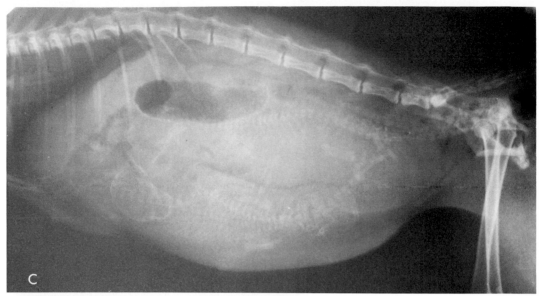

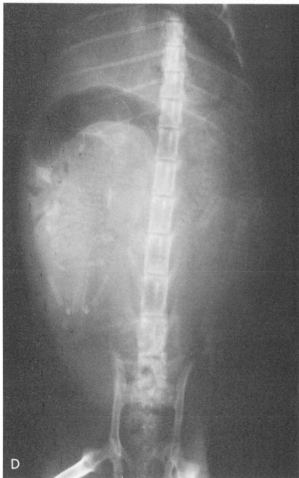

FIGURE 2–58. *Continued. C, D.* A normal pregnancy in a cat.

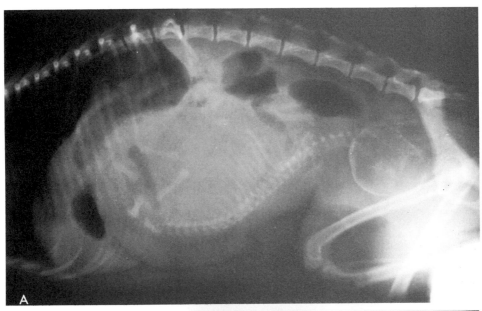

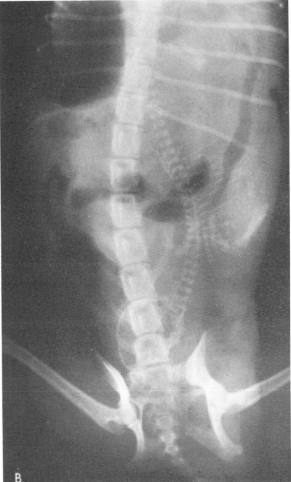

FIGURE 2–59. *A, B*   Dystocia. There is relative oversize and malposition of the fetus.

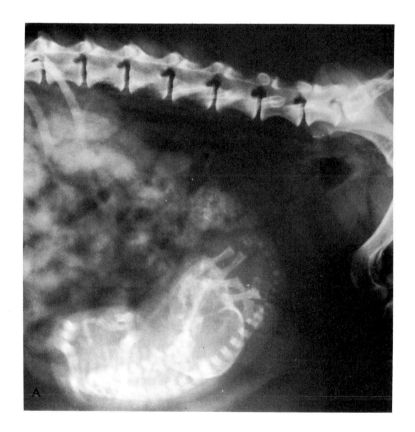

FIGURE 2–60. *A.* Fetal mummification. The fetal bones are much denser than usual and the fetus has a compacted appearance.
(Illustration continued on opposite page.)

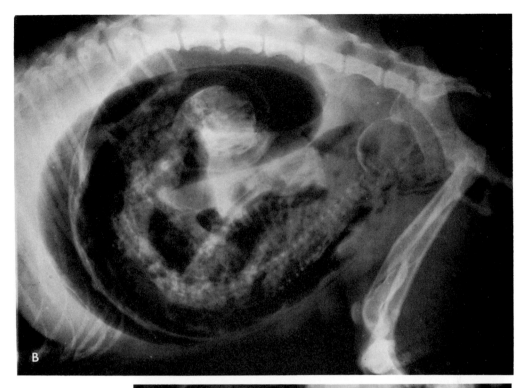

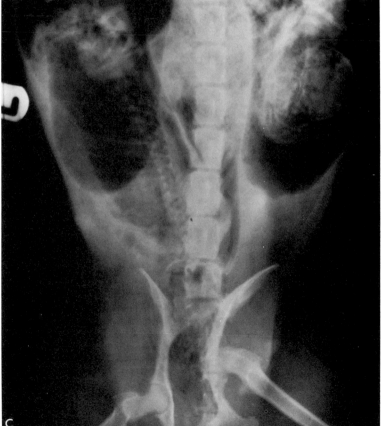

FIGURE 2–60. *Continued. B, C.* Physometra. Normal parturition was not possible because of the gross pelvic damage. The fetuses have died and gas is present within the fetal bodies and in the uterus.

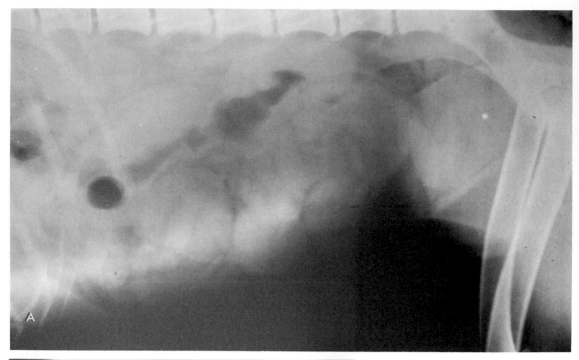

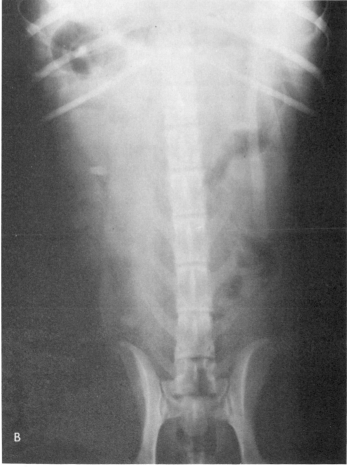

FIGURE 2–61. *A, B.* Pyometra in a bitch Coiled uterine masses can be seen in the caudal abdomen. The lateral view is usually the most helpful.
(Illustration continued on opposite page.)

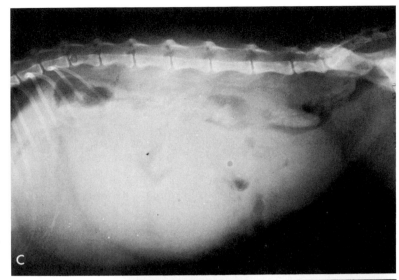

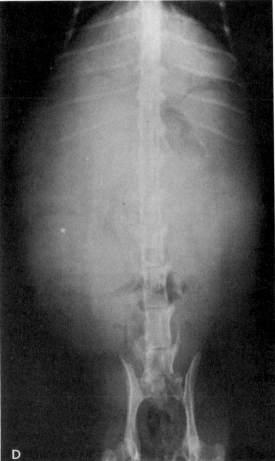

FIGURE 2–61. *Continued. C, D.* Pyometra in a cat.

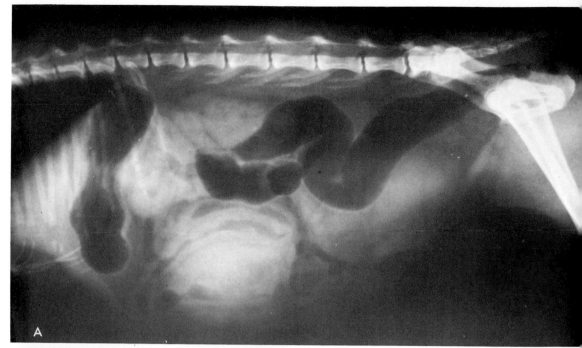

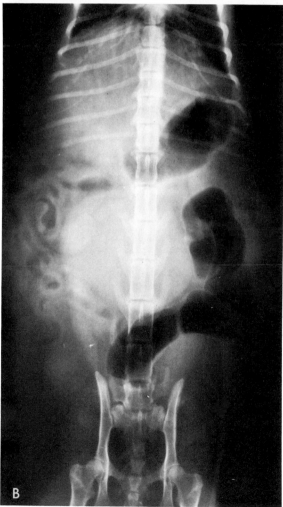

FIGURE 2–62. *A, B.* This intra-abdominal mass in an eleven year old cat was due to a uterine leiomyosarcoma. It is impossible to determine the origin of the mass from the plain radiographs. The bladder can be identified in the caudal abdomen.

OVARIAN MASSES. Ovarian masses can be seen on plain radiographs. They may displace coils of the small intestine in the cranial abdomen. A left ovarian mass may displace the descending colon. Ovarian masses, though rare, should be considered in the differential diagnosis of intra-abdominal masses. They can be demonstrated by pneumoperitonography.

REFERENCES

Allan, G. S. and Dixon, R. T. (1975). Cholecystography in the dog. The choice of contrast media and optimum dose rates. J. A. V. R. S. XVI. 3. 98.

Archibald, J. and Sumner-Smith, G. (1974). In Canine Surgery. 2nd ed. American Veterinary Publications, Inc. Santa Barbara, California.

Barber, Don L. (1975). Renal Angiography in Veterinary Medicine. J. A. V. R. S. XVI. 6. 187.

Barrett, R. B. and Kittress, J. E. (1966). Congenital peritoneopericardial hernia in a cat. J. Amer. Vet. Rad. Soc. VII. 21.

Bartels, J. E. (1972). How to delineate canine and feline hernias radiographically. Mod. Vet. Pract. 53. 2. 27.

Berg, P., Rhodes, W. H. and O'Brien, J. B. (1964). Radiographic diagnosis of gastric adenocarcinoma in a dog. J. Amer. Vet. Rad. Soc. V. 47.

Brodeur, A. E., Goyer, R. A. and Melick, W. (1965). A potential hazard of barium cystography. Radiology. 85. 1080.

Carlson, W. D. (1977) Veterinary Radiology. Gillette, E. L., Thrall, D. E. and Lebel, J. L. Editors. 3rd Ed. Lea and Febiger. Philadelphia.

Clifford, D. H., Lee, M. O., Lee, D. C. and Ross, J. N. (1976). Classification of congenital neuromuscular dysfunction of the canine esophagus. J. A. V. R. S. XVII. 3. 98.

Cornelius, L. M., Wingfield, W. E., Anderson, N. V., Lorenz, M. D. and Hardy, R. M. (1975). In Textbook of Veterinary Internal Medicine of the Dog and Cat. W. B. Saunders Co. Philadelphia.

DeHoff, W. D. and Greene, R. W. (1974). Gastric dilatation-torsion complex. Current Veterinary Therapy, R. W. Kirk, Editor. Vol. V. W. B. Saunders Co. Philadelphia.

Douglas, S. W. (1968). Lesions involving the pyloric region of the canine stomach. J. A. V. R. S. IX. 89.

Douglas, S. W. and Williamson, H. D. (1972). Principles of Veterinary Radiography. 2nd ed. Williams and Wilkens Co. Baltimore.

Douglas, S. W. and Williamson, H. D. (1970). Veterinary Radiological Interpretation. Lea and Febiger. Philadelphia.

Ettinger, S. (1975). Editor. Textbook of Veterinary Internal Medicine of the Dog and Cat. W. B. Saunders Co. Philadelphia.

Ettinger, S. A. and Suter, P. F. (1970). Canine Cardiology. W. B. Saunders Co. Philadelphia.

Ewing, G. O., Suter, P. F. and Bailey, C. S. (1974). Hepatic insufficiency associated with congenital anomalies of the portal vein in dogs. J. Amer. An. Hosp. Assoc. 10. 5. 463.

Farrow, C. S., Morgan, J. P. and Story, E. C. (1976). Late term fetal death in the dog. Early radiographic diagnosis. J. A. V. R. S. XVII. 1. 11.

Gibbs, C., Denny, H. R., Minter, H. M. and Pearson, H. (1972). Radiological features of inflammatory conditions of the canine pancreas. J. Sm. Anim. Pract. 13. 531.

Gomez, J. A. (1974). The gastrointestinal contrast study. Methods and Interpretation. The Veterinary Clinics of North America. Radiology. Nov., 1974. W. B. Saunders Co. Philadelphia.

Grandage, J. (1974). The radiology of the dog's diaphragm. J. Sm. Anim. Pract. 15. 1. 17.

Grandage, J. (1975). Some effects of posture on the radiographic appearance of the kidney of the dog. J. A. V. M. A. 166. 2. 165.

Kleine, L. J. (1973). Radiographic diagnosis of urinary tract trauma. J. A. V. M. A. 163. 10. 1185.

Kneller, S. K. (1976). Radiographic interpretation of the gastric dilatation-volvulus complex in the dog. J. Amer. An. Hosp. Assoc. 12 (2) 154.

Lane, J. G. (1973). Canine ectopic ureter. Two further case reports. J. Sm. Anim. Pract. 14. 555.

Ljunggren, G. (1964). The radiological diagnosis of some acute abdominal disorders in the dog. J. A. V. R. S. V. 5.

Lord, P. F. and Wilkins, J. (1972). Emphysema of the gall bladder in a diabetic dog. J. A. V. R. S. XIII. 49.

Miller, M. E., Christensen, G. C. and Evans, H. E. (1964). Anatomy of the Dog. W. B. Saunders Co. Philadelphia.

Morgan, J. P. (1964). Normal radiographic anatomy of the gastrointestinal tract of the dog. Scientific Proceedings. American Veterinary Medical Association. 101st Annual Meeting. 155.

Morgan, J. P., Silverman, Sam and Zontine, W. J. (1975). Techniques of Veterinary Radiography. Veterinary Radiology Associates, Davis, California.

Murray, M., McKeating, F. J. and Lauder, I. M. (1972). Peptic ulceration in the dog. A clinicopathlogical study. Vet. Rec. 91. 441.

O'Brien, T. R. (1978). Radiographic Diagnosis of Abdominal Disorders in the Dog and Cat. W. B. Saunders Co. Philadelphia.

Olsson, S. E. (1973). The Radiological Diagnosis in Canine and Feline Emergencies. Lea and Febiger. Philadelphia.

Osborne, C. A., Engen, M. H., Yano, B. L., Brasmer, R. M., Jessen, C. R. and Blevins, W. E. (1974). Congenital urethrorectal fistula in two dogs. J. A. V. M. A. 165. 999.

Osborne, C. A. and Jessen, C. R. (1971). Double contrast cystography in the dog. J. A. V. M. A. 159. 1400.

Osborne, C. A., Low, D. G. and Finco, D. R. (1972). Canine and Feline Urology. W. B. Saunders Co. Philadelphia.

Osborne, C. A., Low, D. G. and Perman, V. (1968). Neoplasms of the canine and feline urinary bladder. Clincal findings, diagnosis and treatment. J. A. V. M. A. 152. 247.

Pearson, H. (1970). Differential diagnosis of persistent vomiting in the young dog. J. Sm. Anim. Pract. 11. 403.

Pollock, S. (1968). Urethral carcinoma in the dog. A Case Report. J. A. V. R. S. IX. 95.

Pollock, S. and Rhodes, W. H. (1970). Gastroesophageal intussusception in an Afghan Hound. A Case Report. J. A. V. R. S. XI. 5.

Rhodes, W. H. and Brodey, R. S. (1965). The differential diagnosis of pyloric obstructions in the dog. J. A. V. R. S. VI. 65.

Rhodes, W. H. and Biery, Darryl (1967). Pneumocystography in the dog. J.A.V.R.S. VIII. 45.

Roenigk, W. J. (1971). Radiography of gastrointestinal diseases. Proc. American Animal Hospital Association. 496.

Root, C. R. (1971). Steatitis in cats. The radiographic appearance. J. A. V. R. S. XII. 60.

Root, C. R. (1974). Abdominal Masses. The radiographic differential diagnosis. J. A. V. R. S. XV. 2. 26.

Root, C. R., Gomez, J. A., Kneller, S. K. and Park, R. D. (1974). In The Veterinary Clinics of North America. Radiology. Nov., 1974. W. B. Saunders Co. Philadelphia.

Root, C. R. and Lord, P. F. (1971). Peritoneal carcinomatosis in the dog and cat. Its radiographic appearance. J. A. V. R. S. XII. 54.

Root, C. R. and Lord, P. F. (1971). Linear radiolucent gastrointestinal foreign bodies in cats and dogs. Their radiographic appearance. J. A. V. R. S. XII. 45.

Root, C. R. and Morgan, J. P. (1969). Contrast radiography of the upper gastrointestinal tract in the dog. J. Sm. Anim. Pract. 10. 279.

Rosin, G. and Hanlon, G. F. (1972). Canine Cricopharyngeal Achalasia. J .A. V. M. A. 160. 1496.

Schnelle, G. B. (1950). Radiology in Small Animal Practice. 2nd ed. The North American Veterinarian, Inc.

Scwartz, A., Ravin, C.E., Greenspan, R. H., Schoemann, R. S. and Burt, J. K. (1976). Congenital neuromuscular esophageal disease in a litter of Newfoundland puppies. J. A. V. R. S. XVII. 3. 101.

Seward, C. O. (1951). The use of barium in studying the digestive tract of the dog. J. A. V. M. A. 119. 125.

Small, E. (1971). Diseases of the esophagus. In Current Veterinary Therapy. R. W. Kirk, Editor. Vol. IV. W. B. Saunders Co. Philadelphia.

Sokolovsky, V. (1967). Cricopharyngeal achalasia in a dog. J. A. V. M. A. 150. 281.

Suter, P. F. (1975). Portal vein anomalies in the dog. Their angiographic diagnosis. J. A. V. R. S. XVI. 3. 84.

Suter, P. F. and Olsson, S. E. (1969). Traumatic hemorrhagic pancreatitis in the cat. A report with emphasis on the radiological diagnosis. J. A. V. R. S. X. 4.

Thrall, D. E. (1973). Esophagobronchial fistula in a dog. J. A. V. R. S. XIV. 1. 22.

Ticer, J. W. (1975). Radiographic Technique in Small Animal Practice. W. B. Saunders Co. Philadelphia.

Tiedeman, K. and Henschel, E. (1973). Early radiographic diagnosis of pregnancy in the cat. J. Sm. Anim. Pract. 14. 9. 567.

Van Kruiningen, H. J., Gregoire, K. and Meuten, D. J. (1974). Acute gastric dilatation. A review of comparative aspects by species and a study in dogs and monkeys. J. Amer. Anim. Hosp. Assoc. 10. 3. 294.

Watters, J. W. (1970). Radiography of the canine colon using different contrast agents. J. A. V. M. A. 165. 423.

Zeskov, Borislav., Petrovic, Branislav and Dragnovic, Borislav (1976). J. A. V. R. S. XVII. 23.

Zontine, W. J. (1973). Effect of chemical restraint drugs on the passage of barium sulphate through the stomach and duodenum of dogs. J. A. V. M. A. 162. 878.

THE THORAX

The air-filled lungs provide good contrast for the demonstration of intrathoracic structures.

RADIOGRAPHY

For routine examinations two views are necessary, a lateral and a dorsoventral (DV) or a ventrodorsal (VD).

LATERAL VIEW. The animal is placed in lateral recumbency and the forelimbs are drawn cranially and held parallel to one another. The sternum should be on the same level as the thoracic vertebrae so that there is no rotation of the thorax. The beam is centered at the level of the fifth rib. Right lateral recumbency is preferred to left, because the phrenicopericardial ligament inhibits movement of the cardiac apex towards the dependent side in this position. Standing lateral views are occasionally useful if pleural fluid is suspected. For this view, the cassette is positioned along the left chest wall with the animal in a standing position. A horizontal beam is used, centered on the fifth rib. A lateral view with the animal in dorsal recumbency is an alternative.

DV OR VD VIEW. There is likely to be less distortion of the cardiac outline on the DV view, since the heart may move away from the sternum when the animal is in dorsal recumbency. However, better inspiratory films can be obtained on the VD view and positioning is easier. The DV view is preferable if the cardiac shadow is the main item of interest.

To obtain a DV view the animal is placed in sternal recumbency with the elbows abducted and the forelimbs drawn slightly forward. The hindlimbs are flexed with the hocks resting on the table. The thoracic vertebrae should overlie the sternum. The head is held low between the forelimbs. The beam is centered at the level of the sixth rib.

For the VD view the animal is placed in dorsal recumbency with the forelimbs pulled forward and the beam centered at the level of the sixth rib. The sternum should overlie the thoracic vertebrae. Occasionally, placing an animal on its back may increase distress in cases of respiratory embarrassment.

OBLIQUE VIEW. This view is sometimes helpful in demonstrating areas of lung tissue that are obscured by the cardiac silhouette in the more conventional views.

Radiographs of the thorax should be made at the end of inspiration. On films made at expiration, the lung fields appear dense and most of the pulmonary vasculature detail is lost. The beam should be collimated to include the entire thorax from a point about 2 cm cranial to the first rib to a point just caudal to the first lumbar vertebra. Accuracy of technique is vital to the production of consistent and comparable films. The chest thickness should be measured with calipers, and the technique chart exposure recommendations should be adhered to. A grid should be used if the thorax measures 15 cm or more in thickness. A machine with a capability of at least $^1/_{30}$ (or better, $^1/_{60}$) of a second is desirable. Slower speeds do not effectively exclude motion unless the animal is anesthetized and artificially ventilated. Underexposure gives the impression of increased lung density. Overexposure blackens out normal vascular patterns and may mask pathologic changes. A good technique will barely outline the spinous processes of the cranial thoracic vertebrae on the lateral view. (Fig. 3–1).

THE RESPIRATORY SYSTEM

The Larynx and Hyoid Apparatus

ANATOMY

The larynx is composed of a number of cartilages, namely the epiglottis, the thyroid, the cricoid, and two arytenoids. In addition, there is a small oval sesamoid cartilage cranial to the cricoid lamina between the arytenoid cartilages and a small flat interarytenoid cartilage caudal to the sesamoid.

The hyoid apparatus is a bony structure that suspends the tongue and the larynx. It is attached to the skull dorsally and to the tongue and the larynx ventrally. It is composed of a single basihyoid bone in the base of the tongue

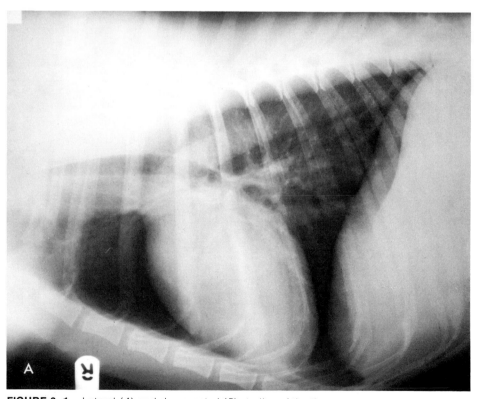

FIGURE 3–1. Lateral (*A*) and dorsoventral (*B*) studies of the thorax.

(*Illustration continued on opposite page*)

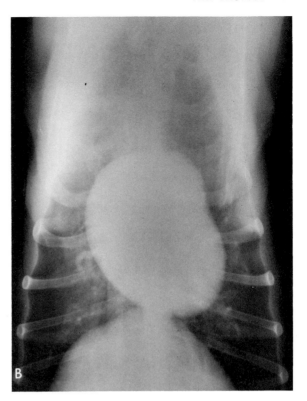

FIGURE 3-1 *Continued.*

and several other small bones. These are the thyrohyoid, the keratohyoid, the epihyoid, and the stylohyoid.

NORMAL APPEARANCE

The larynx is readily identifiable on properly exposed lateral views of the neck. In VD projections, the larynx overlies the cervical vertebrae and most of its detail is lost. Good radiographs will show the soft palate, the hyoid apparatus, the epiglottis, and the cricoid cartilage. (Fig. 3–2).

ABNORMALITIES

Abnormalities of the larynx are usually diagnosed by methods other than radiologic. Displacement of the larynx, compression, or calcification may result in visible radiologic signs.

The Trachea

ANATOMY

The trachea extends from the level of the body of the axis to about the fifth thoracic vertebra, where it bifurcates over the base of the heart. The apex of the partition between the openings of the primary bronchi is called the carina.

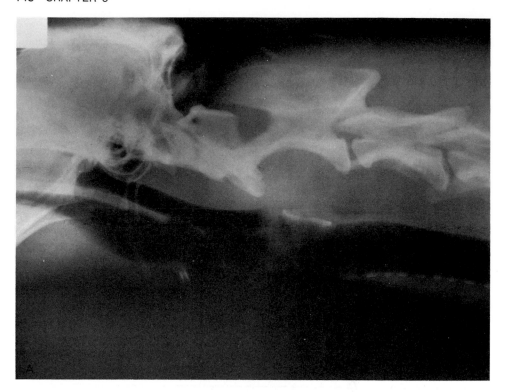

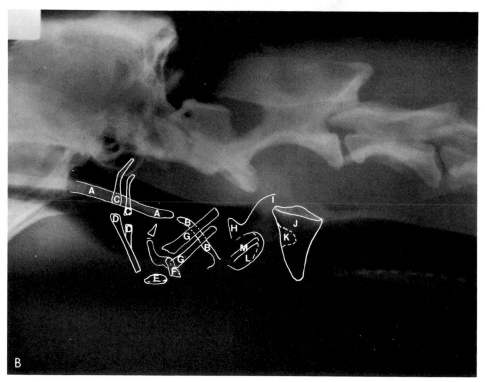

FIGURE 3–2. *A, B*. The Larynx. *A*. Soft palate. *B*. Epiglottis. *C*. Stylohyoid bones. *D*. Epihyoid bones. *E*. Keratohyoid bones. *F*. Basihyoid bone. *G*. Thyrohyoid bones. *H*. Cranial cornu of the thyroid cartilage. *I*. Corniculate process of the arytenoid cartilage. *J*. Cricoid cartilage. *K*. Muscular process of the thyroid cartilage. *L*. Lateral ventricle. *M*. Vocal cord.

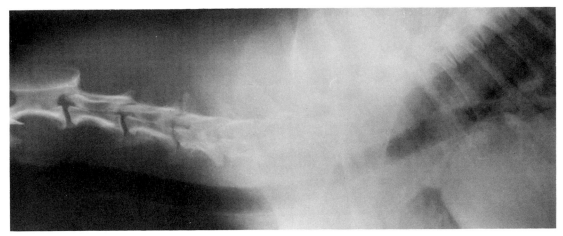

FIGURE 3–3. The trachea.

RADIOGRAPHY

Lateral and VD views of the neck and thorax are required for routine examination of the trachea and bronchi. Oblique views are helpful in demonstrating the trachea without superimposition of the vertebrae and sternum. Care must be taken that no rotation is present on lateral views, as this will cause an apparent displacement of the trachea.

NORMAL APPEARANCE

The trachea is visualized more clearly on lateral views. The air within it acts as a contrast medium. In the VD or DV view the trachea is more difficult to see because of the superimposed vertebrae and sternum. The trachea, in the cranial mediastinum, lies to the right of the midline, becoming centrally placed at the carina. In the lateral view it forms an acute angle with the line of the thoracic vertebrae. A dark circular shadow over the base of the heart marks the point of bifurcation. The trachea curves somewhat ventrally as it bifurcates between the fifth and sixth ribs. Only the primary bronchi near the bifurcation are recognizable on radiographs. Smaller bronchi cannot be distinguished from vascular shadows. (Fig. 3–3).

ABNORMALITIES

DISPLACEMENT OF THE TRACHEA. The trachea may be displaced by cervical or mediastinal masses or by an enlarged heart. Before making a diagnosis of tracheal displacement, one must be sure that the animal has been positioned correctly. Unusual positioning of the trachea may be the result of having the head and neck flexed during radiography. Rotation of the thorax on the lateral view will cause an apparent elevation of the trachea. Intrathoracic masses may displace the carina forward. (Fig. 3–4 *A*).

TRACHEAL COLLAPSE. The usual type of collapse is in the dorsoventral plane. Both cervical and thoracic portions may be affected. Lateral radiographs are the most informative. The lumen of the trachea is seen to be markedly

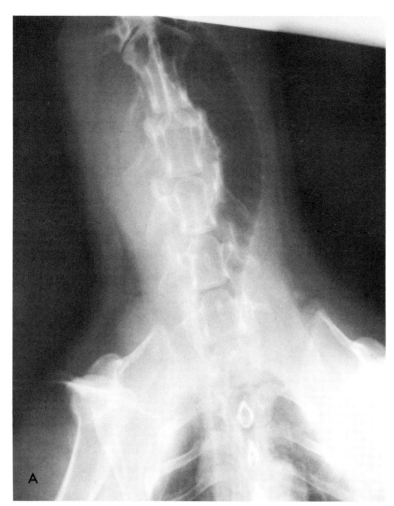

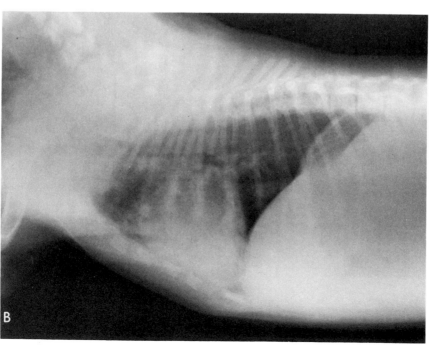

FIGURE 3–4. *A.* The trachea is displaced to the left by a mass in the neck. *B.* A congenitally narrowed trachea. A three month old female French bulldog had severe gagging and respiratory distress. At autopsy there was a congenitally narrowed trachea and pneumonia. Patchy infiltrates are seen in the lung fields and the trachea is very narrow.

(Illustration continued on opposite page)

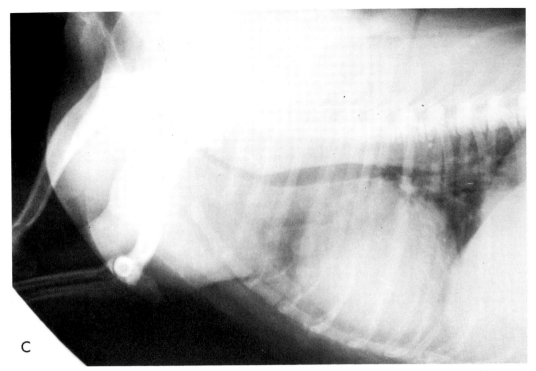

C

FIGURE 3–4 *Continued.* *C.* A seven year old Cairn terrier had a history of persistent coughing over several months. A lateral radiograph shows marked narrowing of the trachea at the thoracic inlet. On fluoroscopy the thoracic portion of the trachea was seen to collapse with each expiratory movement. The cervical portion was not affected.

narrowed. Some obese animals may appear to have a narrowed trachea on radiographic examination due to overlying fat. Excessive extension of the neck may produce an apparent narrowing of the trachea.

Tracheal collapse is most often seen in the smaller breeds of dog in middle and old age. Fluoroscopic examination is very useful in confirming the diagnosis. If the collapse is intrathoracic, the trachea will be seen to collapse at each expiration. If the collapse is in the cervical trachea, then the collapse occurs at each inspiration. Induced coughing may help to make the collapse visible. A normal appearance of the trachea on plain radiographs does not exclude the possibility of tracheal collapse. Fluoroscopy is necessary if the clinical signs suggest the diagnosis.

Tracheal collapse has to be distinguished from hypoplasia of the trachea, in which the lumen size is also narrowed but there is no variation in diameter during fluoroscopy. In fat animals, the trachea is less clearly visualized than in thinner ones. (Fig. 3–4 *B, C*).

CALCIFICATION OF THE TRACHEA. Calcification of the tracheal rings is sometimes seen in older dogs, particularly in the chondrodystrophoid breeds. It does not appear to be of significance. (Fig. 3–5).

OBSTRUCTION OF THE TRACHEA. Foreign body obstruction of the trachea is not common. The air-filled trachea provides a good contrast background against which the foreign body can usually be seen. If the foreign body passes into a bronchus the resulting atelectasis may obscure it.

The trachea may be narrowed because of pressure from an extrinsic mass. The point of narrowing is visible radiographically.

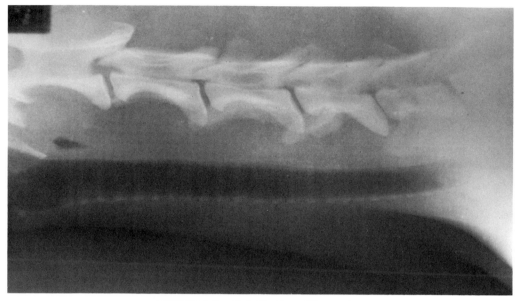

FIGURE 3–5. Calcification of the trachea.

NEOPLASIA OF THE TRACHEA. Neoplasia of the trachea is rarely seen. The neoplastic mass can be seen projecting into the tracheal lumen. Extraluminal masses, such as enlarged mediastinal or hilar lymph nodes, tend to displace the trachea rather than compress it.

The use of contrast medium is helpful in differentiating intra- and extraluminal masses. The contrast material will demonstrate the integrity, or lack of integrity, of the lining mucosa.

FILAROIDES OSLERI.   Irregularities in the outline of the tracheal shadow at and cranial to the carina have been described in *Filaroides osleri* infestation. Diagnosis is more readily achieved by other methods.

RUPTURE OF THE TRACHEA.   If the trachea ruptures, air escapes into the peritracheal tissues and subcutaneous emphysema can be recognized on radiographs. Pneumomediastinum may result if the rupture is within the thorax.

The Bronchi

The trachea divides into left and right primary, or main stem, bronchi. The left primary bronchus divides into cranial and caudal secondary bronchi. The cranial secondary bronchus supplies the cranial (apical) and the caudal (cardiac) segments of the cranial lung lobe. The caudal secondary bronchus supplies the caudal (diaphragmatic) lung lobe. The right primary bronchus divides into four secondary bronchi: cranial (apical), middle (cardiac), caudal (diaphragmatic), and accessory (intermediate or azygous).

RADIOGRAPHY

Lateral and VD or DV views of the thorax are required for routine examination of the bronchi.

NORMAL APPEARANCE

Plain radiographs give little information about the normal bronchi. Only the larger bronchi in the hilar region are regularly seen. Widespread disease changes associated with the bronchi will be manifested as decreased lucency of the lung fields, an increase in nonvascular linear markings, and peribronchial infiltration seen as "ring" shadows in end-on views of individual bronchi. The pattern is not readily distinguishable from the changes seen associated with advancing age. (Fig. 3–6).

ABNORMALITIES

BRONCHITIS. Acute bronchitis may be present without radiographic evidence of disease. Chronic bronchitis frequently shows an interstitial pattern. (See page 165).

BRONCHIECTASIS. In early cases, radiography may reveal little change in normal pulmonary pattern. As the disease progresses, a bronchial pattern develops with peribronchial infiltration and thickened bronchial walls. Pneumonia, with its associated alveolar changes, may complicate the picture. Atelectasis or consolidation may occur and air bronchograms are seen within the consolidated masses. (See pages 157 to 171.)

Bronchography is sometimes employed to demonstrate bronchiectasis, especially in suspected early cases. It is not without hazard, as general anesthesia is necessary in an animal with compromised respiratory function.

The anesthetized patient is intubated and the contrast material is introduced by means of a catheter through the endotracheal tube. The catheter is passed down the trachea to a point just cranial to its bifurcation and the contrast agent is deposited. The animal is positioned so that gravity carries the contrast material into the bronchi that are to be examined — left lateral recumbency for the left lung and right lateral recumbency for the right lung. Sternal recumbency is necessary to fill the right middle lobe bronchus. Selective bronchography can be done under fluoroscopic control.

Oily contrast material is preferred to water-soluble agents, since it does not enter the alveoli as readily. (Dionosil. Picker). One to 2 mls are adequate for each lung. A 50 to 60 per cent w/v suspension of barium in a carboxymethylcellulose base (Redi-Flow 100% w/v. Flow Pharmaceuticals, Inc.) at a rate of ½ to 1 ml per bronchus has been recommended.

One lung should be studied at a time. All of the agents used are irritant to some extent and may provoke varying degrees of reaction. (Fig. 3–7).

BRONCHIAL FOREIGN BODY. A radiopaque foreign body will be visible on

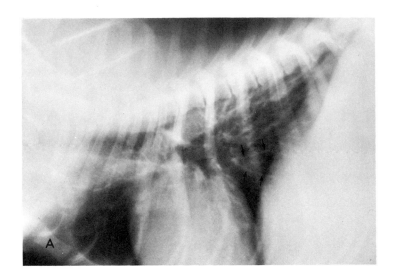

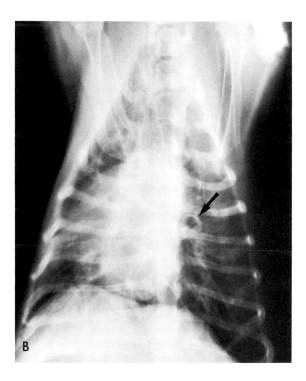

FIGURE 3-6 *A, B.* Nonvascular linear marks and peribronchial infiltration. On the lateral view (*A*) arrows indicate some of the many nonvascular line marks. Vascular detail is obscured by the interstitial infiltration. A large bronchus with peribronchial infiltration (arrow) is seen on the ventrodorsal view (*B*). Sometimes the blood vessel accompanying the bronchus is seen giving a "signet ring" appearance to the bronchus and blood vessel. The ventrodorsal view is rotated, giving a clearer view of the left lung.

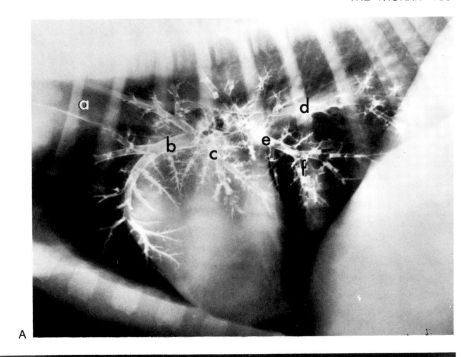

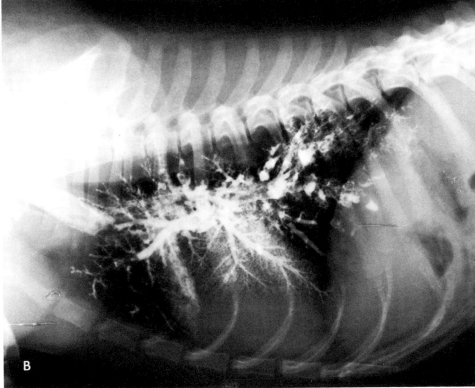

FIGURE 3–7 *A.* Bronchogram of the left lung, lateral view. *a.* Trachea; *b,* left cranial lobe bronchus; *c,* left middle lobe bronchus; *d,* left caudal lobe bronchus; *e,* right caudal lobe bronchus; *f,* accessory lobe bronchus. (From Ticer, J. W. 1975. Radiographic Technique in Small Animal Practice. W. B. Saunders Co. Philadelphia.) *B.*   The left cranial lobe bronchus appears dilated. Bronchiectatic dilatations are seen in the caudal lung lobe area. Alveolization of the contrast material is evident around the secondary bronchus supplying the caudal (cardiac) segment of the cranial lung lobe.

plain radiographs, although it may appear to be in the esophagus. A localized bronchopneumonia develops following foreign body inhalation. The caudal lung lobe is the most commonly affected. Obstruction of a bronchus will result in atelectasis of the lung lobe supplied by that bronchus.

BRONCHIAL ASTHMA. Radiologic signs of bronchial asthma include increased lucency of the lung fields with an increase in size of the lung fields themselves. They may extend beyond the costal arch. There is also some flattening of the diaphragm and unusually clear visibility of the bronchovascular markings. It is not common; cats appear to be affected more frequently than dogs.

The Lungs

ANATOMY

The left lung has two lobes, a cranial and a caudal. The cranial lobe is divided into cranial (apical) and caudal (cardiac) segments. The right lung has four lobes: cranial (apical), middle (cardiac), caudal (diaphragmatic), and accessory (intermediate, or azygous). The lobes are separated from one another by interlobar fissures. The left cranial lobe projects a little into the right side of the thorax at its cranial extremity. The hilus is that part of the lung at which the bronchi, the pulmonary vessels, the bronchial vessels, and the nerves enter.

NORMAL APPEARANCE

A radiograph of the lung fields is a composite shadow of many structures. These include the pulmonary vasculature, the alveoli, the alveolar interstitial tissue, the alveolar ducts, the bronchi and the bronchioles, the lymphatics, and the pleurae. Air in the alveoli and bronchial tree provides a good contrast medium against which the pulmonary vasculature can be seen. Only the larger bronchi, near the hilus, are seen on normal films. Interlobar fissures are not normally visible. The composite lung shadows are often referred to as bronchovascular markings.

The most prominent feature in the lung fields is the pulmonary vasculature. The clarity with which the vessels are seen varies with the degree of inspiration, the age of the animal, its posture, and radiographic technique. Films made at expiration show an apparent increase in lung density. This is due to the fact that the reduced air mass decreases contrast and expiration compresses the lung structure. Older animals show poorer contrast than young ones. The pulmonary vasculature may be obscured by other structures in improperly positioned studies.

In the VD or DV view the pulmonary vasculature is best seen in the middle areas of the lung fields. Near the hilar area vessels are obscured by the cardiac shadow, while at the periphery vascular shadows are small and few. In most DV or VD radiographs of the thorax a thin, dense line is seen extending from the apex of the cardiac shadow to the left hemidiaphragm. This has been called the phrenicopericardial ligament, the diaphragmaticopericardial ligament, or the cardiophrenic ligament. It represents the mediastinum and pleura at the line where the accessory and left caudal lung lobes meet.

In the lateral view the vessels of the right and left lungs are superimposed on one another. Cranial to the heart two pairs of vessels can usually be distinguished. The dorsal pair are the left cranial lobar artery and vein, while the ventral pair are the right cranial lobar artery and vein. On lateral views arteries lie dorsal to the corresponding veins. Caudal to the heart, the right and left pulmonary arteries branch out toward the periphery of the thorax.

The pulmonary vasculature seen on normal radiographs is made up, for the most part, of branches of the pulmonary arteries. If one traces the vascular shadows cranially it can be seen that they originate from the area of the pulmonary artery trunk. Veins, when seen, can be traced to the area of the left atrium. In the VD or DV view arteries lie lateral to the corresponding bronchi, while veins lie medial to them. Arteries are somewhat sharper in outline than are veins and are noticeably denser.

The thoracic aorta can be seen through the pulmonary shadow on lateral views and through the cardiac shadow on well-penetrated VD or DV views. The great vessels in the cranial thorax form part of the mediastinal shadow. (Fig. 3–8).

ABNORMALITIES

Many difficulties are encountered in distinguishing pathologic densities within the lungs and in classifying them satisfactorily. The pulmonary vasculature in normal lungs is seen with a considerable degree of clarity owing to the background air-filled lungs. Anything that causes loss of alveolar air will make the vascular pattern less distinct. The vascular pattern will also be obscured by changes in the interstitial tissues. The increased density associated with such changes decreases contrast between the vessels and the lungs. Disease processes affecting the vessels themselves may reduce their visibility or distort their normal pattern. Pleural effusions mask normal lung shadows. Affections of the bronchial tree will be reflected in thoracic radiographs. Consequently, pulmonary disease may manifest itself in a variety of ways.

The lungs of aged animals frequently present a different appearance to those of younger ones. The changes associated with advanced age include an increase in linear markings in the lungs, these markings being unassociated with blood vessels. They are referred to as nonvascular linear marks. They probably represent an increase in connective tissue within the lungs. They often do not follow the course of blood vessels and they may fade out after a short distance. Discrete, small nodular densities may be present with some degree of tracheal or bronchial calcification. Emphysematous bullae are rarely seen. Similar changes are often seen in city dogs at a relatively early age.

Pathologic changes in basic lung patterns can be classified according to the structures primarily involved, namely alveoli, interstitial tissue, bronchi, and blood vessels. A mixed pattern may also be found.

THE ALVEOLAR PATTERN. An alveolar pattern results when the alveoli become filled with fluid or cellular debris or when they collapse.

RADIOLOGIC SIGNS

(a) Ill-defined "fluffy" lung densities that fade gradually into adjacent, more normal lung tissue.

(b) The areas of increased density tend to merge with one another.

(c) The areas of increased density affect a lobe or portion of a lobe. Lobar borders, not normally seen, often become visible; that is, interlobar fissures are visualized.

Text continued on page 163

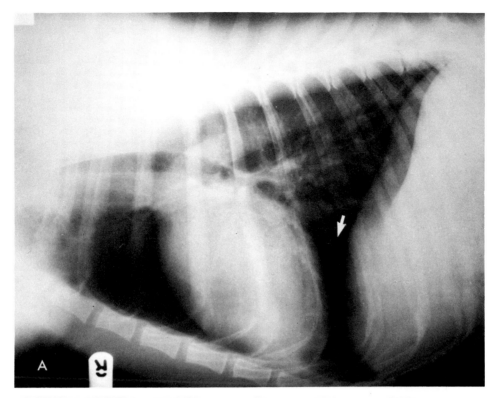

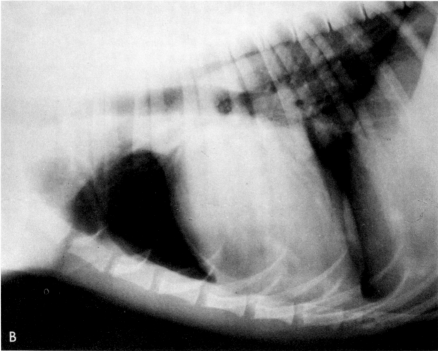

FIGURE 3–8.   *A, B.* Lateral views of the thorax taken at inspiration (*A*) and expiration (*B*). At inspiration the ribs are more widely separated and the lung fields appear more lucent. Greater vascular detail can be seen especially in the caudal lung lobes. Much more of the accessory lung lobe area caudal to the heart (arrow) can be seen on inspiration. At expiration the caudal vena cava is toward the dorsal third of the thorax and it has a ventrocranial direction. At inspiration it is more centrally placed and almost horizontal. The diaphragm does not overlie the cardiac shadow on the inspiratory film.

(*Illustration continued on opposite page*)

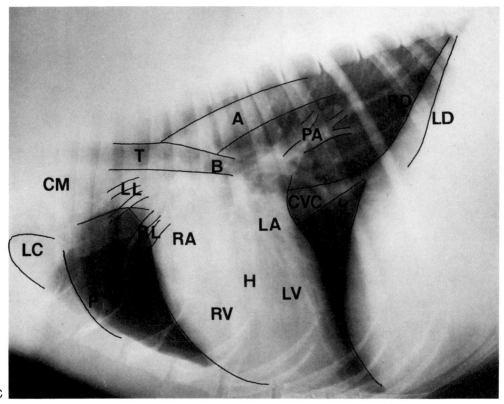

FIGURE 3–8 *Continued.* C. Some structures visible on the lateral thoracic radiograph.

A: Thoracic aorta.
T: Trachea.
B: Origin of the left cranial lobe bronchus.
PA: Branches of the pulmonary artery.
RD: Right diaphragm crus.
LD: Left diaphragm crus.
CVC: Caudal vena cava.
H: The heart.
RL: Artery and vein for the right cranial lung lobe.
LL: Artery and vein for the left cranial lung lobe.
CM: Cranial mediastinum.
P: Fold of pleura marking the cranial limit of the right cranial lung lobe. Caudal to this fold the right and left cranial lung lobes are superimposed on one another.
LC: Cranial portion of the left cranial lung lobe viewed end-on.
CL: Right cranial lung lobe and part of the left cranial lobe superimposed.
LA: Left atrium.
LV: Left ventricle.
RA: Right atrium.
RV: Right ventricle.

(*Illustration continued on following page*)

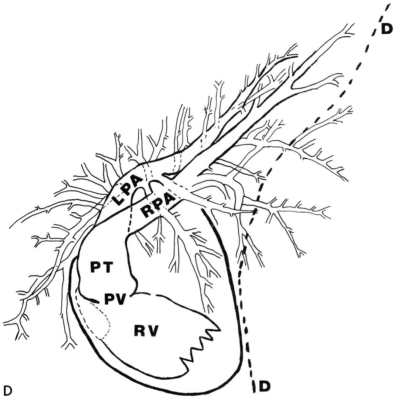

D

FIGURE 3–8 *Continued. D.* Distribution of the pulmonary arteries within the lungs as seen on the lateral view.

        RV: Right ventricle.
        PV: Pulmonic valve.
        PT: Pulmonary artery trunk.
        RPA: Right pulmonary artery.
        LPA: Left pulmonary artery.
        DD: The diaphragm.

(Illustration continued on opposite page)

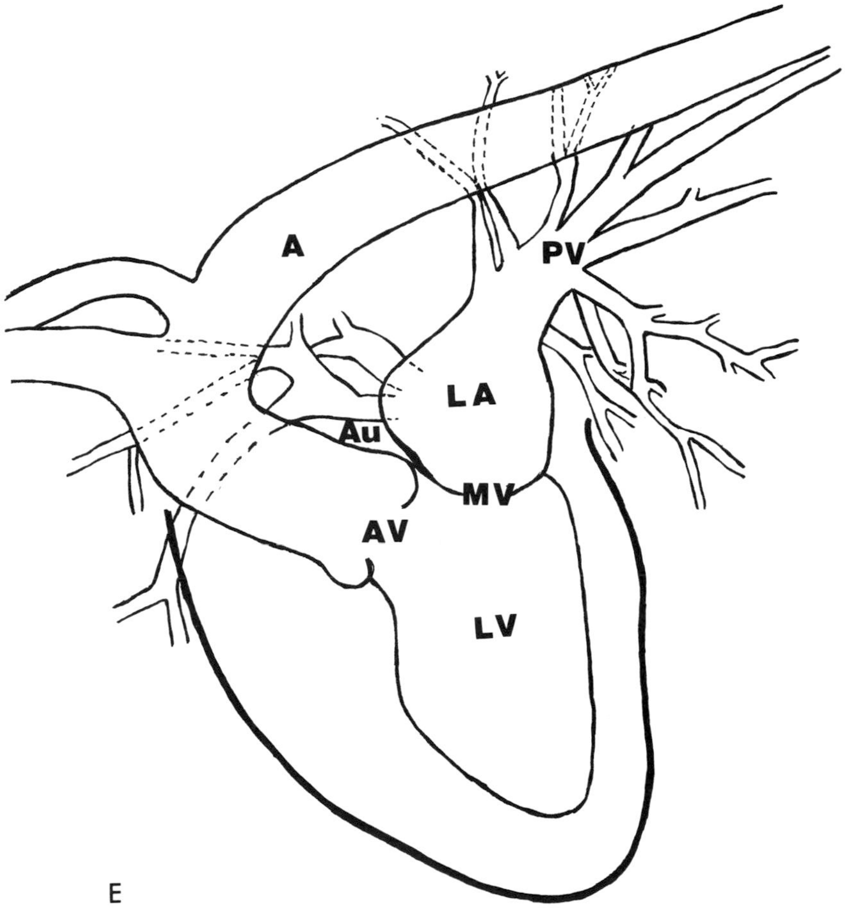

E

FIGURE 3–8 *Continued. E.* The larger pulmonary veins as seen on the lateral view.
LV: Left ventricle.
AV: Aortic valve.
A: Aorta.
PV: Pulmonary veins entering the left atrium.
LA: Left atrium.
MV: Mitral valve.
Au: Left auricle.

(Illustration continued on following page)

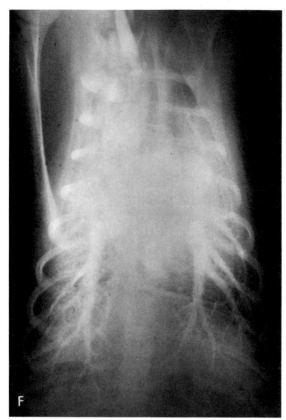

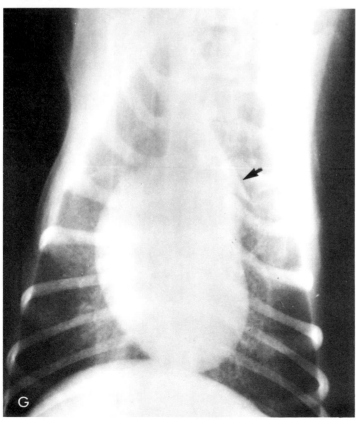

FIGURE 3–8 *Continued.* *F.* An angiocardiogram showing the distribution of the pulmonary arteries as seen on the ventrodorsal view. *G.* The thymus gland (arrow) is sometimes seen in the left thorax on the VD or DV view. Because of its shape it is sometimes referred to as the "thymic sail."

(See also Fig. 3–25)

(d) Bronchi, which contain air, become visible against the denser infiltrated lung tissue. These are referred to as "air bronchograms." The spaces between the cranial lobar arteries and veins should not be mistaken for air bronchograms.

(e) Dispersed among the infiltrated alveoli are groups of alveoli that contain air. This gives the lung fields a mottled appearance. The radiolucent air-filled groups of alveoli are referred to as "air alveolograms."

(f) The alveolar pattern often undergoes rapid change. It appears soon after the onset of symptoms and tends to disappear rapidly if successful therapy is being employed.

Conditions that show an alveolar pattern include pulmonary edema, pulmonary hemorrhage, pneumonia, atelectasis, allergies, obstruction of a bronchus, and chronic alveolar disease. (Fig. 3–9).

THE INTERSTITIAL PATTERN. The interstitium of the lung is the supporting structure that includes the walls of the alveoli; alveolar sacs and ducts; the walls of the bronchioles; the interlobular septa; and the tissues that support the lymphatics, the bronchi, and the pulmonary vessels. Interstitial disease is often more difficult to evaluate than alveolar disease. Indeed, interstitial disease may affect the alveoli before it becomes detectable on radiographs.

RADIOLOGIC SIGNS

(a) Nodular densities with discrete margins. The nodules vary in size and outline. These densities must not be confused with the circular densities that

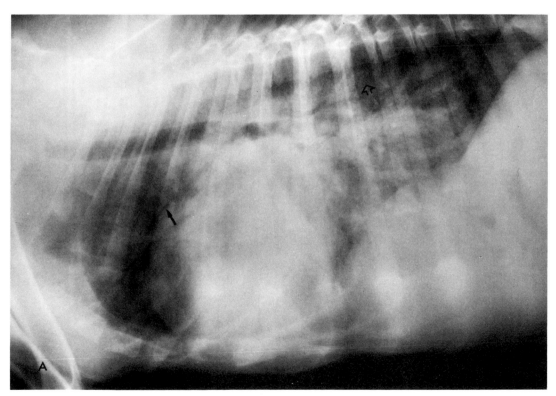

FIGURE 3–9. *A* and *B* show the fluffy type of infiltration characteristic of an alveolar pattern. The densities are irregular in outline and frequently coalesce. Air bronchograms (black arrows) and areas showing air alveolograms (some indicated by open arrows) are seen.

(*Illustration continued on following page*)

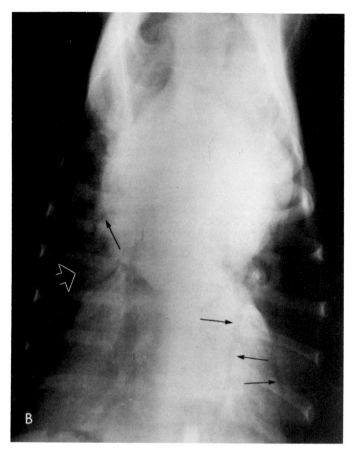

FIGURE 3–9 *Continued.* *B.* See legend on preceding page.

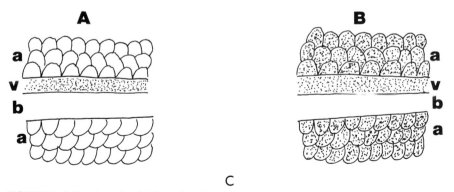

C

FIGURE 3–9 *Continued.* *C.* The principle of the air bronchogram.
A, a represents air filled groups of alveoli, **b** is a bronchus and **v** a pulmonary vessel. Air in the alveoli and bronchus provides a contrast for the soft tissue density (fluid density) of the vessel and so the vessel can be seen on a radiograph. The bronchus is not seen as it has the same radiographic density as the alveoli. In **B**, the alveoli have been infiltrated. They now have the same density as the vessel. Contrast is lost and the vessel can no longer be seen. However, the bronchus now becomes visible as it contrasts with the fluid density in the alveoli and blood vessel.

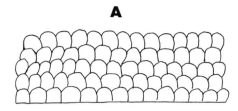

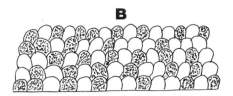

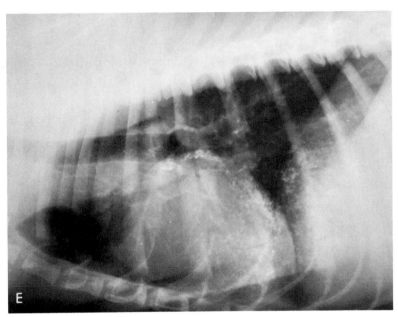

FIGURE 3–9 *Continued.* *D.* The principle of the air alveologram. **A** represents groups of air filled alveoli. They all have the same degree of radiolucency and will be seen as a dark area on the radiograph. **B**. If some groups of alveoli become infiltrated while others retain air, then a mottled effect is produced on the radiograph. The fluid density in some alveoli contrasts with the air density in others. *E.* Barium in the lungs showing an alveolar distribution.

are exhibited by blood vessels when seen end-on. These are not usually numerous and they are larger toward the hilus.

(b) Nonvascular line markings are seen throughout the lung fields. Rarely, chronic interstitial disease produces a honeycomb appearance on radiographs.

(c) There may be an overall increase in lung density with loss of contrast between the pulmonary vasculature and the lungs.

Diseases that show an interstitial pattern include neoplasia, edema, pneumonia, lung granuloma, fungal diseases, and lymphosarcoma. The interstitial pattern resulting from disease changes has to be distinguished from the changes frequently seen in the lungs of aging animals. The case history is of value in making the distinction. (Fig. 3–10). See also Figure 3–6.

THE BRONCHIAL PATTERN. Whether or not bronchi can be seen depends on their relative densities when contrasted with the air-filled lung tissue. Except for the larger bronchi near the hilus, the bronchial tree cannot be recognized under normal conditions except when a bronchus is seen end-on.

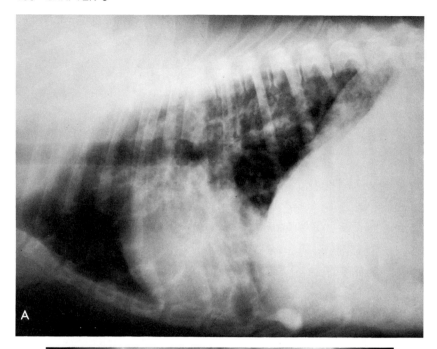

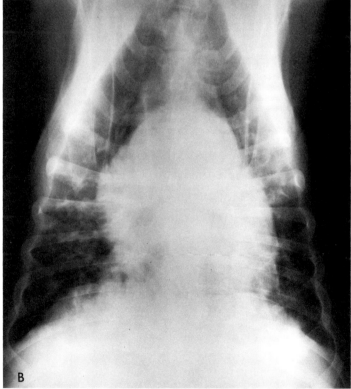

FIGURE 3–10. *A, B.* Extensive interstitial disease is present both in left and right lungs. The pulmonary vasculature has been almost completely obliterated. Numerous nonvascular line marks give an almost reticulated appearance to the lung fields. Numerous small nodular densities are present. An air bronchogram can be seen in the right caudal lung lobe indicating alveolar infiltration in that area. This is a mixed pattern with interstitial changes predominating.

RADIOLOGIC SIGNS

(a) Calcification of the bronchial cartilage.

(b) Peribronchial infiltration. In chronic inflammatory conditions an irregular infiltrate may surround the bronchi. This can be clearly seen in end-on views as a cuff around the affected bronchus. Affected bronchi appear as ring-like structures. Thick cuffs suggest an acute condition, while thin cuffs suggest chronicity.

(c) Thickened bronchial walls give rise to a linear pattern within the lungs that follows the outline of the bronchial tree. Branching pairs of parallel lines may be seen. This is sometimes referred to as a "railway line" or "tramline" effect. The pulmonary vasculature will be somewhat obscured.

Diseases that show a bronchial pattern include chronic bronchitis and bronchiectasis. (Fig. 3–11).

THE VASCULAR PATTERN. Abnormalities may affect the pulmonary vessels in a number of ways.

RADIOLOGIC SIGNS

(a) Hypovascularization: There is a scarcity of pulmonary vessels within the

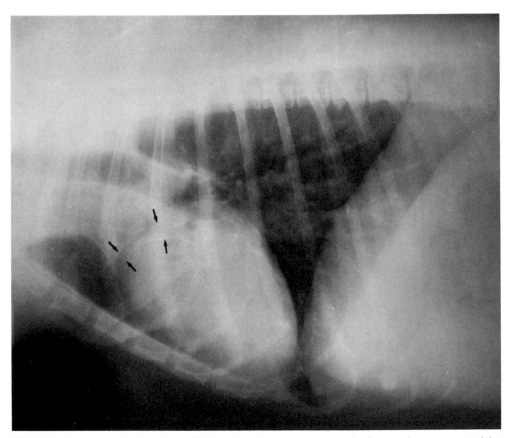

FIGURE 3–11. A bronchial and interstitial pattern. Numerous nonvascular line marks are seen and the interstitial infiltration obscures details of the pulmonary vasculature. Calcified bronchi can be seen in the cranial lung lobe area (arrows). The parallel calcified bronchial walls are sometimes said to give a "tramline" or "railway line" effect. Thin peribronchial infiltrates are seen. There are some nodular densities. (A blood vessel seen end on gives a nodular density but few are seen in the normal thorax. They are largest at the hilus and smallest at the periphery.)

lung fields. Vessels are seen to taper off more rapidly than usual and the periphery of the lung fields is excessively radiolucent.

(b) Hypervascularization: There is an increase in the number and size of the vessels visualized. Vessels are seen to extend further into the periphery of the lung fields than is usual.

(c) Dilatation and tortuosity of vessels, particularly of the pulmonary arteries, is a feature of some conditions.

(d) Vessels not normally seen, particularly the pulmonary veins, may become prominent.

Diseases that may show a vascular pattern include various cardiac conditions, dirofilariasis, angiostrongyliasis, and arteriovenous fistula. Pulmonic hypoplasia or agenesis may cause distortion of the normal vascular pattern in the opposite lung. (Fig. 3–12).

THE MIXED PATTERN. In many conditions, the patttern seen will be a mixed one because the structures of the lung are in contact with one another. Hence, disease processes in one structure may affect surrounding tissues. Thus, congestive heart failure, while showing a vascular pattern, may also show an alveolar pattern if alveolar edema develops.

The significance of changes seen within the lungs may often be very difficult to evaluate. Clinical findings and the results of other diagnostic procedures must be taken into account in arriving at a diagnosis. There is a tendency to

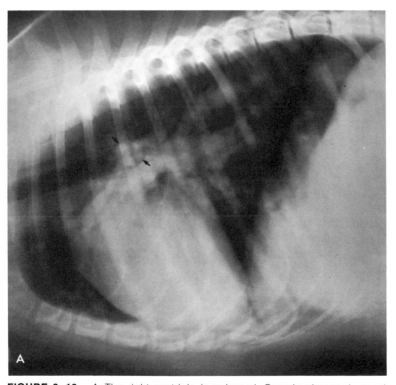

FIGURE 3–12. *A.* The right ventricle is enlarged. Grossly abnormal vessels are seen in the caudal lung fields. A large abnormal vessel is seen end-on (arrows) overlying the trachea. (Dirofilaria immitis infestation). See Figs. 3–39 and 3–40.

(*Illustration continued on opposite page.*)

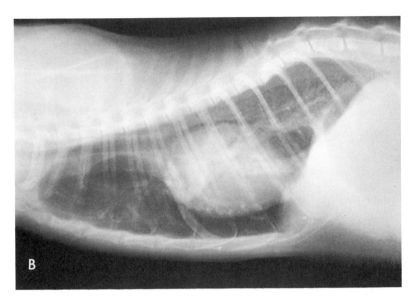

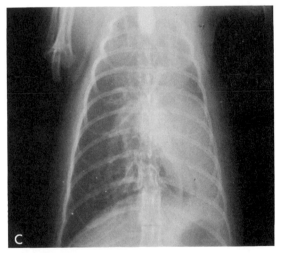

FIGURE 3–12 *Continued. B–F.* An eight month old Siamese cat had respiratory difficulty when stressed. There was poor weight gain. *B.* A lateral radiograph shows the heart in an unusual position. Pulmonary vessels are seen but their distribution is abnormal. *C.* A ventrodorsal radiograph shows the heart on the left side of the thorax. Unusual pulmonary vessels are seen in the right lung. *D, E.* A nonselective angiocardiogram through a jugular vein shows an abnormal distribution of the pulmonary vessels. On the lateral view the contrast medium seems to "stain" the caudal lung lobe area through a mass of fine capillaries. On the dorsoventral view no left pulmonary artery is seen. There is some reflux into the caudal vena cava.

(Illustration continued on following page.)

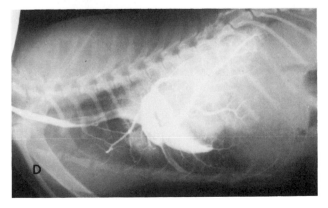

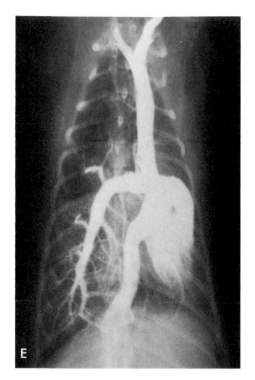

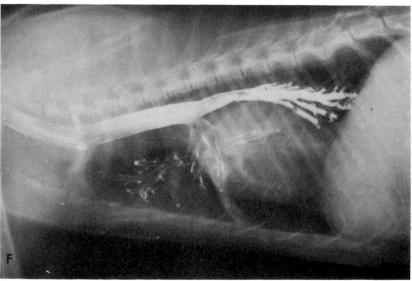

FIGURE 3–12 *Continued.* *F,* A bronchogram shows an abnormal bronchial distribution. At autopsy the diagnosis was hypoplasia of the left lung, which was virtually entirely absent.

Pulmonary Patterns

Alveolar	Interstitial	Bronchial	Vascular	Mixed
Fluffy densities.	Nonvascular line markings.	Calcification of cartilages.	Hypovascularization.	Shows features of two or more of the other patterns.
Areas of increased density tend to merge.	Nodular densities.	Peribronchial infiltration.	Hypervascularization.	
Interlobar fissures become visible.	Loss of clarity in the outline of vessels.	Linear pattern of thickened bronchial walls.	Dilated and tortuous vessels.	
Air bronchograms.			Prominent pulmonary veins.	
Air alveolograms.				
Rapid changes.				

overread chest radiographs, attaching pathologic significance to normal variations. The recognition of a particular pattern of change, however, limits the possible range of diagnoses and facilitates a correlation between the changes seen and basic pathologic processes.

THE SILHOUETTE SIGN

A lesion within the thorax that touches the heart, aorta, or diaphragm will cause obliteration of the border of the structure it touches at the area of contact. This is known as the silhouette sign. A lesion within the thorax that does not touch the heart, aorta, or diaphragm will not obliterate the borders of any of these structures. This is based on the fact that air-filled lung between a lesion and a structure acts as a contrast agent outlining both lesion and structure. Thus the aorta can be seen through the cardiac shadow in the VD or DV view because of the interposed lung tissue.

It has been suggested that where there is uniformity of thickness, atomic number, and density in superimposed structures, the silhouette sign will occur irrespective of whether or not the structures are in contact. Anatomically, this is probably unlikely to occur frequently (Fig. 3–13).

Specific Conditions

PNEUMONIA. Acute bacterial pneumonias produce an alveolar pattern with fluffy infiltrates. The exudative process results in the obliteration of air in groups of alveoli and alveolar ducts. In acute pneumonia radiologic changes become evident soon after the onset of symptoms. Pneumonic infiltrates are usually patchy in distribution with irregular, indistinct borders. Bronchopneumonia commonly affects the dependent parts of the lungs in the middle and cranial lobes. Serial radiographs made over a number of days show changes in the pattern, either progressive or regressive.

Interstitial pneumonitis is characterized by loss of clarity of the vascular pattern. This is because the interstitial structures become denser, the overall air volume is reduced, and contrast with the vessels is lost. Because air is present in the alveoli, the densities seen in the alveolar pattern are not apparent in interstitial pneumonia.

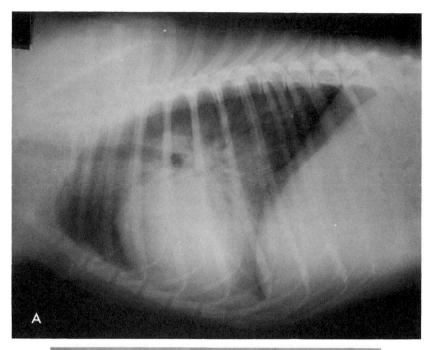

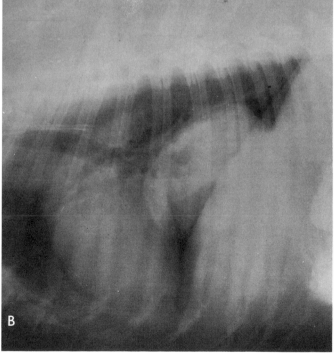

FIGURE 3–13. The Silhouette Sign: *A.* The caudal cardiac outline has been lost owing to infiltration of the adjacent lung. (Positive silhouette sign). *B.* The caudal cardiac border can be clearly seen through the superimposed intrathoracic mass. This indicates that the mass is not in contact with the heart. (Negative silhouette sign).

Viral pneumonia usually causes little visible radiographic change unless accompanied by exudation or atelectasis. Diminished contrast between the pulmonary vasculature and the lungs and some peribronchial infiltration may be noted.

Inhalation pneumonia usually affects the caudal part of the left cranial lobe and the right middle lobe or the dependent parts of the caudal lobes. A mixed pattern is frequently seen. Atelectasis may occur. Bronchial foreign bodies may result in bronchopneumonia, bronchiectasis, lung abscess, atelectasis, or a granulomatous pneumonia.

Fungal pneumonias, most commonly seen in the southwestern United States, show mainly an interstitial pattern. Nodular densities of varying size are usual. The picture may simulate metastatic lung disease. The history and origin of the patient are helpful in the differential diagnosis. Hilar lymphadenopathy is a common feature. Nocardiosis is frequently accompanied by pleural effusion. Coccidioidomycosis may be present without any visible pulmonary abnormality.

SPECIFIC PNEUMONIAS

CANINE DISTEMPER. An interstitial pattern is frequently observed with reduced contrast between the pulmonary vasculature and the lung parenchyma. There may be peribronchial infiltration. Should a secondary bacterial pneumonia supervene an alveolar pattern will become evident.

TOXOPLASMOSIS. In dogs, the radiographic pattern is variable with frequently some degree of pleural effusion. In cats an alveolar pattern, particularly prominent in the caudal lobes, is the main radiologic finding.

ALEUROSTRONGYLOSIS. The worms live in the bronchioles of affected cats. Ill-defined nodular densities are seen widely distributed throughout the lung fields. The caudal lobes are most severely affected. Some pleural effusion is common.

PARAGONIMIASIS. Lung fluke worms in dogs are common in some parts of the United States and in Eastern Asia. Radiographic findings comprise nodular densities, linear and peribronchial infiltration, and intrapulmonary cystic lesions.

EOSINOPHILIC PNEUMONIA (Pulmonary Infiltration of Eosinophils. PIE.). The changes seen on radiographs are not characteristic, being usually those of a mixed pattern. It may simulate bronchopneumonia. (Fig. 3–14).

PULMONARY EDEMA

Pulmonary edema may affect the alveoli, the respiratory ducts, and the interstitium of the lung. Edema may, therefore, be alveolar or interstitial. Alveolar edema is usually preceded by interstitial edema. Pulmonary edema is usually associated with left heart failure. It may also be seen in allergic conditions (responses), electrocution, the inhalation of noxious gases, and advanced uremia.

RADIOLOGIC SIGNS

The radiologic pattern in alveolar edema is the alveolar pattern. If the edema is associated with cardiac failure, the following may be observed:
  (a) Enlargement of the heart, particularly the left atrium.
  (b) Elevation of the trachea.

Text continued on page 180

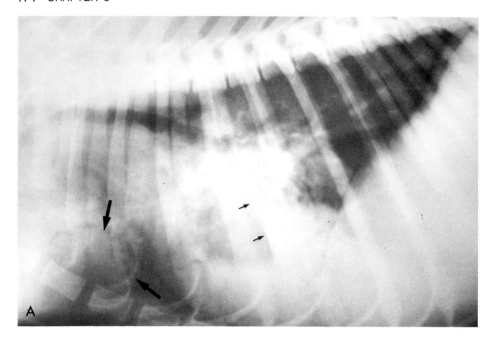

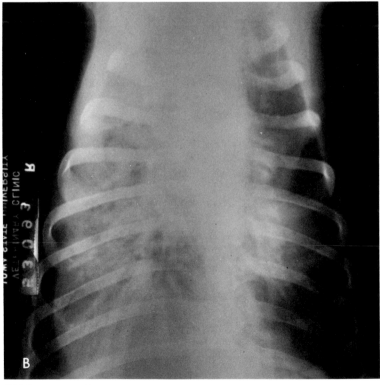

FIGURE 3–14. Pneumonia. *A, B.* Both lungs show patchy infiltration. The right is the more severely affected. Air alveolograms and air bronchograms are seen (large arrows). An interlobar fissure (small arrows) is also visible. This was a one year old English Pointer with conjunctivitis and ocular and nasal discharges. At autopsy there was rhinitis and bronchopneumonia. The right middle lung lobe is often first affected in bronchopneumonia.

(Illustration continued on opposite page.)

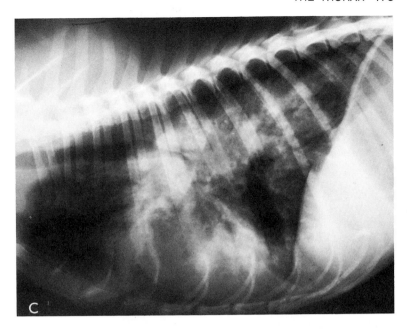

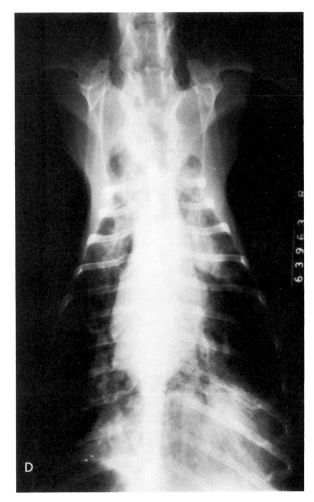

FIGURE 3–14 *Continued.* *C, D.* Both lungs show patchy infiltration. Air bronchograms and peribronchial infiltrates are seen. Nonvascular linear markings are present. The increased density at the hilus is due to hilar lymphadenopathy. This is a mixed pattern. At autopsy there was a chronic granulomatous pneumonia with lymphadenitis. No etiologic agent was isolated.

(Illustration continued on following page.)

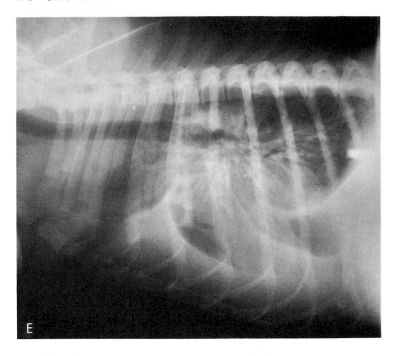

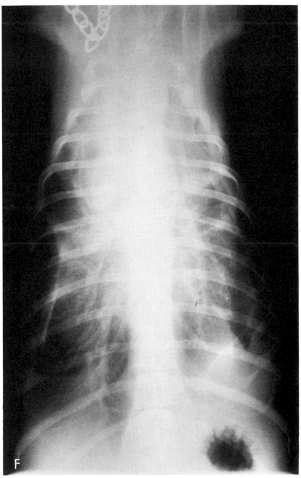

FIGURE 3–14 *Continued. E, F.* The lateral radiograph shows intrathoracic fluid obscuring the cardiac shadow and outlining interlobar fissures. Fluid is seen in the costophrenic angles on the ventrodorsal view. The visible lungs are infiltrated. The ventrodorsal view shows hypervascularization of the lungs. The apparent elevation of the trachea is partly due to rotation. This was a three year old female Labrador referred to the clinic with a diagnosis of pneumonia. The animal was emaciated and very depressed. At autopsy there was a granulomatous mass in the thorax with hyperplasia of the tracheobronchial lymph nodes and focal atelectasis. The diagnosis was granulomatous pleuritis and pyothorax due to actinomycosis.

(*Illustration continued on opposite page.*)

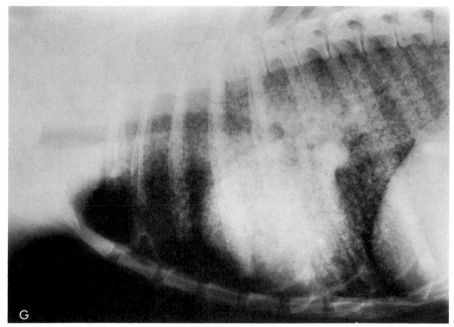

FIGURE 3–14 *Continued. G.* Fungal pneumonia. Widespread miliary infiltration of the lungs was due to coccidioidomycosis. The increased density in the hilar region is due to hilar lymphadenopathy.

(*Illustration continued on following page.*)

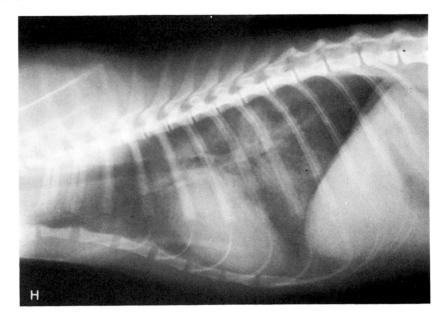

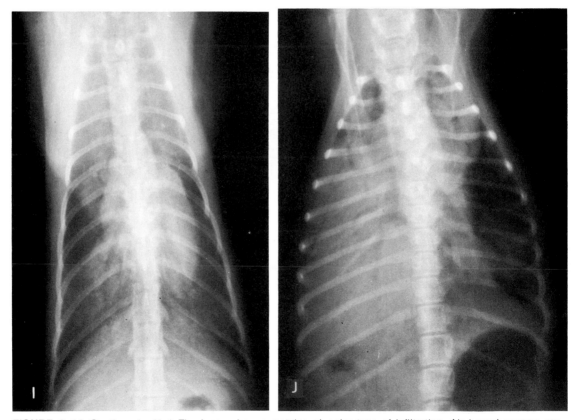

FIGURE 3–14 *Continued.* *H, I.* The lungs show a patchy, alveolar type of infiltration. Air bronchograms are seen on the ventrodorsal view. This was a one year old domestic cat, spayed one month earlier, presented with respiratory difficulty. The clinical diagnosis was pneumonia. *J.* This dog developed respiratory distress following surgery for the removal of a cystic calculus. It died 36 hours later. The right lung is completely infiltrated and air bronchograms are seen. There is also some infiltration of the left caudal lung lobe. Part of the density in the left cranial lung lobe area is due to overlying of the scapula. The diagnosis was Klebsiella pneumonia.

(*Illustration continued on opposite page.*)

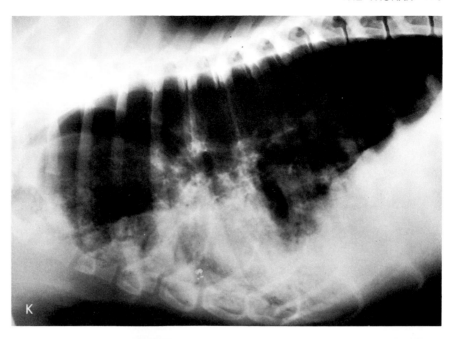

FIGURE 3–14 *Continued.* *K, L.* A purulent pneumonia of long standing. The dependent lung fields are grossly infiltrated
and partly obscure the cardiac shadow. A
distorted interlobar fissure is seen caudal
to the heart. The trachea is distorted owing
to adhesions. The ventrodorsal view shows
widespread infiltration of the lungs, numerous air bronchograms, hypervascularization, and peribronchial infiltration.

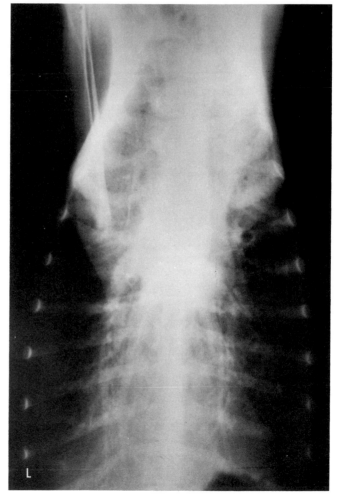

(c) An increase in interstitial markings with loss of the normal contrast between the lungs and the pulmonary vasculature (interstitial edema).

(d) Pulmonary vascular dilatation, particularly affecting the pulmonary veins.

(e) An alveolar pattern that spreads out from the hilus in a symmetrical fashion (so-called "butterfly pattern"), obscuring the interstitial changes (alveolar edema). The periphery of the lung fields appears normal.

(f) The radiographic pattern may change rapidly on successive radiographs.

Edema due to causes other than cardiac failure is not usually symmetric and the heart shadow will probably be normal in outline.

Animals that have been in prolonged recumbency may show pulmonary edema on the dependent side. (Fig. 3–15).

PULMONARY HEMORRHAGE

Pulmonary hemorrhage is usually the result of trauma, though it may occur in cases of poisoning with anticoagulant agents. The radiologic pattern is alveolar with patchy infiltration and often some bronchial consolidation. Concomitant injuries, such as a broken rib, are frequently seen. There is usually a rapid resolution of the radiographic changes over a period of days in recovering cases. Discrete densities that appear to remain as the general lung pattern clears represent hematomas. (Fig. 3–16).

PULMONARY NEOPLASIA

Primary lung neoplasms are relatively rare in the dog. Metastatic lung disease is common in dogs, less common in cats.

A single nodular density is more likely to be associated with a primary lung tumor. Other conditions, however, may cause solitary nodular densities, for example lung abscess, infarction, cyst, or granuloma. The signs of metastatic lung disease are mainly those of an interstitial pattern.

RADIOLOGIC SIGNS

(a) Multiple, sharply defined nodular densities.

(b) The size of individual lesions varies considerably; several different sizes are seen in the one lung.

(c) The lesions are usually widely distributed throughout the lungs.

(d) Superimposition of masses on one another, when they are very numerous, may give the impression that their margins are not discrete. Lesions should be examined toward the edges of the areas of greatest infiltration or at the lung periphery. The absence of air bronchograms helps to exclude the presence of an alveolar pattern.

(e) A diffuse interstitial pattern is seen with some primary lung tumors, such as bronchiolar cell carcinoma. Lymphosarcoma may show nodular densities but there will be concomitant hilar lymph node enlargement, or enlarged sternal and mediastinal lymph nodes, or both of these conditions.

It should be remembered that negative radiographic findings do not exclude the possibility that lung metastases are present. Widespread metastatic disease may be present although the chest films appear normal. This is because the lesions are below the size at which they can be visualized, which is about 1 cm in diameter. (Fig. 3–17).

Text continued on page 192

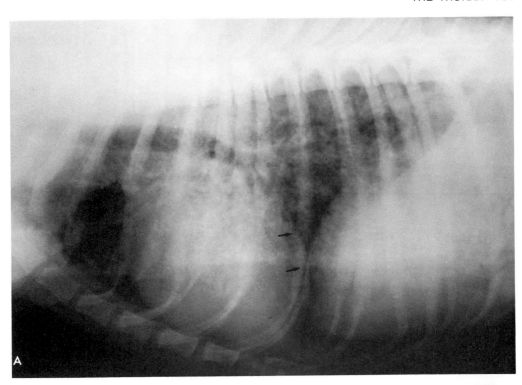

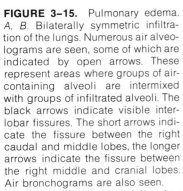

FIGURE 3–15. Pulmonary edema. *A, B.* Bilaterally symmetric infiltration of the lungs. Numerous air alveolograms are seen, some of which are indicated by open arrows. These represent areas where groups of air-containing alveoli are intermixed with groups of infiltrated alveoli. The black arrows indicate visible interlobar fissures. The short arrows indicate the fissure between the right caudal and middle lobes, the longer arrows indicate the fissure between the right middle and cranial lobes. Air bronchograms are also seen.

(*Illustration continued on following page*)

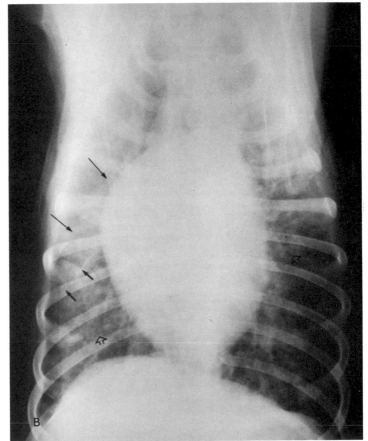

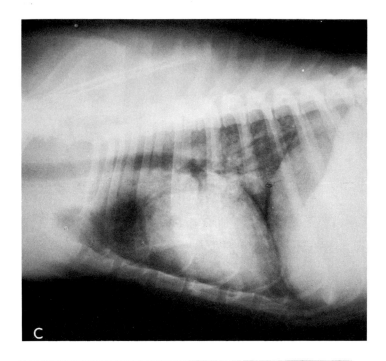

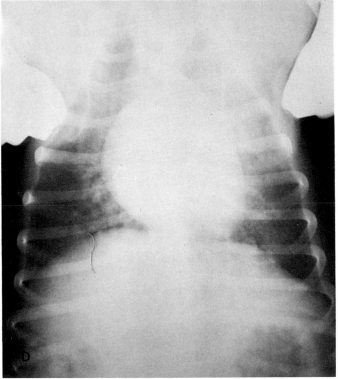

FIGURE 3-15 *Continued. C, D.* A widespread, ill-defined, symmetric, fluffy infiltration is seen both in right and left lungs. Air bronchograms are evident. There is some right heart enlargement. (*Illustration continued on opposite page.*)

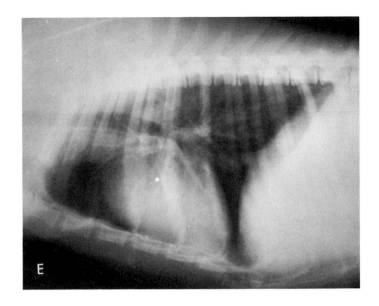

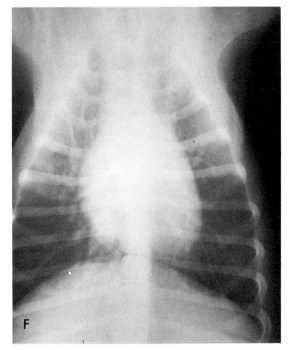

FIGURE 3-15 *Continued. E, F.* Seven days later the lungs have assumed a more normal appearance. Alveolar changes disappear rapidly when successful therapy is employed.

(Illustration continued on following page.)

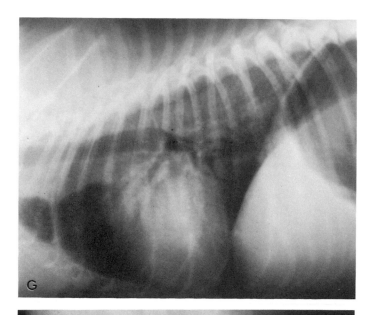

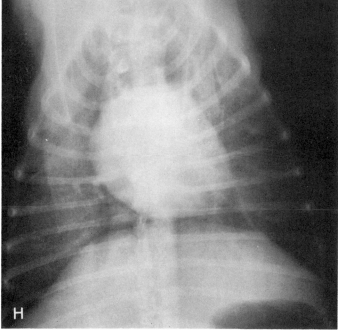

FIGURE 3–15 *Continued.* *G, H.* This evenly distributed, mainly reticular type pattern suggests interstitial, rather than alveolar, edema. Interlobar fissures are seen both on the left and right sides. Some alveolar densities are present as indicated by air bronchograms.

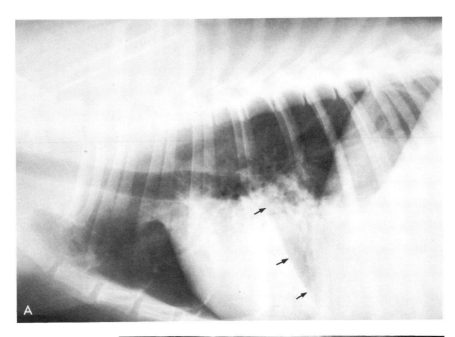

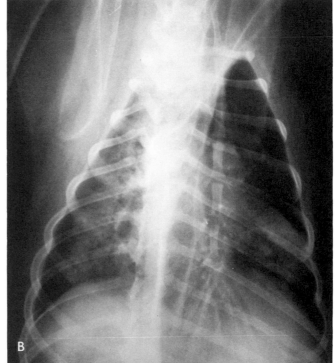

FIGURE 3-16. Pulmonary hemorrhage.
A, B. A six year old female Shetland sheep-
dog was hit by an automobile. There is
widespread patchy infiltration of the right
and left lungs. An interlobar fissure is seen
on the lateral view (arrows). (The ventrodorsal view is rotated.)

(*Illustration continued on following page.*)

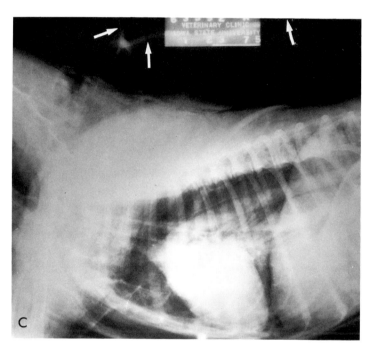

C

FIGURE 3-16 *Continued. C, D.* On the lateral radiograph the trachea and aorta are unusually well outlined owing to air in the mediastinum, which acts as a contrast agent. A large amount of gas (air) is present between the skin (arrows) and the body wall. Patchy, fluffy densities due to pulmonary hemorrhage are seen in both lungs.

(Illustration continued on opposite page)

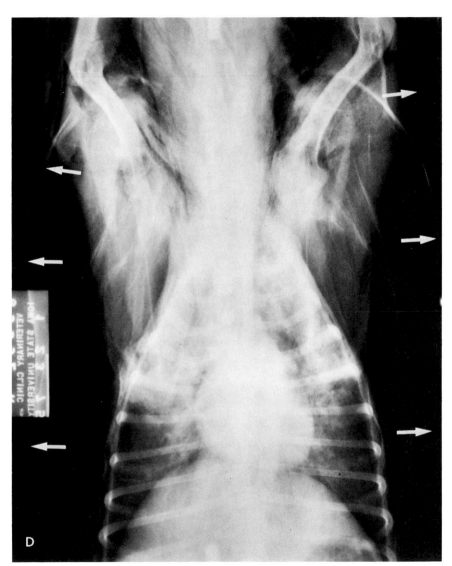

FIGURE 3–16 *Continued. D, See legend on opposite page.)*

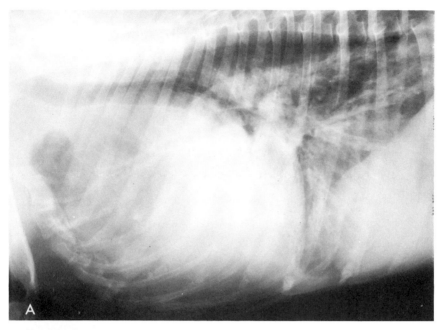

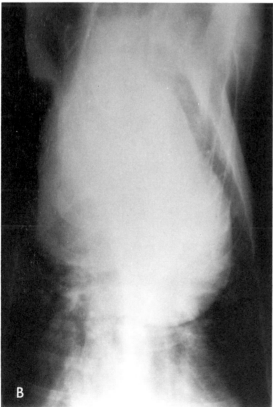

FIGURE 3–17. Pulmonary neoplasia. *A, B.* A seven year old female Doberman suffered weight loss for a month. She was emaciated, incoordinate, and had a small moveable lump on the left chest wall. There was nonproductive retching for 5 weeks. The right cranial hemithorax is occupied by a homogeneous soft tissue mass that is displacing the heart and deforming the sternum. The visible lungs show marked interstitial infiltration. At autopsy the right cranial lobe was filled with a large mass that contained pus and necrotic tissue. The diagnosis was primary bronchogenic carcinoma.

(Illustration continued on opposite page.)

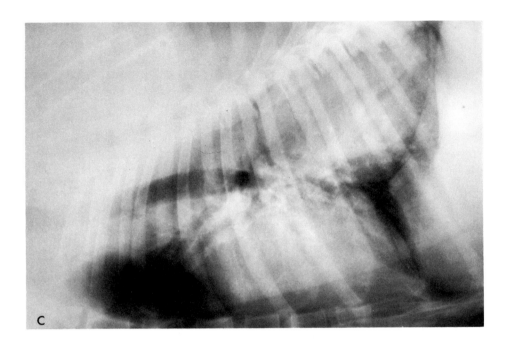

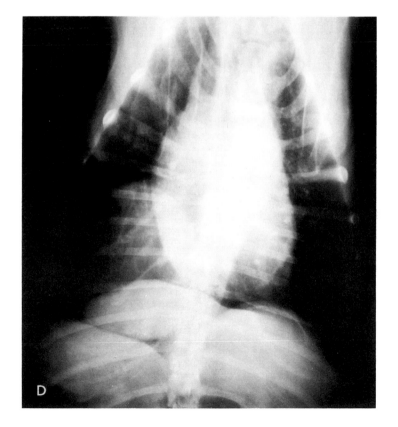

FIGURE 3–17 *Continued. C, D.* A 12 year old Brittany spaniel had labored breathing and depression. The lateral radiograph shows a large mass in the caudal thorax. On the ventrodorsal view the mass can be seen in the right caudal lung lobe partially overshadowing the heart (negative silhouette sign). The lung lobe was resected. It contained a large hematocyst surrounded by a granulomatous reaction with focal areas of bronchogenic carcinoma. Part of the diaphragm is displaced caudally by the mass, giving a double diaphragmatic outline on the right side.

(Illustration continued on following page.)

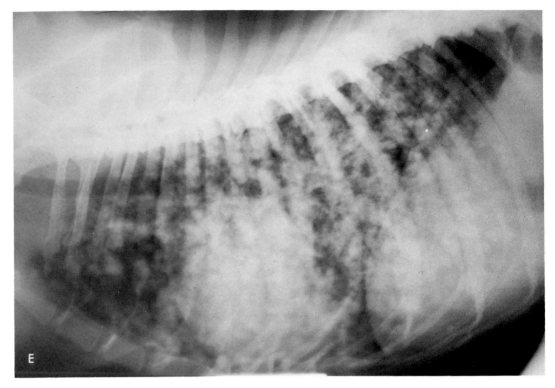

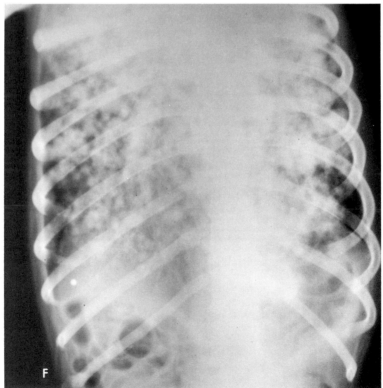

FIGURE 3–17 *Continued.* *E, F.* Metastatic disease. Multiple metastases are seen in both lungs. While individual lesions have sharply demarcated edges, superimposition of numerous lesions may give an overall fluffy appearance. Lesions should be examined at the periphery of the lungs, where detail may be more readily appreciated. Miliary lesions of this nature may indicate lymphatic spread of a tumor.

(*Illustration continued on opposite page*)

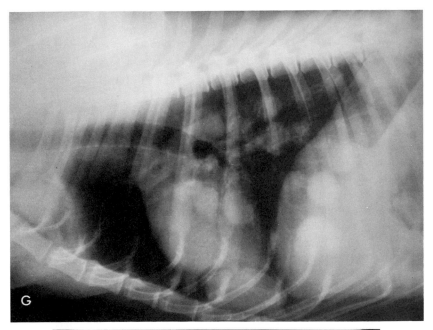

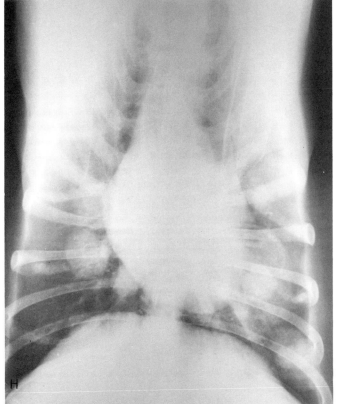

FIGURE 3–17 *Continued.   G, H.* So-called "cannon ball" metastases, which are frequently seen associated with osteosarcoma.

TORSION OF A LUNG LOBE

Torsion of lung lobes has been reported both in cats and dogs. The right middle lobe is the most commonly affected. The principal radiologic signs are pleural effusion, with the fluid trapped about the rotated lobe, an alveolar pattern, and eventual lobar consolidation.

The Diaphragm

ANATOMY

The diaphragm is a musculotendinous sheet that separates the abdominal and thoracic cavities. It projects into the thorax like a dome. It consists of a centrally located cupula and right and left crura, sometimes referred to as hemidiaphragms. Between the crura there is an intercrural cleft.

NORMAL APPEARANCE

The appearance of the diaphragm varies depending on several factors: the position of the animal, the phase of the respiratory cycle, the position of the central ray of the x-ray beam, and the conformation of the animal.

In lateral recumbency the crus on the dependent side appears cranial to the uppermost crus. In right lateral recumbency the crura appear more or less parallel to one another, while in left lateral recumbency they appear to intersect at about the level of the caudal vena cava. The vena cava pierces the right hemidiaphragm.

On VD or DV views, deep-chested animals clearly show left and right crura, while shallow-chested animals frequently show a single diaphragm line. The right crus often appears marginally cranial to the left. The cupula may be indented at its point of contact with the heart.

At inspiration, the position of the diaphragm may vary by about the length of two vertebral bodies from its position at expiration. The cranial crus usually crosses the ventral edge of the vertebral column between the eleventh and the thirteenth thoracic vertebrae. It may, however, be as far cranial as the ninth thoracic vertebra and as far caudal as the first lumbar vertebra. At rest the diaphragmatic movement may be the length of one vertebra or less.

The position of the central x-ray beam affects the diaphragmatic shadow, particularly in the VD or DV view. If the beam is centered over the abdomen, separate shadows may be cast by each crus, the cupula, and the intercrural cleft. (Fig. 3–18).

ABNORMALITIES

DIAPHRAGMATIC HERNIA. The radiographic appearance of diaphragmatic hernia varies depending on the site of rupture, the degree of rupture, and the volume and nature of the herniated contents.

In most cases there is an interruption or loss of the normal diaphragmatic shadow. Because of the increased intrathoracic density, contrast between the diaphragm, the liver shadow and the lungs is lost or partially lost. If stomach

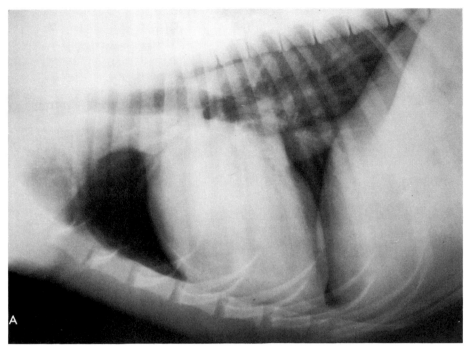

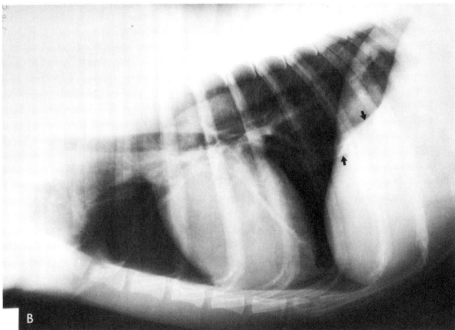

FIGURE 3–18. The Diaphragm. *A.* In right lateral recumbency the right hemidiaphragm lies cranial to the left. The caudal vena cava can be seen to emerge through it. Left and right crura lie parallel to one another. *B.* In left lateral recumbency the left hemidiaphragm lies cranial to the right. The caudal vena cava (arrows) can be seen crossing it. The right and left crura intersect at the intercrural cleft.

(*Illustration continued on following page*)

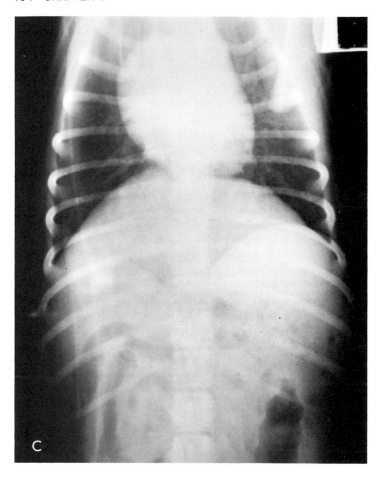

FIGURE 3–18 *Continued. C.* More than one diaphragm outline may be seen if the tube is not accurately positioned over the thorax. The crura and the cupula are seen.

or intestine is present within the thorax, abdominal gas shadows may be seen within the chest. Pneumothorax may be seen in the cranial thorax. Barium is often useful in identifying the position of the stomach and small intestine.

If the liver is displaced into the thorax, the stomach will be displaced forward. This can often be appreciated because of the gas within the stomach. Incarceration of the liver tends to provoke transudation into the thorax because of impairment of the venous return to the heart. Herniation of a small portion of liver may escape radiographic detection.

Compression of the lung or collapse, and in unilateral cases a mediastinal shift toward the unaffected side, are commonly seen. If the hernia has been present for some time fluid may obscure all detail within the thorax.

Pneumoperitonography in the upright position using a horizontal beam will usually show air (gas) under the diaphragm if it is intact. Cholecystography has been recommended to demonstrate the position of the liver.

Diaphragmatic hernia may be accompanied by other abnormalities such as fractured ribs, and intrathoracic or intrapulmonary hemorrhage. (Fig. 3–19).

Loss of Outline.   Fluid within the thorax or masses in the caudal lung lobes may cause partial or complete loss of the diaphragmatic shadow. Smaller amounts of fluid cause blurring of the costophrenic angles. (Fig. 3–20).

Text continued on page 198

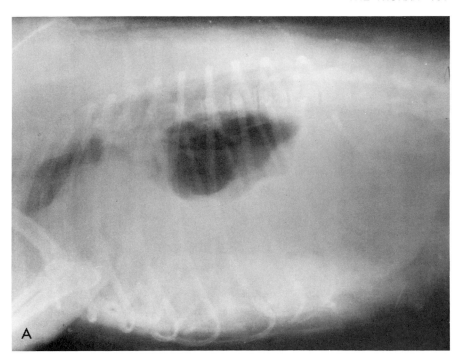

FIGURE 3-19. Diaphragmatic hernia. *A–D*. The plain radiographs show loss of the diaphragm shadow on the left side. The heart and mediastinum are displaced towards the right. An unusual gas density is seen caudal to the heart. Intrathoracic detail is lost on the lateral view. A barium study shows the stomach and some of the small intestine within the left hemithorax. A large amount of gas is present within the stomach. There are fractures of the 12th and 13th ribs on the left side.
(Illustration continued on following page.)

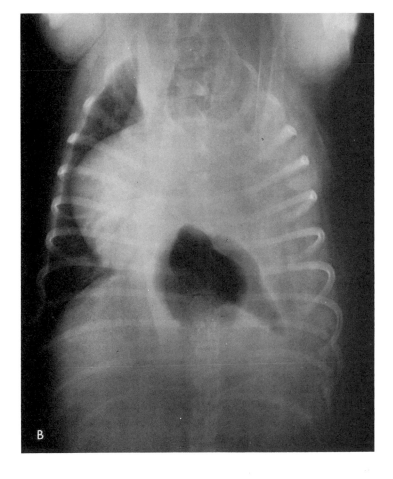

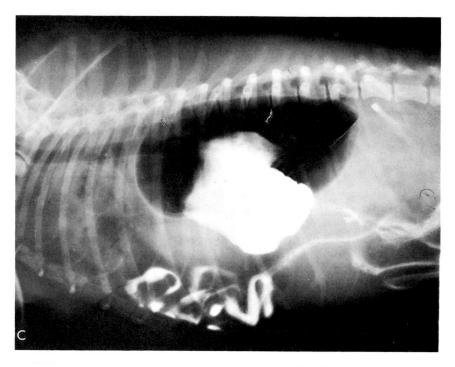

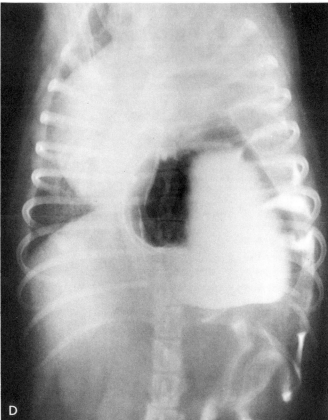

FIGURE 3–19 *Continued.* *C, D.* See legend on page 195.

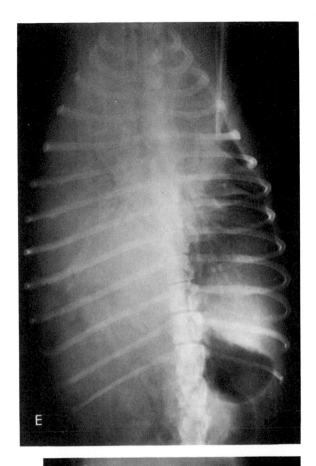

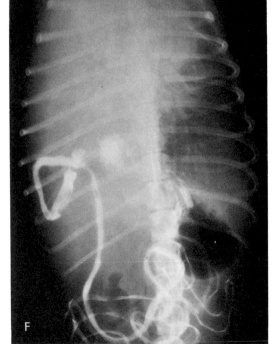

FIGURE 3–19 *Continued. E, F.* The plain radiograph shows obliteration of the diaphragm lines. A fluid density fills the right thorax. Fluid is seen in interlobar fissures on the left side. A barium study shows a loop of small intestine and part of the stomach within the thorax. The fundus of the stomach, outlined by gas, remains within the abdomen. (See Fig. 2–6).

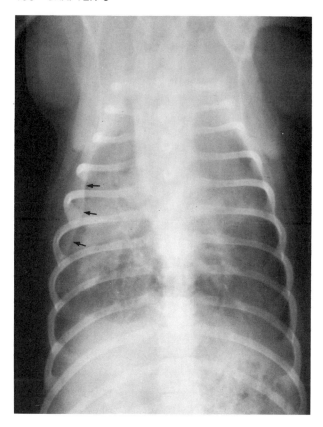

FIGURE 3-20. Fluid within the thorax obliterates the diaphragmatic outline. The fluid obscures the cardiac outline. Fluid can be seen in the pleural space separating the lung edge from the right thoracic wall (arrows). The normally sharp costophrenic angles are blunted. Air bronchograms can be seen through the fluid. See Fig. 3-21.

The Pleurae and Mediastinum

ANATOMY

The pleurae are membranes that cover the lungs and line the thoracic cavity. They form two sacs within the thorax, one covering each lung. The sacs are known as the pleural cavities or pleural space. The visceral pleura covers the lung; the parietal pleura lines the thoracic cavity. Each pleural cavity contains a thin film of fluid.

The mediastinum is the space between the two pleural sacs; it contains the thymus gland, the heart, the trachea, the esophagus, lymph nodes, vessels entering and leaving the heart, and nerves. The mediastinum is in potential communication with the tissues of the neck cranially and with the retroperitoneal space caudally through the aortic hiatus. Since the mediastinal structures all have a soft tissue density, they are not distinguishable from one another under normal conditions. The caudal vena cava is within a separate pleural fold.

The mediastinum may be divided into three areas, cranial, middle, and caudal. The cranial mediastinum is cranial to the heart. The middle mediastinum is the part that contains the heart. The caudal mediastinum is the part that is caudal to the heart.

NORMAL APPEARANCE

The pleurae are not normally seen on radiographs. Fluid within the pleural space can be seen. It separates the lung edges from the thoracic wall and outlines the interlobar fissures of the lungs. Pleural thickening due to fibrosis may also make the pleura visible. Pleurography, that is, the injection of a contrast medium into the pleural space, is occasionally used to demonstrate the pleural space and outline structures within it.

The mediastinum is seen because of the structures within it. On the dorsoventral or ventrodorsal view the left border is formed by the left subclavian artery and the right border by the cranial vena cava. On the lateral view the cranial mediastinum can be seen ventral to the trachea.

ABNORMALITIES

PLEURAL FLUID.   Pleural fluid means fluid within the pleural space.

RADIOLOGIC SIGNS

(a) A homogeneous density in the ventral thorax that often has a scalloped appearance on the lateral view. This appearance is due to fluid tracking into the interlobar fissures.

(b) Partial or complete obliteration of the cardiac shadow.

(c) Visualization of interlobar fissures due to the fluid within them.

(d) Loss of the normal sharp angles at the costophrenic junctions.

(e) In the VD or DV views a fluid density can be seen between the thoracic wall and the lung edges. The fluid density may extend into the interlobar fissures. On the lateral view fluid may be seen dorsal to the caudal lung lobes.

(f) If much fluid is present the diaphragmatic shadow may be obscured.

Standing lateral views are sometimes helpful in demonstrating fluid within the thorax. Small amounts of fluid may be difficult to detect in conventional lateral or ventrodorsal radiographs. If much fluid is present the underlying pathologic changes may become evident only after thoracocentesis.

Fluid within the thorax, unless it is trapped, can be made to vary its position with changes in posture of the animal.

Any fluid within the thoracic cavity may cause the changes mentioned. Thus, it is not possible to distinguish radiologically between hydrothorax, hemothorax, chylothorax, and pyothorax. A unilateral effusion is suggestive of inflammatory change. (Fig. 3–21).

PLEURAL THICKENING.   Pleural thickening is a term given to conditions in which the pleurae become visible but without any significant amount of pleural fluid being present. It is characterized by a thin opacity between the lung edges and the thoracic wall. Interlobar fissures may become visible. It is usually due to fibrosis.

PLEURAL NEOPLASIA.   Primary neoplasms of the pleura are rare in the dog and cat. They are called mesotheliomas and are not readily seen on radiographs. Secondary neoplasms are also difficult to demonstrate.

Masses originating outside the pleurae are usually accompanied by periosteal reaction on the ribs or lysis of the ribs. They protrude into the thorax and have well-defined margins.

PNEUMOTHORAX.   Pneumothorax is free air within the pleural cavity. As a result of loss of the vacuum that normally is present between the parietal and visceral pleurae, the lungs undergo a degree of collapse. Pneumothorax is usually the result of trauma to the lung, though spontaneous pneumothorax may occur in

Text continued on page 203

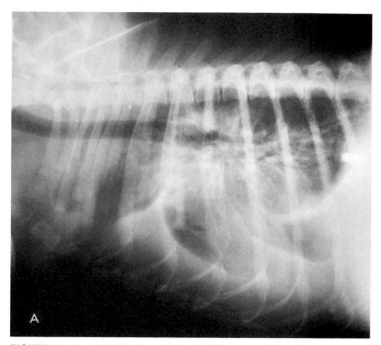

FIGURE 3–21. Hydrothorax. *A*. The leaf-like, or scalloped, appearance of fluid within the pleural cavity is seen on the lateral radiograph. The appearance results from the presence of fluid in the interlobar fissures.

(*Illustration continued on opposite page.*)

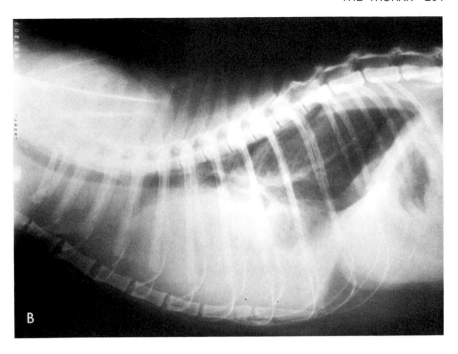

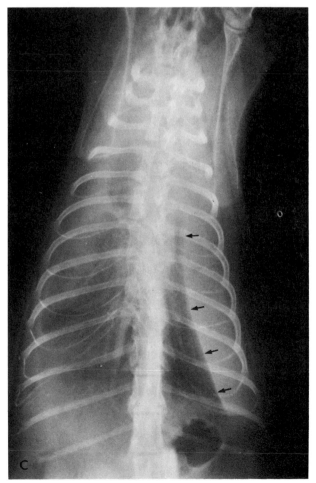

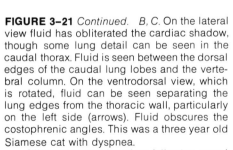

FIGURE 3–21 *Continued.* *B, C.* On the lateral view fluid has obliterated the cardiac shadow, though some lung detail can be seen in the caudal thorax. Fluid is seen between the dorsal edges of the caudal lung lobes and the vertebral column. On the ventrodorsal view, which is rotated, fluid can be seen separating the lung edges from the thoracic wall, particularly on the left side (arrows). Fluid obscures the costophrenic angles. This was a three year old Siamese cat with dyspnea.

(Illustration continued on following page.)

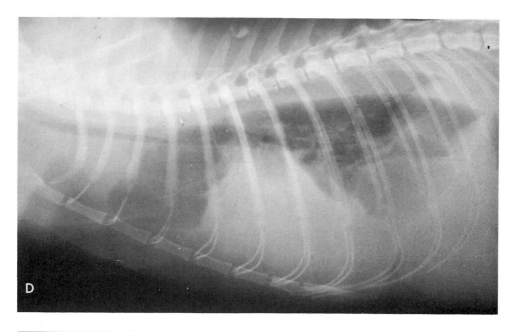

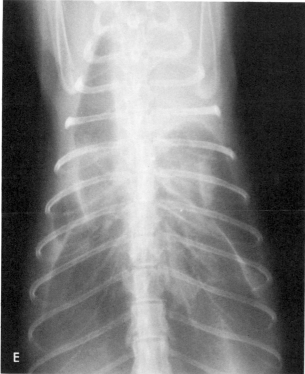

FIGURE 3–21 *Continued. D, E.* A three year old domestic cat presented with labored breathing and depression. The radiologic diagnosis is fluid in the thorax. The cardiac shadow is obscured and the diaphragm outline is lost. Fluid is seen between the dorsal edges of the caudal lung lobes and the vertebral column. On the ventrodorsal view fluid can be seen between the lung edges and the thoracic wall and in the interlobar fissures. There is fluid in the left cranial thorax. At autopsy there was a pleuritis due to *Pasteurella multocida.*

(Illustration continued on opposite page)

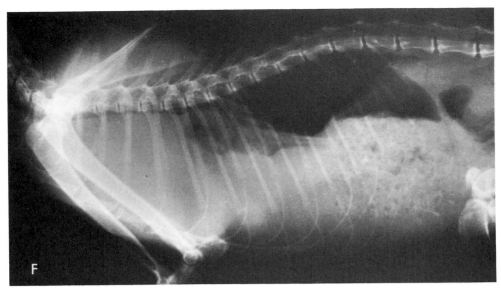

FIGURE 3–21 *Continued.* *F.* A standing lateral view of a cat's thorax. Fluid has collected in the ventral and middle thorax and a fluid line is seen. A fluid line is seen only when there is both free air and fluid in the pleural space. (pneumohydrothorax).

dogs and cats. Rupture of the esophagus, trachea, or bronchi may also result in pneumothorax.

RADIOLOGIC SIGNS

(a) On the lateral view the apex of the heart is lifted away from the sternum.

(b) The thorax appears to have increased radiolucency, particularly at the periphery.

(c) The edges of the caudal lung lobes may be seen to be separated from the ventral aspect of the thoracic vertebrae or from the diaphragm.

(d) Air is sometimes seen in the interlobar fissures of the lungs.

(e) The lungs have an increased density due to atelectasis or partial atelectasis.

(f) In the VD or DV view air can usually be seen in each hemithorax between the lung edges and the thoracic wall.

Tension pneumothorax occurs when a wound in the chest wall or in the bronchial tree acts as a valve, allowing air to be forced into the pleural space at inspiration that cannot escape at expiration. Pressure builds up in the pleural cavity, causing the diaphragm to be displaced caudally and flattened. The condition is accompanied by collapse of the lungs. If unilateral, there is a mediastinal shift away from the affected side. It may be rapidly fatal. (Fig. 3–22).

PNEUMOMEDIASTINUM. This may result from rupture of the esophagus, the intrathoracic trachea, bronchi, or bronchioles. Air may track into the neck and into the retroperitoneal area. Subcutaneous emphysema is common.

RADIOLOGIC SIGNS

(a) Mediastinal structures not normally seen are clearly visualized. Thus, one may see the great vessels in the cranial mediastinum and the esophagus. The dorsal and ventral tracheal walls are well outlined. The thoracic aorta is outlined by air.

(b) Air is often seen in the tissues of the neck with subcutaneous emphysema, which may extend cranially as far as the head.

Text continued on page 207

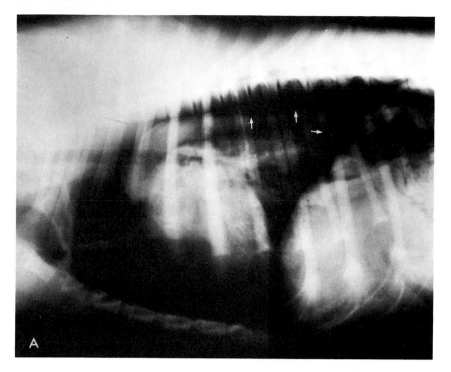

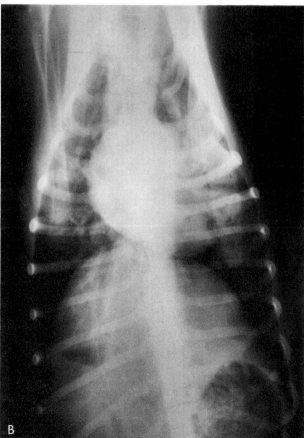

FIGURE 3–22. Pneumothorax. *A, B.* The heart is displaced dorsally from the sternum. There is increased radiolucency of the thorax at the periphery. A lung edge (arrows) can be seen separated from the vertebral column and from the diaphragm. The caudal lung lobe area is increased in density owing to partial atelectasis. On the dorsoventral view the partially collapsed lung is seen on the left side. The costophrenic angles are deep. This is the classic appearance of pneumothorax.

(Illustration continued on opposite page.)

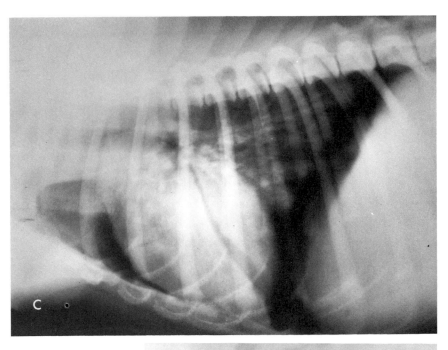

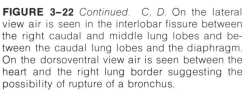

FIGURE 3–22 *Continued. C, D.* On the lateral view air is seen in the interlobar fissure between the right caudal and middle lung lobes and between the caudal lung lobes and the diaphragm. On the dorsoventral view air is seen between the heart and the right lung border suggesting the possibility of rupture of a bronchus.

(*Illustration continued on following page*)

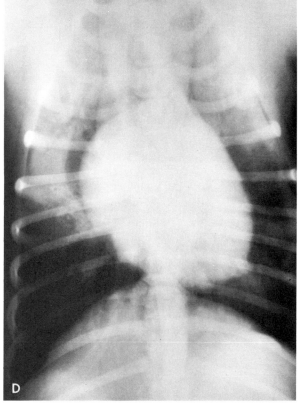

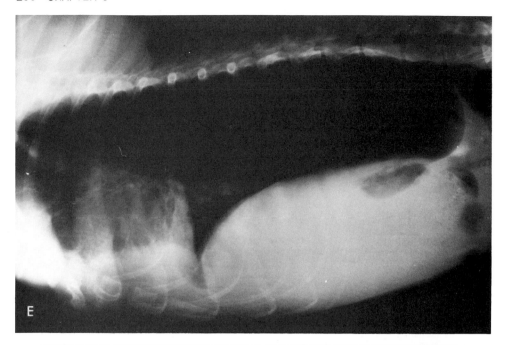

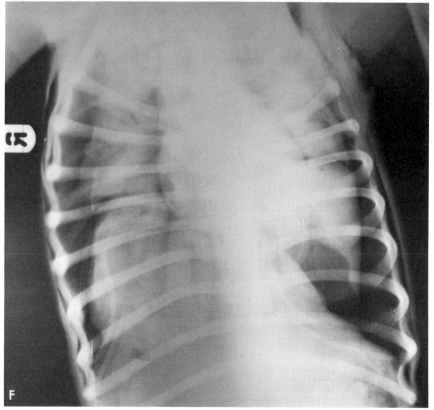

FIGURE 3–22 *Continued. E.* A tension pneumothorax. A large amount of air is present within the thorax. The diaphragm is displaced caudally, flattened, and shows a reverse dome. The heart retains its sternal contact. Owing to the large amount of air present the film appears overexposed and no lung detail can be seen. Air is seen in the sublumbar area indicating pneumomediastinum. *F,* Bilateral atelectasis due to pneumothorax. The lung edges are clearly seen and there is an absence of bronchovascular markings at the periphery of the thorax.

(Illustration continued on opposite page.)

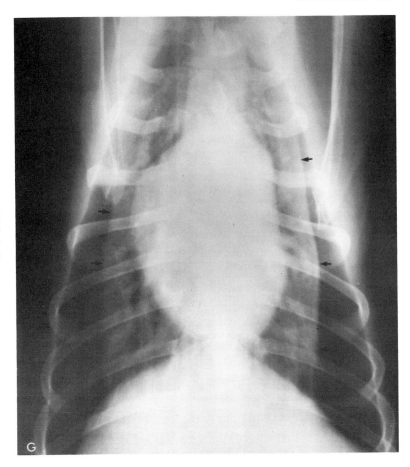

FIGURE 3–22 *Continued.* G. On the ventrodorsal view skin folds (arrows) may simulate lung edges leading to a false diagnosis of pneumothorax. They can usually be traced beyond the confines of the thorax.

(c) Air may pass through the aortic hiatus and be seen in the retroperitoneal space under the lumbar vertebrae. The kidneys may be outlined. (Fig. 3–23).

MEDIASTINAL MASSES.   Masses within the mediastinum may be diffuse or discrete. Diffuse masses cause a widening of the mediastinal shadow, and an accurate assessment of the underlying pathologic changes is usually difficult. Pleural fluid may cause widening of the mediastinum.

Small discrete masses are usually visualized only in the ventral pericardial area or in the dorsocaudal mediastinum behind the heart. Masses in the cranial mediastinum cause an increase in density of the mediastinum and may produce a positive silhouette sign with the heart. If ventrally located, they displace the trachea dorsally. Dorsal mediastinal masses displace the trachea ventrally. Masses in the hilar area cause an increased density at the tracheal bifurcation and may displace the primary bronchi. Masses in the caudal mediastinum produce well-defined densities superimposed on the caudal lung lobes.

Conditions that may produce masses in the cranial mediastinum include mediastinitis, abscess formation, neoplasia, enlarged thymus, lymphadenopathy, esophageal abnormalities, and anomalies of the great vessels. Mediastinal lymphoma is common in cats and is frequently accompanied by pleural effusion.

Perihilar masses in the middle mediastinum may be due to lymphadenopathy, neoplasia such as heart base tumors, esophageal masses, enlarged pulmonary arteries or veins, or enlarged left or right atria.

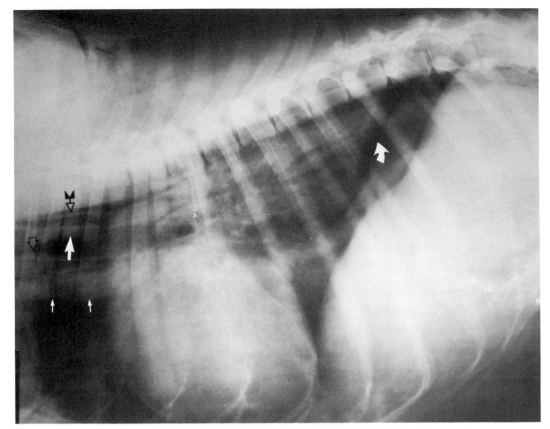

FIGURE 3–23. Pneumomediastinum. Air in the mediastinum acts as a contrast agent outlining structures within the mediastinum. On this radiograph, the left subclavian artery (large white arrow), the brachiocephalic trunk (open arrow), and the cranial vena cava (small white arrows) are all well outlined in the cranial mediastinum. The esophagus (winged arrow) partly overlies the left subclavian artery. There is some degree of pneumothorax as evidenced by the separation of the lung edge (curved arrow) from the diaphragm shadow. The descending aorta is more clearly seen in the caudal thorax partly owing to the pneumothorax and partly to the pneumomediastinum. An interlobar fissure can be seen through the caudal cardiac shadow. Subcutaneous emphysema is seen along the back. The aorta is outlined behind the diaphragm by air in the retroperitoneal space. Air in the mediastinum may track cranially into the neck and subcutaneous tissues or caudally into the retroperitoneal space through the aortic hiatus. (See also Fig. 3–16C)

Caudal mediastinal masses may be due to esophageal lesions, such as foreign bodies, *Spirocerca lupi* infestation, megaesophagus, gastroesophageal intussusception, neoplasms, granulomas, or abscess formation. Masses in the caudal mediastinum may be difficult to distinguish from intrapulmonary masses.

Fluid within the thorax may mask mediastinal lesions particularly in the cranial mediastinum. A standing lateral film using a horizontal beam is occasionally helpful. In the standing position fluid moves into the ventral thorax, allowing visualization of mediastinal lesions. Contrast studies, such as barium studies of the esophagus, angiography, and pleurography, are also used. (Fig. 3–24).

MEDIASTINAL DISPLACEMENT (SHIFT). Displacement of the mediastinum is usually indicative of an abnormality in one or other of the pleural cavities. It may be due to collapse or removal of a lung or lung lobe, pneumothorax, diaphragmatic hernia, or adhesions. The heart displaces with the mediastinum.

Text continued on page 213

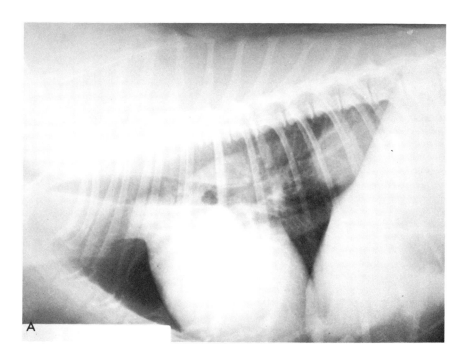

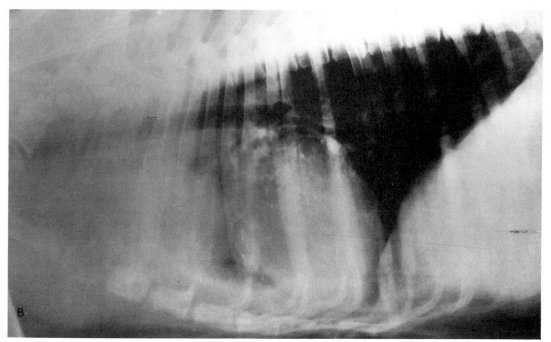

FIGURE 3–24. Intrathoracic masses. A specific diagnosis of the cause of a solitary mass lesion in the thorax is usually not possible on plain radiographs. *A.* A 12 year old dog, of mixed breed, had been coughing for a month. A circumscribed density is seen in the caudal thorax. The left caudal lung lobe, containing the mass, was removed surgically. An impression smear revealed inflammatory cells but no bacteria. In *B,* a large mass in the cranial mediastinum obscures the cranial lung lobes in the lateral view. There is lysis of a rib and part of the sternum.

(Illustration continued on following page.)

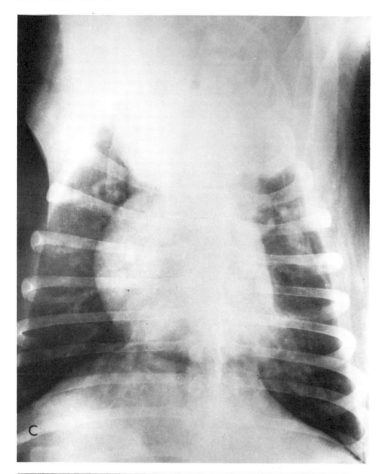

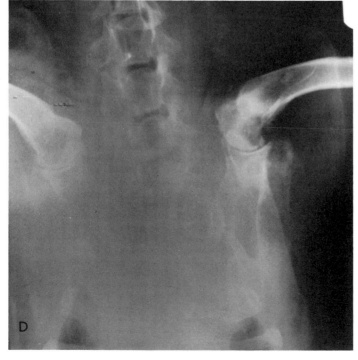

FIGURE 3–24 *Continued.* *C, D.* The dorsoventral view shows a widened cranial mediastinum. *D.* The left scapula and left and right humeri are involved in the destructive process. This was a fibrosarcoma.

(*Illustration continued on opposite page.*)

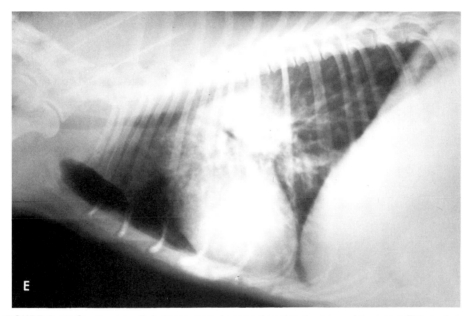

FIGURE 3–24 *Continued.   E.* A dense mass is seen dorsal to the base of the heart. This is due to enlargement of lymph nodes. The terminal trachea is narrowed and depressed. (Left atrial enlargement elevates the trachea. Enlarged lymph nodes above and caudal to the trachea depress it.) The cranial mediastinum is widened owing to lymphadenopathy, which narrows the trachea by extrinsic pressure. This was a mycotic lymphadenitis in a one and one-half year old dog of mixed breed.

(Illustration continued on following page.)

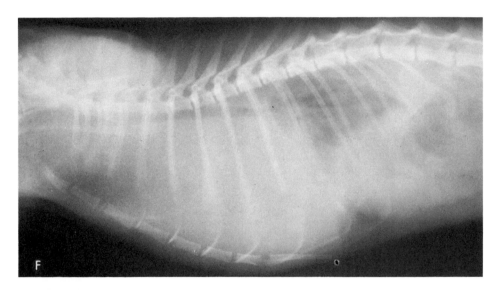

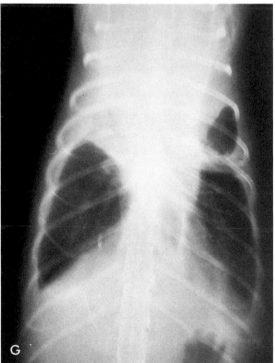

FIGURE 3-24 *Continued.* *F, G.* A nine month old female Siamese cat had a history of "breathing hard." The lateral radiograph shows a fluid density within the thorax obscuring the cardiac shadow. The trachea is elevated. The ventrodorsal view, made after paracentesis, shows widening of the cranial mediastinum suggestive of a mediastinal mass. The visible lung fields are small and fluid is apparent in the fissure in the left cranial lung lobe. At autopsy the diagnosis was thymic lymphosarcoma.

THE CARDIOVASCULAR SYSTEM

ANATOMY

THE HEART.   The normal heart is cone shaped. It lies obliquely in the thorax with its base, or hilus, facing dorsocranially and its apex ventrocaudally. A transversely curved, longitudinal, obliquely placed septum divides the heart into cranioventral and caudoventral parts. The cranioventral part is customarily referred to as the right heart and the caudodorsal part as the left heart.

The right heart is composed of the right atrium and the right ventricle. The atrium has, in addition to its main chamber, a blind pouch that projects cranioventrally, called the auricle. The cranial and caudal venae cavae and the coronary sinus open into the atrium. The azygos vein usually empties into the cranial vena cava but may empty directly into the right atrium. The right atrium drains into the right ventricle through the atrioventricular opening. Backflow of blood is prevented by the right atrioventricular, or tricuspid, valve. The right ventricle, having received blood from the atrium, pumps it into the pulmonary circulation through the pulmonary artery trunk. The part of the ventricle that leads into the pulmonary artery trunk is called the conus arteriosus. The pulmonary artery valve prevents regurgitation of blood from the pulmonary artery into the right ventricle.

The left heart is composed of the left atrium and the left ventricle. The left atrium forms the dorsocaudal part of the base of the heart. It also has a blind pouch, or auricle, in addition to the main chamber. The left atrium receives blood from the pulmonary veins, three veins from the left lung and two or three veins from the right lung. The pulmonary artery trunk separates the left and right auricles. The interatrial septum separates the left and right atria.

The left atrium empties into the left ventricle. Regurgitation of blood from the ventricle into the atrium is prevented by the atrioventricular, or mitral, valve. The ventricle pumps blood to most parts of the body through the aorta. Regurgitation of blood from the aorta into the ventricle is prevented by the aortic valve. The left ventricle is cone shaped and its apex forms the apex of the heart. The wall of the left ventricle is several times the thickness of the right ventricular wall. The interventricular septum separates the left and right ventricles.

THE PULMONARY ARTERIES.   The pulmonary artery trunk arises at the conus arteriosus of the right ventricle. After a short course to the left of the midline it divides into right and left pulmonary arteries. The right pulmonary artery travels obliquely across the base of the heart to reach the right side of the thorax. Its first branch supplies the cranial lobe of the right lung. Just distal to the first branch it divides into several branches that supply the cranial (apical), middle (cardiac), caudal (diaphragmatic), and accessory (intermediate, or azygous) lung lobes. The left pulmonary artery divides into two branches, the smaller of which supplies the cranial part (apical) of the cranial lung lobe and the larger branch divides to supply the caudal part of the cranial lung lobe (cardiac) and the caudal (diaphragmatic) lobe. The pulmonary veins from each lung lobe empty separately into the left atrium, though variations in this arrangement are common. (See Fig. 3–8).

THE AORTA.   The aorta leaves the left ventricle near its center. The initial part lies within the pericardium and is called the ascending aorta. It then makes a U-turn dorsocaudally and to the left. This part is called the aortic arch. The remainder of the aorta, from the arch to its terminal branches, is called the descending aorta. The thoracic aorta is that portion of the aorta that lies within the thorax, while the abdominal aorta is the part that lies within the abdomen. The aortic valve lies at the origin of the aorta. The aortic sinus, or bulb of the aorta (Sinus of Valsalva), is a dilatation of the aorta at its origin, from which the coronary arteries arise. The aorta gives off two large branches in the cranial mediastinum, the brachiocephalic trunk and the left subclavian artery.

THE PERICARDIUM.   The pericardium is a strong fibroserous sac that surrounds the heart. In young animals it is in contact with the thymus gland cranially. It contains a small amount of fluid. The pericardium blends with the adventitia of the great vessels leaving and entering the heart. It is not seen on normal radiographs unless there is pericardial fat.

RADIOGRAPHY

Routine lateral and dorsoventral (or ventrodorsal) views of the thorax give much information about the status of the heart and great vessels. The dorsoventral view is preferred to the ventrodorsal, as there may be some distortion of the cardiac outline when the animal is radiographed in dorsal recumbency. The vertebrae should be just visible through the cardiac shadow.

More detailed studies of the heart and great vessels require the use of angiocardiography. Contrast medium is introduced into the heart, either directly or indirectly, and rapid serial radiographs are made to demonstrate its passage through the heart, vessels, and lungs. Suitable contrast agents include Hypaque 50% and Hypaque 75% (Winthrop Laboratories); Renovist 69% (Squibb), Renografin 76% (Squibb); Conray and Angioconray (Mallinckrodt).

Selective angiocardiography means the introduction of contrast medium through a catheter, the tip of which is placed in a preselected position either within a chamber of the heart or in a blood vessel. Fluoroscopy is desirable to facilitate placement of the catheter and to determine its exact location before an injection is made. Catheters with side holes are preferred to those with end openings only, as the latter tend to recoil when the injection is made. The contrast medium must be injected rapidly as a bolus, otherwise it will be rapidly diluted by the circulating blood and the structures under examination will be poorly outlined. The reader is referred to standard works on radiographic technique for details of the procedure.

A catheter may be introduced into the right atrium, right ventricle, and pulmonary artery trunk through a jugular or cephalic vein. The left atrium, left ventricle, and aorta can be entered through a carotid artery or a femoral artery. It is usually more satisfactory to expose a vessel surgically before introducing a catheter. Percutaneous introduction is not always easy and it makes accurate positioning of the canula carrying the catheter more difficult.

Nonselective angiography is done by rapidly injecting contrast medium into a jugular vein and making serial radiographs following the injection. The injection should be made through a wide bore needle (14 gauge or 50 mm) so that a good bolus of contrast medium can be injected in a short space of time. The amount of the contrast medium to be injected is from 0.5 ml to 1 ml per pound body weight. Some reflux into the caudal vena cava is common with this method. The larger doses are used with the less concentrated agents. (See these Chapter 3 References: Ticer, Ettinger and Suter, Morgan et al.).

Nonselective studies using relatively modest equipment can produce valuable information. A single film made a few seconds following injection of contrast material into the jugular vein can give a good picture of the status of the pulmonary artery tree. A simple hand-operated cassette changer can be made to produce four or five radiographs at the rate of about one per second. Even with sophisticated equipment, a rate of two films per second is rarely exceeded.

Direct needle puncture of the left ventricle through the thoracic wall can be used for selective study of the left ventricle and aorta. Its use should be reserved for cases that cannot be studied by more acceptable methods. It may result in cardiac tamponade or improper injection of contrast material into the heart muscle or pericardium. Pneumothorax, ventricular fibrillation, or damage to the coronary artery are also hazards of the technique.

NORMAL APPEARANCE

In the lateral view, the cardiac outline varies considerably in the different breeds or types of dogs. Dogs with a deep thorax, such as the greyhound or the Irish setter, show a more upright cardiac silhouette than dogs with a barrel-shaped thorax, such as the beagle. With a barrel-shaped thorax the heart is wider and more of it lies in contact with the sternum. The heart of the cat is relatively smaller than that of the dog and is more obliquely placed in the craniocaudal plane. Young dogs have relatively larger cardiac outlines than older dogs. A young dog's heart tends to be round in outline.

The cranial, or right, heart border forms a gentle curve that lies about the level of the third intercostal space. Dorsally, the curve is formed by the right atrial border, while the middle and ventral portions are formed by the right auricle and right ventricle. Occasionally, the aortic arch or rarely the pulmonary artery trunk may form the cranial cardiac border dorsally. The cranial vena cava forms a small depression where it joins the right atrium. This is called the cranial cardiac waist.

The caudal, or left, heart border is not as curved as the right. It lies at about the seventh or eighth rib. It is formed by the left atrium caudodorsally and the left ventricle at its middle and ventral thirds. A small depression is present where the atrium meets the ventricle. This is called the caudal cardiac waist and is at the level of the atrioventricular groove. The dorsal edge of the caudal vena cava lies at about the level of the caudal cardiac waist. The distance between the diaphragm and the caudal cardiac border varies with inspiration and expiration and with the conformation of the animal. At expiration the diaphragmatic shadow may overlie the caudal cardiac border.

The ventral border of the heart lies along the sternum and is composed of parts of the right and left ventricular walls. The apex is formed by the left ventricle. The dorsal border of the heart, or base, is not clearly defined. It is formed by the right and left atria and the pulmonary arteries and veins. In the lateral view the apicobasilar length of the heart is about two-thirds the length of a line drawn from the cardiac apex through the tracheal bifurcation to the lower border of the thoracic vertebrae. The width of the heart is approximately from 2.5 intercostal spaces in dogs with a narrow thorax to 3.5 spaces in dogs with a wide thorax.

In the dorsoventral view the cranial, or right, heart border is rounded, while the left heart border is only gently curved or almost straight. The long axis of the heart is directed toward the left side. The base lies over the midline, while the apex is to the left of the midline. On the dorsoventral view there is marked foreshortening of the cardiac shadow in animals with an upright heart. The cardiac outline extends from the third to the eighth rib. In this view there is considerable superimposition of thoracic structures. The trachea, esophagus, and great vessels overlie the cardiac shadow. The heart is centrally placed with approximately equal amounts of the lung fields visible on either side of the thorax.

The right cardiac border is composed of the walls of the right atrium and ventricle. The left border is formed by the pulmonary artery trunk as far as the fourth intercostal space, approximately, and by the left ventricular wall caudally. The left atrium is centrally placed in this view and does not form part of the normal cardiac outline.

The cranial border is made up of the aortic arch, the right auricle, the cranial vena cava, the pulmonary artery trunk, the brachiocephalic trunk, and the left subclavian artery. These structures are superimposed on one another in a complex fashion and some cannot be individually distinguished. The aortic arch overlies the right auricle. The cranial vena cava forms the right edge of the cranial mediastinal shadow. The left subclavian artery forms the left border of the cranial mediastinal shadow. The aorta arches caudally running almost parallel to the vertebral column. The pulmonary artery trunk divides into right and left pulmonary arteries to the left of the midline. (Fig. 3–25).

ABNORMALITIES

CARDIAC ENLARGEMENT.   The radiologic diagnosis of cardiac enlargement is based on changes in cardiac size, shape, density, position, or the displacement of adjacent structures. Cardiac disease may also be manifested by changes in the pulmonary vasculature, pulmonary parenchymal changes, pleural effusion, pericardial effusion, hepatomegaly and ascites.

Minimal changes in cardiac outline are difficult to demonstrate or evaluate. The wide variation in normal heart shapes in different types of dogs complicates the problem. Mensuration methods to determine cardiac enlargement have not proved satisfactory in dogs. The variations in cardiac outline and the difficulties encountered in accurate positioning make results unreliable. Determination of cardiac enlargement, therefore, is usually based on experience in looking at thoracic radiographs and, if possible, a study of a series of radiographs of the same animal made over a period of time.

Generalized Cardiac Enlargement.   Generalized cardiac enlargement may be due to hypertrophy of the cardiac muscle or to dilatation. Hypertrophy and dilatation are indistinguishable on plain radiographs. Contrast studies enable one to evaluate the thickness of the ventricular walls.

The signs of cardiac enlargement comprise a rounding of the cardiac outline with loss of the cranial and caudal cardiac waists and an increase in size relative to the rest of the thorax. On the lateral view the right heart border becomes rounder and the left heart border becomes more upright. More of the heart is in contact with the sternum than is usual. The trachea and primary bronchi are elevated so that the angle formed between the trachea and the spine becomes more acute. In severe cases the trachea may run parallel to the spine. Apparent elevation of the trachea may result from improper positioning, that is, rotation of the animal. On the dorsoventral view the diameter of the heart is increased and less of the lung fields is seen than is usual. The cardiac edges approach the thoracic walls.

Generalized cardiac enlargement may be the result of a variety of conditions, including old valvular lesions, myocardial disease, chronic anemia, and infectious or metabolic diseases.

Left heart failure is usually characterized radiologically by pulmonary edema and left atrial and ventricular enlargement. Right heart failure is accompanied by

Text continued on page 223

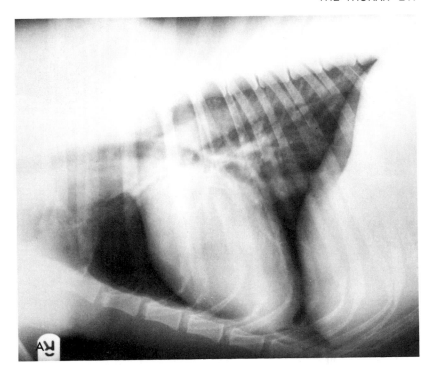

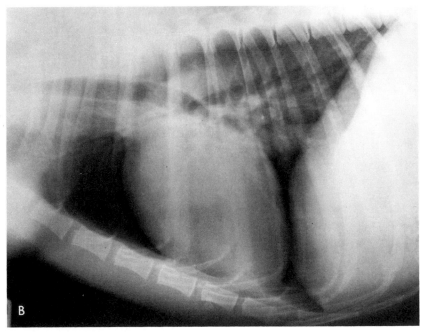

FIGURE 3–25. The Normal Heart. *A, B. A* was taken with the heart in systole and *B* with the heart in diastole. In systole the cardiac shadow appears smaller, the left heart border is straighter and the general outline is sharper. Unless fast exposure times are used (0.05 second or less) the heart usually appears in diastole as the largest shadow cast during the exposure determines the outline.

(Illustration continued on following page.)

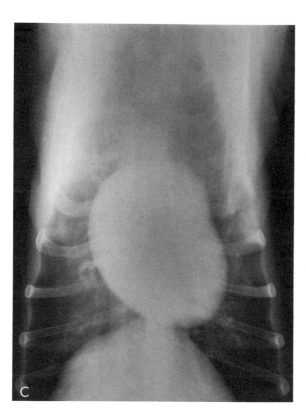
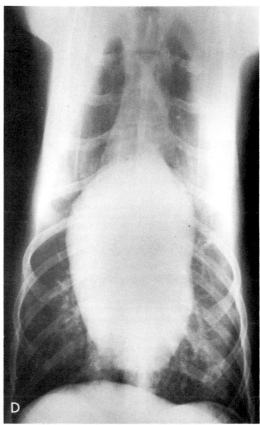

FIGURE 3–25 *Continued.* *C, D. C,* a dorsoventral, and *D,* a ventrodorsal view of the same heart. In the dorsoventral view the heart appears shorter. The dorsoventral view, while more difficult to position accurately, is preferred to the ventrodorsal. Displacement of the heart within the thorax in the ventrodorsal position makes it difficult to produce comparable repeat studies.

(Illustration continued on opposite page.)

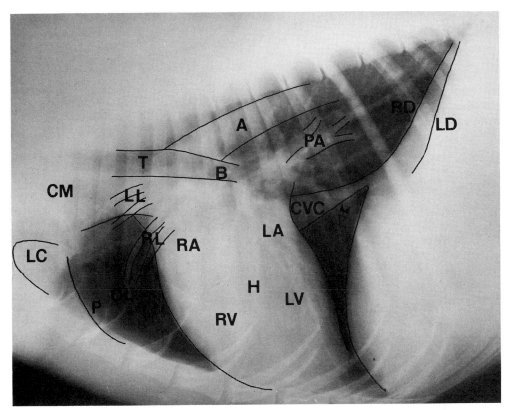

FIGURE 3–25 *Continued.* *E.* A: Thoracic aorta. T: Trachea. B: Origin of the left cranial lobe bronchus. PA: Branches of the pulmonary artery. RD: Right diaphragm crus. LD: Left diaphragm crus. CVC: Caudal vena cava. H: The heart. RL: Artery and vein for the right cranial lung lobe. LL: Artery and vein for the left cranial lung lobe. CM: Cranial mediastinum. PL: Fold of pleura marking the cranial limit of the right cranial lung lobe. Caudal to this fold the right and left cranial lung lobes are superimposed on one another. LC: Cranial portion of the left cranial lung lobe viewed end-on. CL: Right cranial lung lobe and part of the left cranial lung lobe superimposed. LA: Left atrium. LV: Left ventricle. RA: Right atrium. RV: Right ventricle. CVC: Caudal vena cava.

(Illustration continued on following page.)

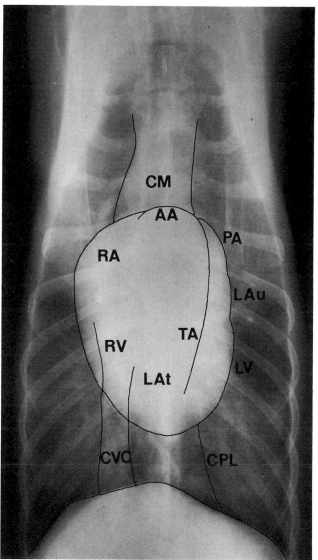

F

FIGURE 3–25 *Continued.* *F.* The dorsoventral
cardiac shadow.

CM: Cranial mediastinum. The right border is formed by the cranial vena cava and the
left by the left subclavian artery.

AA: Aortic arch.

PA: Pulmonary artery segment.

LAu: Left auricle.

LV: Left ventricle.

RA: Right atrium.

RV: Right ventricle.

LAt. Left Atrium. The left atrium is difficult
to demonstrate even on contrast studies as it
overlies the ventricles on this projection.

TA: Aortic trunk.

CVC: Caudal vena cava.

CPL: Cardiophrenic   ligament.   This
shadow represents the fold of pleura where
the accessory lobe contacts the left caudal
lobe.

(*Illustration continued on opposite page*)

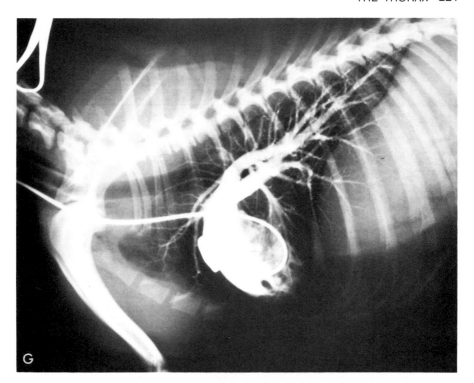

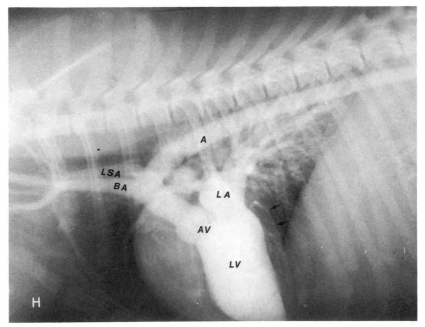

FIGURE 3–25 *Continued.* G. A selective angiocardiogram with the catheter placed in the right ventricle through a jugular vein. The right auricle, right ventricle, and pulmonary artery distribution are demonstrated. *H.* A nonselective angiocardiogram in which the contrast medium was given in a bolus through a jugular vein. The contrast medium outlines the left side of the heart. LA: Left atrium. LV: Left ventricle. AV: Aortic valve. The dilatation cranial to the valve is the aortic sinus (Sinus of Valsalva). BA: Brachiocephalic trunk. LSA: Left subclavian artery. A: Aorta. Arrows indicate the outer edge of the left ventricular wall and so the thickness of the wall can be evaluated. Pulmonary veins are seen entering the left atrium.

(*Illustration continued on following page*)

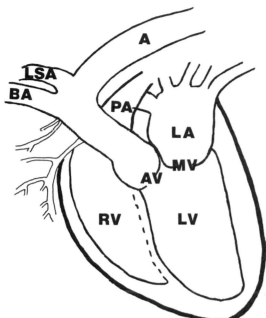

FIGURE 3-25 Continued. I. Diagrammatic representation of superimposition of the left and right angiocardiograms. The drawing was made from a contrast study.

LA: Left atrium. LV: Left ventricle. MV: Mitral valve. AV: Aortic valve. RV: Right ventricle. BA: Brachiocephalic trunk. LSA: Left subclavian artery. A: Aorta. PA: Pulmonary artery. J. Contrast medium may remain in the right auricle long after the right atrium and ventricle have cleared. (See also Fig. 3-8).

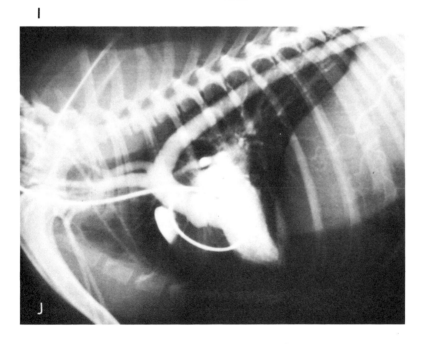

right atrial and ventricular enlargement, venous engorgement, ascites, and pleural and pericardial effusions. Right atrial enlargement is often difficult to evaluate. The term "cor pulmonale" is frequently used to describe changes occurring in the heart as a result of pulmonary disease, whether vascular or parenchymal. (Fig. 3–26).

Enlargement of Individual Chambers. Because of the interrelationship between the actions of the right and left sides of the heart, marked enlargement of an individual chamber is rare. If it does occur it will be short-lived, as compensatory mechanisms will produce enlargements elsewhere.

RIGHT-SIDE ENLARGEMENT

THE VENTRICLE. On the lateral view the cranial border of the heart becomes rounder in the area of the ventricle. This may cause the angle formed between the cardiac shadow and the mediastinum to become more acute; that is, the cranial cardiac waist becomes more prominent; later, it may be lost. More of the heart than normal is in contact with the sternum. The trachea is not elevated but the craniocaudal diameter of the heart is increased.

On the dorsoventral view, in the early stages of right ventricular enlargement, the pulmonary artery segment appears excessively prominent. The right heart border is rounded and comes closer to the right thoracic wall. The enlarged ventricle gives the right side of the heart the appearance of an inverted "D." The cardiac apex may be displaced to the left and the left ventricle may appear closer to the left thoracic wall, mimicking left ventricular enlargement. In fact, the left ventricle is displaced to the left by the enlarged right heart. A considerable degree of hypertrophy may be present with minimal changes in cardiac contour. (Fig. 3–27).

THE ATRIUM. Right-atrial enlargement is rarely encountered as a single entity. There is usually an associated right-ventricular enlargement. The trachea is elevated cranial to the carina and the right primary bronchus is elevated so that both primary bronchi can be seen end-on. The cranial cardiac waist becomes less prominent. Enlargement of the right auricle may cause disappearance or accentuation of the cranial cardiac waist, depending on its position.

On the dorsoventral view the enlarged atrium may cause a bulging of the cardiac silhouette craniolaterally (in the 9 to 11 o'clock position). The caudal vena cava is usually enlarged, as is the cranial mediastinum, owing to engorgement of the cranial vena cava.

LEFT-SIDE ENLARGEMENT

THE VENTRICLE. On the lateral view, in early cases, the caudal border of the heart loses its inward curve at the caudal cardiac waist. Later, the caudal border becomes more upright, that is, more perpendicular to the sternum. The elongation of the left ventricle causes a dorsal shift of the terminal trachea.

On the dorsoventral view, the left cardiac border and the apex become rounder. The left cardiac border approaches the left-chest wall.

THE ATRIUM. On the lateral view, the left atrial enlargement causes a dorsal shift of the terminal trachea. The left primary bronchus is elevated and separated from the tracheal shadow, which it normally overlies. Sometimes the left atrium can be visualized dorsally between the left and right caudal bronchi. It may appear as a density extending into the caudal lung fields. The caudal cardiac waist is lost. The pulmonary veins are prominent as they enter the left atrium.

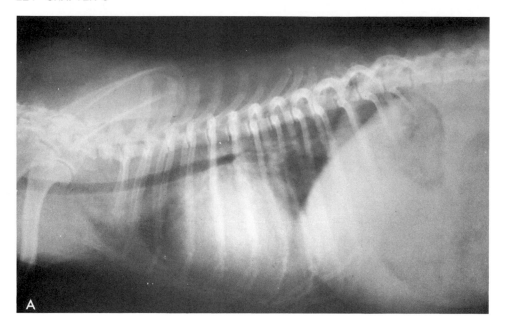

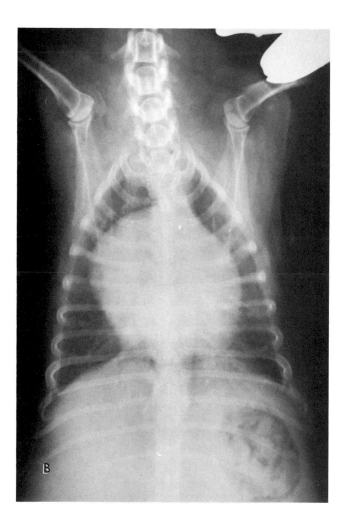

FIGURE 3–26. *A, B.* Generalized Cardiac Enlargement. Both sides of the heart are enlarged. The trachea is elevated. The right heart border is rounded and more of the heart than usual contacts the sternum. On the dorsoventral view both right and left cardiac borders approach the thoracic wall.

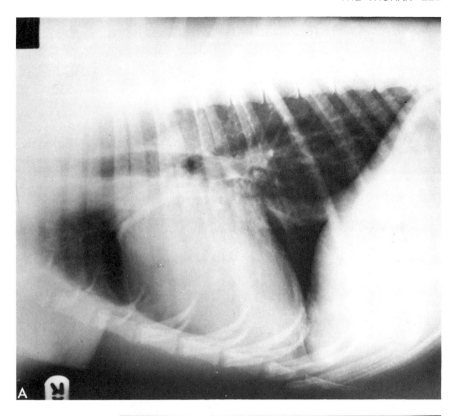

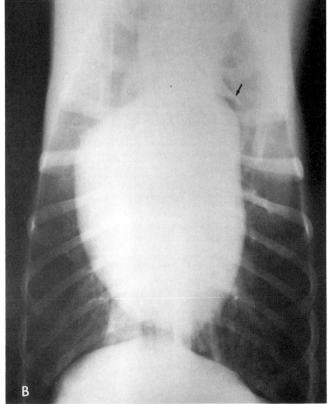

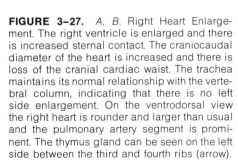

FIGURE 3-27. *A, B.* Right Heart Enlargement. The right ventricle is enlarged and there is increased sternal contact. The craniocaudal diameter of the heart is increased and there is loss of the cranial cardiac waist. The trachea maintains its normal relationship with the vertebral column, indicating that there is no left side enlargement. On the ventrodorsal view the right heart is rounder and larger than usual and the pulmonary artery segment is prominent. The thymus gland can be seen on the left side between the third and fourth ribs (arrow).

On the dorsoventral view the left auricle may extend beyond the left cardiac border in the central part of the cardiac oultine. The enlarged left atrium often causes a double shadow where it is superimposed on the right ventricle so that the edge of the atrium may be seen within the cardiac shadow as a line paralleling the border of the right ventricle. The enlarged atrium may be seen to separate and to spread the primary bronchi. (Fig. 3–28).

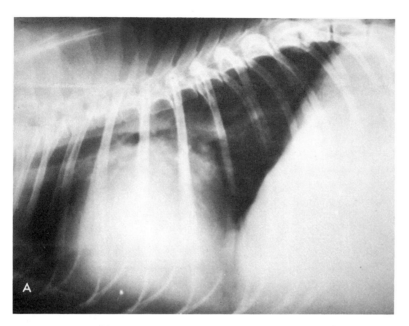

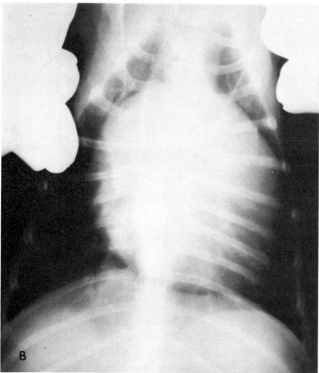

FIGURE 3–28. *A, B.* Left Ventricular Enlargement. On the lateral view the left heart is enlarged. The trachea is displaced dorsally. It is difficult to evaluate the right heart, as it has been displaced cranially by the enlarged left side. On the dorsoventral view there is obvious enlargement of the left ventricle, which approaches the left thoracic wall. (Gloved hands are seen on the dorsoventral view. Hands, even when gloved, should not be in the x-ray beam.)

(Illustration continued on opposite page.)

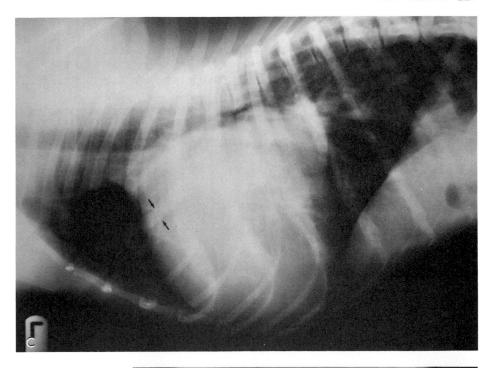

FIGURE 3-28 *Continued.* *C, D.* Left Atrial Enlargement. The trachea is elevated on the lateral view. The atrium is extending into the caudal lung fields which show early edematous changes. The atrium pushes up between the bronchi, supplying the caudal lung lobes. The right cranial lobar vein (arrows) is seen to be distended as it crosses the cardiac shadow. Distended pulmonary veins are seen in the caudal thorax. On the dorsoventral view the margin of the enlarged left atrium (arrows) can be seen within the cardiac shadow. There is marked prominence of left cardiac border in the area of the left auricle.

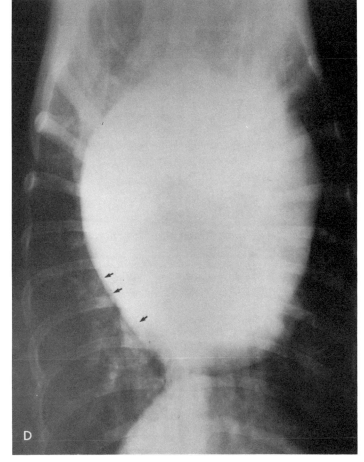

PULMONARY ARTERY ENLARGEMENT

An enlarged pulmonary artery trunk causes a bulging of the right cardiac border dorsally, on the lateral view. On the dorsoventral view, the pulmonary artery segment becomes more prominent.

AORTIC ENLARGEMENT

The aorta, when enlarged, may form part of the cranial cardiac border at the level of the auricle, in the lateral view. It extends into the cranial mediastinum. On the dorsoventral view, it causes an apparent increase in the length of the heart.

Pericardial Effusion.   Marked pericardial effusion causes the cardiac shadow to enlarge and become rounded in outline both on the lateral and the dorsoventral or ventrodorsal views. Individual prominences are lost and the cardiac outline may appear flattened where it contacts the thoracic wall. The trachea is elevated. (Fig. 3–29). Pneumopericardium may be the result of trauma or may follow pneumothorax or pneumomediastinum. A radiolucent zone is seen to surround the heart. A fluid level may be observed within the pericardial sac. The condition is rare.

SPECIFIC CONDITIONS

MITRAL INSUFFICIENCY.   This is the most common acquired cardiac abnormality in the dog. It results in regurgitation of blood from the ventricle into the atrium at systole. It is due to valvular fibrosis. It may also occur in the cat. Coughing is frequently noted and there may be varying degrees of respiratory distress. The course of the disease may be prolonged over several years.

RADIOLOGIC SIGNS

(a) The left ventricular border becomes more upright and the caudal cardiac waist is lost.

(b) Right ventricular enlargement is usually present and the heart size is increased in the craniocaudal diameter.

(c) The left atrium enlarges, causing the trachea to be elevated dorsally. The atrium may extend beyond the left ventricular border.

(d) The enlarged atrium extends upward between the left and right primary bronchi into the caudal lung fields.

(e) The pulmonary veins are engorged and prominent as they enter the left atrium.

(f) The vessels frequently have a hazy indistinct appearance due to pulmonary edema. If alveolar edema develops, fluffy infiltrates and air bronchograms are seen.

(g) On the dorsoventral view the left ventricle is enlarged and approaches the left thoracic wall.

(h) The enlarged left atrium is sometimes seen as a double shadow paralleling the outline of the right ventricular border.

(i) The enlarged atrium spreads the primary bronchi apart on the dorsoventral view.

(j) Advanced cases show alveolar edema, pleural effusion, hepatomegaly, and ascites. The left atrial wall may split, resulting in hemopericardium. This, when it occurs, gives the heart a globular appearance, as in hydropericardium. (Fig. 3–30).

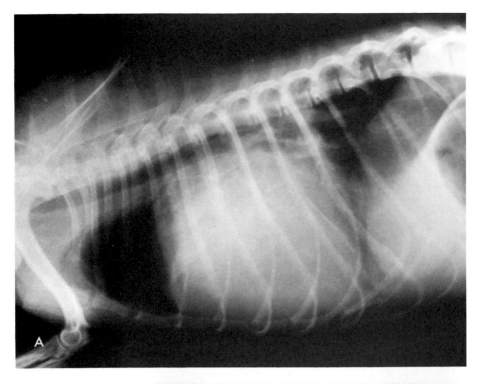

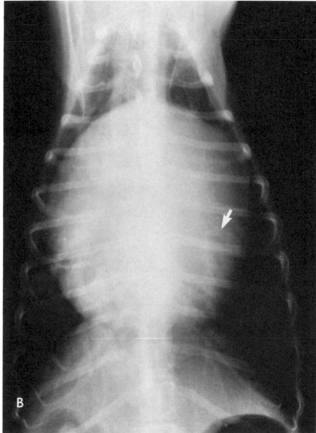

FIGURE 3–29. *A, B.* Hydropericardium. The heart is globular in outline and on the dorso-ventral view appears to fill almost the entire thorax. The trachea is elevated. An interlobar fissue is seen on the left side through the cardiac shadow (arrow).

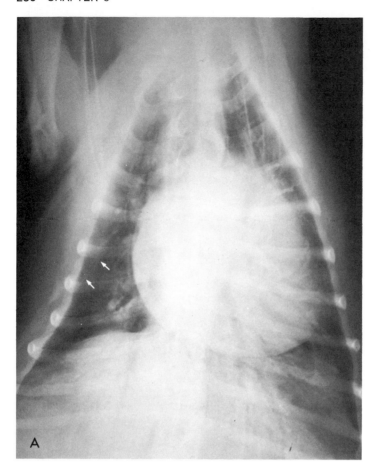

FIGURE 3-30. *A, B.* Mitral Insufficiency. On the lateral view the left atrium, left ventricle, and right ventricle are enlarged. The trachea is elevated. The dorsoventral view, though slightly rotated, shows marked left ventricular enlargement. Air bronchograms are seen. The caudal lung fields show edematous infiltration (alveolar pattern). Arrows indicate a visible interlobar fissure.

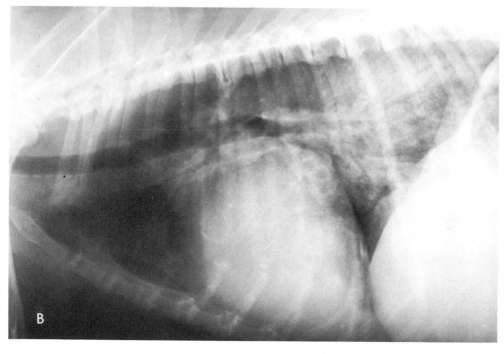

PULMONIC STENOSIS.   Pulmonic stenosis is a narrowing of the outflow tract from the right ventricle that interferes with the passage of blood from the right ventricle into the pulmonary artery. The stenosis may affect the infundibulum, the pulmonary artery valve, or the pulmonary artery distal to the valve. In dogs, the valve is most commonly affected. Valvular stenosis is rare in cats. Infundibular stenosis may develop secondarily to valvular stenosis due to hypertrophy of the ventricular muscle. Supravalvular stenosis is rare. Pulmonic stenosis usually causes no clinical signs. A poststenotic dilatation develops on the pulmonary artery.

RADIOLOGIC SIGNS

(a) Some degree of rounding of the right heart border is seen both on the lateral and dorsoventral views.

(b) On the lateral view the cranial cardiac waist is obliterated owing to protrusion of the poststenotic dilatation of the pulmonary artery, which forms part of the cranial cardiac border.

(c) The cardiac apex, on the lateral view, is displaced caudodorsally owing to the right ventricular hypertrophy.

(d) The dilated pulmonary artery may be seen in the cranial mediastinum overlying the tracheal shadow.

(e) The trachea is usually elevated over the right heart region but dips again ventrally at its extremity.

(f) On the dorsoventral view the right heart border approaches the right thoracic wall and the cardiac apex may be displaced toward the left side. The pulmonary artery segment is prominent.

(g) Selective angiocardiography through the right ventricle will outline the stenosis and the extent of the poststenotic dilatation. Nonselective angiocardiography through a jugular vein can also give useful information, though dye in the right atrium may obscure the area of the pulmonary valve. The poststenotic dilatation will, however, be well demonstrated.

(h) The pulmonary vasculature beyond the bifurcation of the pulmonary artery trunk is usually normal.

The pulmonary artery trunk may increase in diameter as a result of increased blood flow through it. Dilatation of the pulmonary artery, therefore, does not necessarily mean that there is a pulmonic stenosis. (Fig. 3–31).

AORTIC STENOSIS.   Aortic stenosis is a narrowing of the outflow tract from the left ventricle in the area of the aortic valve. It interferes with the passage of blood from the left ventricle to the aorta. It may affect the valve (valvular stenosis), the aorta (supravalvular stenosis), or the ventricular outlet (subaortic stenosis). Subaortic stenosis is the more common form of the condition in dogs, while supravalvular stenosis occurs congenitally in cats. Affected animals may show no clinical signs of disease, though syncope, coughing, pulmonary edema, and sudden death have been described. Congenital aortic stenosis has been described in the Boxer and the German Shepherd.

RADIOLOGIC SIGNS

Radiologic signs are frequently absent. When present they include the following:

(a) Absence of the cranial cardiac waist due to protrusion of the poststenotic dilatation beyond the cardiac border.

(b) The caudal left heart border is straighter than usual on the lateral view owing to ventricular hypertrophy.

(c) Mitral insufficiency may develop secondarily to the stenosis and the ven-

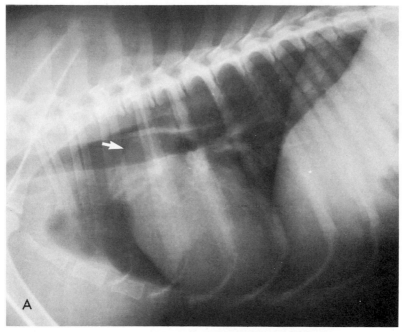

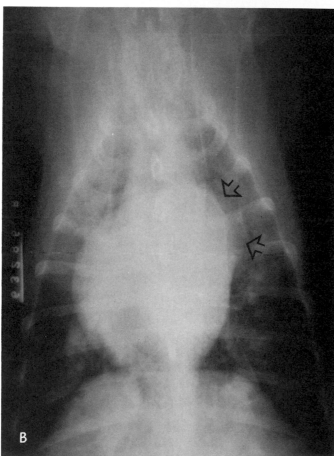

FIGURE 3–31. *A–C.* Pulmonic Stenosis. This laboratory dog, of unknown age, showed no clinical signs of disease. A murmur was detected over the pulmonic valve area during a routine examination. On the plain lateral radiograph an unusual shadow, the pulmonary artery (arrow), crosses the trachea. The dorsoventral view shows an enlarged pulmonary artery segment (arrows). There is some right ventricular enlargement. Selective catheterization of the right ventricle and angiocardiography demonstrate a narrowed valvular outlet from the right ventricle and a large post-stenotic dilatation of the pulmonary artery. The catheter partly overlies the pulmonic valve area.
(Illustration continued on opposite page.)

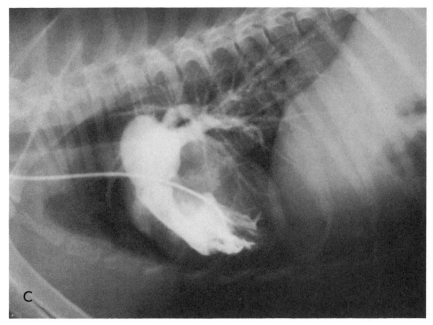

FIGURE 3–31 *Continued. (See legend on opposite page.)*

tricular hypertrophy. This will result in enlargement of the left atrium with elevation of the trachea and prominence of the pulmonary veins entering the left atrium.

(d) On the dorsoventral view the aortic arch is prominent and the cardiac silhouette is increased in length.

(e) Selective angiocardiography through the left ventricle outlines the area of stenosis and the poststenotic dilatation. Nonselective studies are less satisfactory, as residual contrast medium in the right cardiac chambers and pulmonary artery may, at least partially, mask the lesion. The poststenotic dilatation is, however, usually visible. (Fig. 3–32).

PATENT DUCTUS ARTERIOSUS. In the fetus the ductus arteriosus carries blood from the pulmonary artery to the aorta. It normally closes during the first few weeks after birth as the pulmonary circulation becomes functional. If it fails to close, an arteriovenous fistula develops. Signs of cardiac failure may develop early in life or the animal may remain apparently normal for several years. When clinical signs develop they often include inability to exercise, hindlimb weakness, and dyspnea. Cyanosis is not usual, though it may develop if there is reverse shunting of blood due to pulmonary hypertension.

RADIOLOGIC SIGNS

(a) On the lateral view the heart is enlarged, the right ventricle being most obviously affected. The trachea is elevated.

(b) The aorta is dilated and bulges cranially, eliminating the cranial cardiac waist.

(c) There is a generalized increase in density of the lungs due to the left to right shunting of blood from the aorta to the pulmonary artery.

(d) The increased pulmonary circulation is reflected in the size of the cranial lobar arteries and veins. Their diameters may exceed the smallest diameter of the dorsal third of the fourth rib.

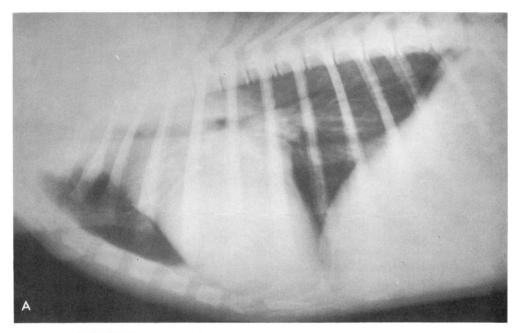

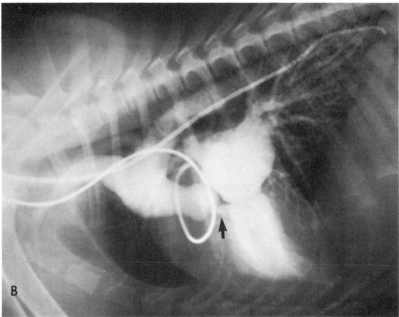

FIGURE 3–32. *A, B.* Subaortic Stenosis. On routine physical examination of a four month old German Shepherd dog, a continuous, systolic, grade 4 murmur was detected. It was of greatest intensity on the right side at the costochondral junction at the third intercostal space. On the left side it was strongest at the fourth intercostal space at the level of the costochondral junction. There was no cyanosis.

On the plain lateral view the right heart border bulges cranially at its dorsal third. The trachea is elevated, the left atrium is prominent, and there is some left ventricular enlargement, though the caudal cardiac waist is preserved. Attempts to pass a catheter into the left ventricle through a carotid artery were not successful. The catheter persistently entered the aorta, where it can be seen. A right side injection was then made. This eventually outlined the left side of the heart and the aorta. A narrowed ventricular outflow tract (arrow), just caudal to the aortic valve, and a large poststenotic dilatation are demonstrated. The left atrium is enlarged. More pulmonary veins than usual are seen, possibly indicating early left heart failure. There is left ventricular hypertrophy as evidenced by the thickness of the left ventricular wall.

(e) On the dorsoventral view the bulge of the aortic arch causes the cardiac shadow to appear elongated.

(f) On the left cardiac border, in the dorsoventral view, three prominences can be detected: the widened descending aorta, the enlarged pulmonary artery segment, and a protrusion of the left auricle beyond the left cardiac border. The left ventricular border is somewhat rounded.

(g) Secondary mitral insufficiency may cause enlargement of the left atrium, elevation of the trachea, and increased prominence of the pulmonary veins entering the left atrium.

(h) Gross enlargement of the cardiac outline is seen in cases of cardiac failure.

(i) Selective angiocardiography, making the injection at the root of the aorta, will demonstrate simultaneous filling of the aorta and the pulmonary artery trunk. The contrast medium should preferably not be injected into the left ventricle, since simultaneous filling of the aorta and the pulmonary artery trunk may also occur in the presence of a ventricular septal defect. In such a case, however, it is probable that some contrast medium would also be seen in the right ventricle. (Fig. 3–33).

TRICUSPID INSUFFICIENCY. Tricuspid insufficiency is often associated with mitral insufficiency. The two conditions may be difficult to distinguish from one another radiologically.

RADIOLOGIC SIGNS

(a) There is right atrial enlargement with elevation of the trachea cranial to the carina.

(b) The caudal vena cava is denser than usual and may be seen within the cardiac shadow.

(c) The right ventricle is enlarged.

(d) Hepatomegaly, ascites, pleural effusion, and pericardial effusion may be seen in cases of right heart failure.

(e) The enlarged right atrium may displace the cranial vena cava to the right on the dorsoventral view.

VENTRICULAR SEPTAL DEFECT. Defects in the interventricular septum most commonly occur in the upper third of the septum. They are the most common congenital cardiac defects found in cats. Affected animals may show no signs. Congestive heart failure may develop. Ventricular septal defect may be associated with other cardiac anomalies. If the defect is severe and the transfer of blood from left to right side is considerable, pulmonary hypertension may develop.

RADIOLOGIC SIGNS

(a) There is some degree of right ventricular enlargement with an enlarged pulmonary artery segment.

(b) Left atrial enlargement is common.

(c) Selective angiocardiography, injecting the contrast material into the left ventricle, will outline the defect or show simultaneous filling of the aorta and pulmonary artery trunk. Usually, the right ventricle will also be visualized. (Fig. 3–34).

ATRIAL SEPTAL DEFECT. This defect, as a single entity, is not common but it may be encountered associated with other cardiac abnormalities.

RADIOLOGIC SIGNS

(a) There is right ventricular hypertrophy due to the increased amount of blood reaching the ventricle from the atrium.

(b) The right atrium enlarges as the blood reaches it from the left atrium.

Text continued on page 239

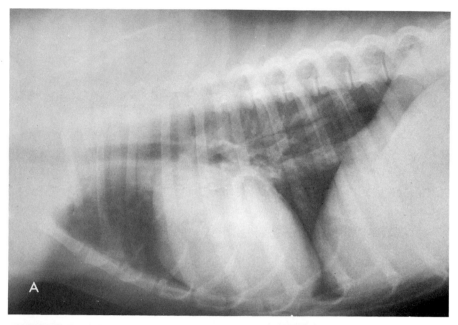

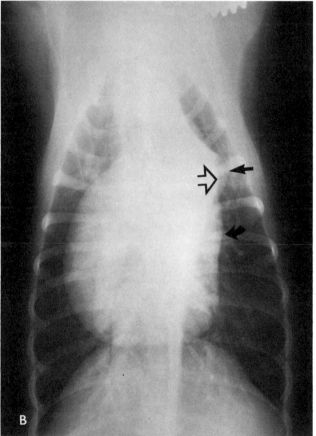

FIGURE 3–33. See legend on opposite page.

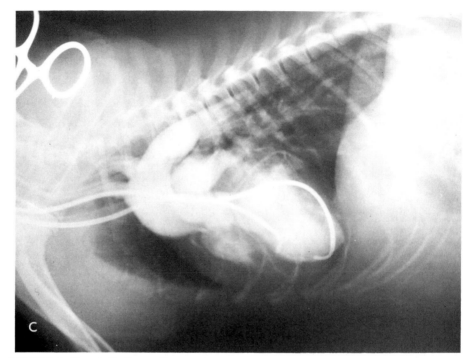

FIGURE 3–33. *A–C.* Patent Ductus Arteriosus. A seven month old Keeshond showed exhaustion after exercise. The condition had been present for several months. A systolic murmur was heard on auscultation, of greatest intensity over the third rib on the left side, near the sternum. The lateral radiograph is somewhat rotated but right ventricular enlargement can be observed. On the dorsoventral view right ventricular enlargement is evident. The pulmonary artery (black arrow) protrudes into the left hemithorax. The aorta (open arrow) is also prominent. A further prominence is present in the area of the left auricle (curved arrow). Selective catheterization of the left ventricle and angiocardiography result in simultaneous filling of the aorta and the pulmonary artery. The dilated aorta is prominent cranially and the enlarged pulmonary artery trunk is well seen. The enlarged pulmonary artery results from increased blood flow. Some contrast material has reached the right ventricle because of pulmonic valve insufficiency. Pulmonic valve insufficiency may be a sequel to pulmonary hypertension associated with patent ductus arteriosus.

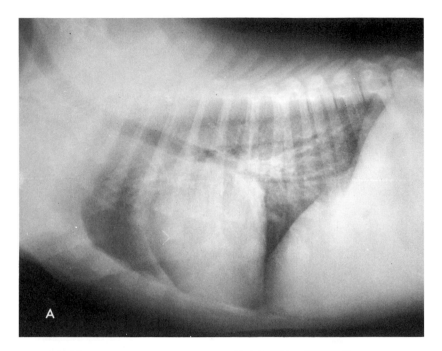

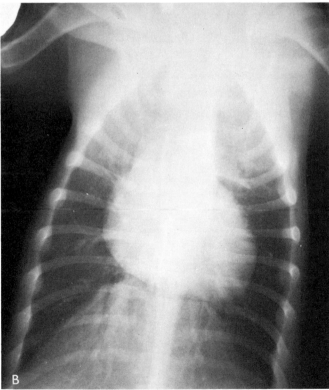

FIGURE 3–34. *A–C* Ventricular Septal Defect. A routine examination of a three month old Doberman revealed a grade 2 systolic murmur over the mitral and aortic valve areas. There was a weak pulse and a split R wave. The plain radiographs show fluid in an interlobar fissure and increased pulmonary vascular markings. The right heart cannot be evaluated on the lateral view because of the fluid. The lateral and dorsoventral views show left ventricular enlargement. Selective catheterization of the left ventricle and angiocardiography show simultaneous filling of the left and right ventricles. The aorta and the pulmonary arteries are also seen. The pulmonary artery appears normal.

(Illustration continued on opposite page.)

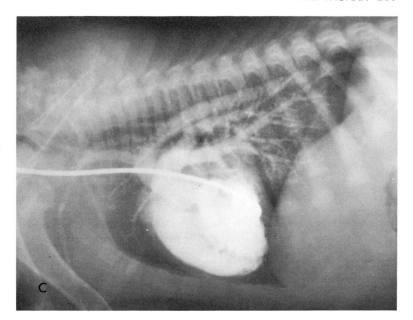

FIGURE 3-34. *C.* See legend on opposite page.

(c) The pulmonary artery trunk increases in size due to increased blood flow through it.

(d) The increased blood flow results in hypervascularization of the lungs.

Patent foramen ovale does not usually produce clinical signs, since shunting of blood, if it occurs at all, is minimal. (Fig. 3-35).

TETRALOGY OF FALLOT. The tetralogy of Fallot is a combination of cardio-vascular anomalies: pulmonic stenosis, right ventricular hypertrophy, ventricular septal defect, and dextroposition of the aorta. The aorta may receive blood both from the right and left ventricles. The radiologic signs are not characteristic. There is enlargement of the right ventricle and hypovascularization of the lungs due to the pulmonic stenosis. The displaced aorta may obliterate the cranial cardiac waist. The left ventricle is not enlarged. (Fig. 3-36).

CARDIOMYOPATHY. Myocardial disease usually manifests itself radiologic-ally as an increase in heart size, irrespective of the cause. There may be an associated hepatomegaly, splenomegaly, ascites, and pleural effusion. Affected animals lose weight rapidly and develop respiratory distress.

Idiopathic cardiomyopathy is occasionally seen in cats. It may develop at any age in the adult. Respiratory distress is a common presenting sign. Posterior paralysis due to thrombosis of the terminal branches of the aorta is not uncommon. Thromboemboli may also occur at other sites, particularly in the renal arteries.

RADIOLOGIC SIGNS

(a) There is marked enlargement of the left atrium. On the dorsoventral view the left atrium bulges on the left cardiac border, giving the heart a so-called "valentine" shape.

(b) The right ventricle is enlarged.

(c) The trachea is elevated.

(d) Pulmonary edema and pleural effusion occur if the heart is failing.

The radiologic signs vary with the stage and nature of the disease in individual cases. (Fig. 3-37).

Text continued on page 244

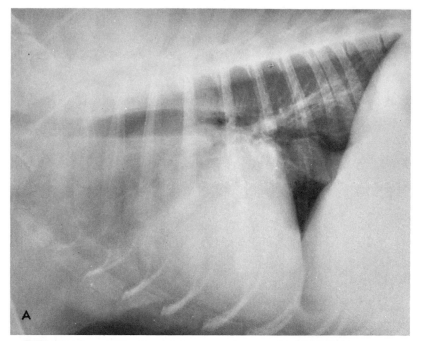

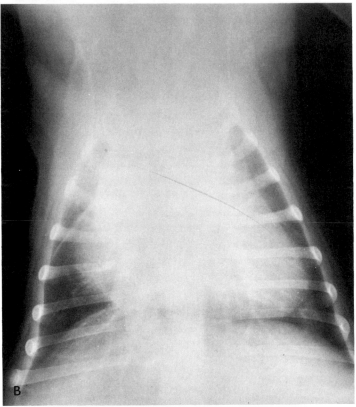

FIGURE 3-35. Atrial Septal Defect. A 10 month old Samoyed had ascites, labored breathing, and a reduced appetite for about one week. A loud systolic murmur was heard on the left side about the middle of the fourth intercostal space.

A, B. The plain radiographs show right heart enlargement. The caudal vena cava is dorsally directed. The left heart appears large on the dorsoventral view and it approaches the left thoracic wall. This is due to displacement by the enlarged right heart. An interlobar fissure is seen in the right lung.

(*Illustration continued on opposite page*)

FIGURE 3–35 *Continued.* *C.* Following injection of contrast medium into the right ventricle (RV), the ventricle was seen to be displaced caudally with an unopacified mass cranial to it. The pulmonary arteries opacified normally. As the contrast material reached the left atrium (LA) the mass cranial to the right ventricle opacified. This proved to be the right atrium (RA), which is grossly distended. *D.* A selective injection into the right atrium (RA) shows the full extent of the dilatation. A little contrast material has reached the right ventricle and there is reflux into the caudal and cranial venae cavae (CVC). At autopsy there was an atrial septal defect. Atrial septal defect as a single entity is rare. It is more usually associated with aortic or pulmonic stenosis.

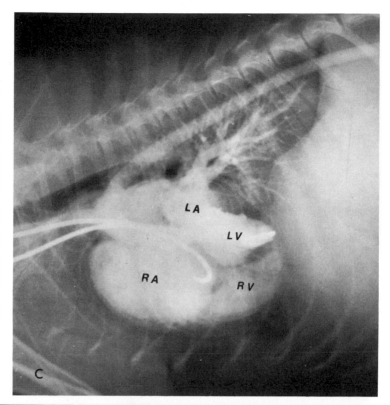

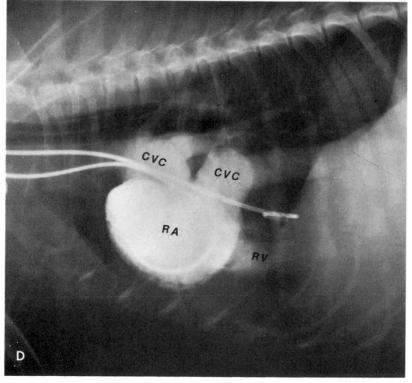

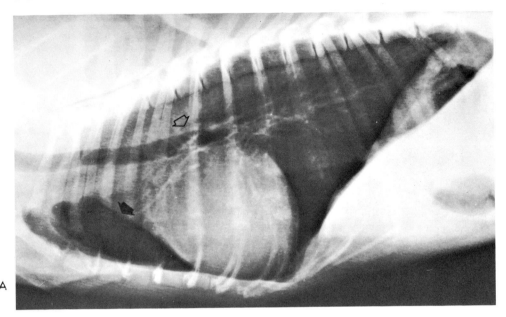

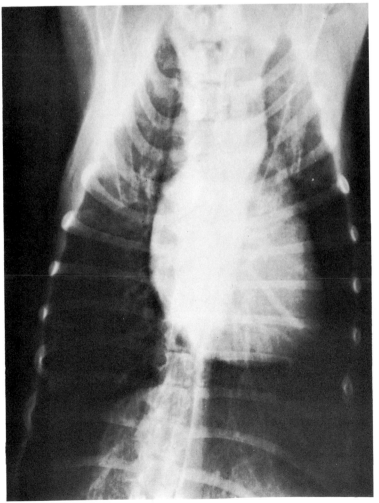

FIGURE 3–36. Tetralogy of Fallot. *A.* Lateral radiograph of an eight-month-old, male dog of mixed breed that had severe dyspnea. The mucous membranes were cyanotic even when the dog was at rest. A loud, pansystolic murmur was auscultated. Blood analysis revealed severe polycythemia (hematocrit, 80 per cent). In spite of treatment, the dog died within a few hours after the initial examination. The right heart is rounded, and the cranial waist has disappeared owing to protrusion of the aortic arch (black arrow). The craniocaudal diameter appears enlarged, but the apicobasilar distance is unaltered, as is further indicated by the normal angle of the trachea with the thoracic spine. The left heart is normal. The lung field is lucent, giving the impression of overinflation or alveolar emphysema. The intrapulmonary vasculature is barely visible. The left pulmonary artery (clear arrow) is smaller than normal. Notice the extreme flattening of the diaphragm caused by the maximal inspiratory effort. In a young dog, right ventricular enlargement, widening of the ascending aorta, undercirculation of the lungs, and cyanosis are characteristic for tetralogy of Fallot. In a ventricular septal defect complicated by pulmonic stenosis, the radiographic appearance may be similar to that seen with tetralogy of Fallot. *B,* Dorsoventral radiograph. (From Ettinger, S. J.: Textbook of Veterinary Medicine of the Dog and Cat. Vol. 2. W. B. Saunders Co. Philadelphia, 1975). The severe dyspnea made it difficult to obtain proper positioning; therefore, the sternum is not exactly superimposed on the thoracic spine. This results in displacement of the cardiac silhouette to the left side. However, the rounded, enlarged right ventricle can still be seen. The left cardiac border looks essentially normal. The lung field is extremely lucent, and the intrapulmonary vascular markings are barely outlined.

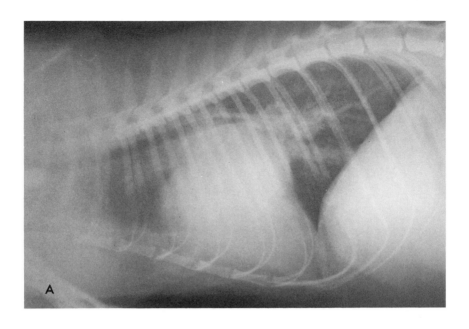

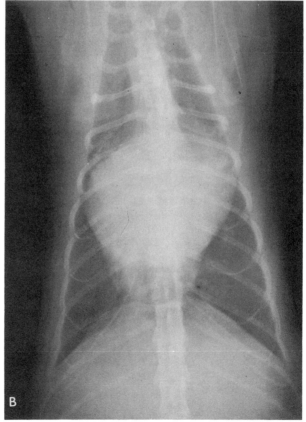

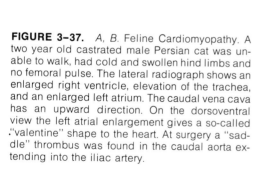

FIGURE 3–37. *A, B.* Feline Cardiomyopathy. A two year old castrated male Persian cat was unable to walk, had cold and swollen hind limbs and no femoral pulse. The lateral radiograph shows an enlarged right ventricle, elevation of the trachea, and an enlarged left atrium. The caudal vena cava has an upward direction. On the dorsoventral view the left atrial enlargement gives a so-called "valentine" shape to the heart. At surgery a "saddle" thrombus was found in the caudal aorta extending into the iliac artery.

HEART BASE TUMOR (CHEMODECTOMA).   Tumors that arise at the base of the heart affect chemoreceptor, thyroid, and parathyroid tissue. Other malignancies, such as lymphomas, may also occur in this area. The radiologic findings are not characteristic. Pericardial effusion is common. A mass may be evident at the base of the heart displacing the trachea or esophagus. The mass may simulate enlarged mediastinal lymph nodes. (Fig. 3–38).

DIROFILARIASIS.   The heart worm of the dog, *Dirofilaria immitis,* has a widespread distribution in North America. It may be encountered anywhere that mosquitoes are found. It is also present in Africa, Asia, and Southern Europe. Occasional cases occur in cats. The worms are found in the right ventricle, right atrium, pulmonary artery, and in the venae cavae. The worms cause obstruction of the pulmonary arteries either by mechanical blockage or by provoking thickening of the vascular intima. Increased pulmonary pressure results in right ventricular enlargement leading to right heart failure. The liver may be enlarged and congested.

Affected dogs may show no signs if the infestation is light. More severely affected dogs show a low exercise tolerance and poor condition. Radiography is useful in demonstrating the extent of damage to the vasculature and pulmonary parenchyma. It may also help in cases in which microfilariae cannot be demonstrated in the blood.

RADIOLOGIC SIGNS

(a) Enlargement of the pulmonary arteries, particularly in the hilar and middle areas of the lung fields.

(b) On the dorsoventral view the pulmonary artery segment of the left heart border is prominent.

(c) The pulmonary artery branches appear tortuous and engorged. They frequently appear to end suddenly — so-called "pruning" of the arteries. The pruning effect is due to occlusion of the arteries.

(d) Thromboembolism gives rise to patchy infiltrates within the lungs. These are circumscribed and irregular in outline. They may simulate neoplastic infiltrates. Areas of atelectasis may be found.

(e) The pulmonary vessels become less sharp in outline because parenchymal infiltration obscures their edges.

(f) Nonvascular linear markings and nodular densities indicate pulmonary fibrosis. Engorged vessels seen end-on should not be mistaken for nodular infiltrates.

(g) In more advanced cases right ventricular enlargement is evident both on lateral and dorsoventral views. The dilated pulmonary artery trunk obliterates the cranial cardiac waist.

(h) The trachea is frequently elevated above the right heart.

(i) Selective and nonselective angiocardiography are both useful in demonstrating abnormalities of the pulmonary vasculature. Heartworms can sometimes be seen as filling defects in the right ventricle and pulmonary arteries. (Fig. 3–39).

ANGIOSTRONGYLIASIS.   The heartworm *Angiostrongylus vasorum* lives in the right ventricle of dogs and foxes. The intermediate host is a mollusk. It is found in Europe, being particularly common in France. Several cases have been encountered in Ireland. The worm produces an anticoagulant substance; spontaneous hematoma formation, particularly on the limbs, is a common presenting sign. Systemic signs are rare, though affected greyhounds lose form. Larvae can be recovered from the feces of affected dogs some 40 days after the primary infestation.

Text continued on page 250

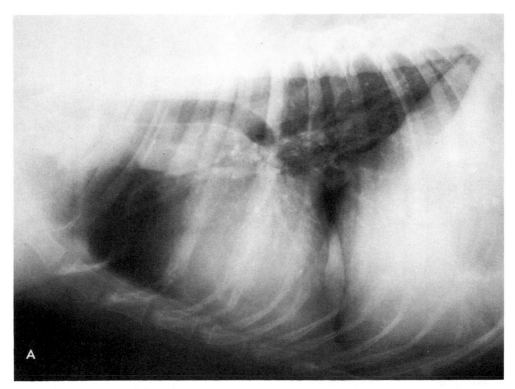

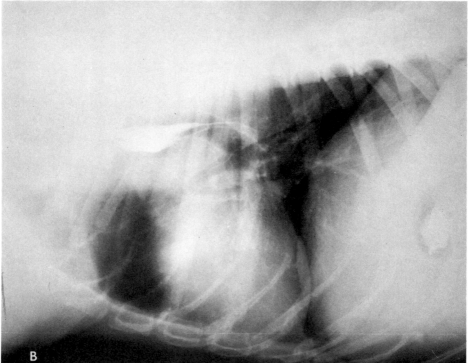

FIGURE 3–38. *A, B.* Heart Base Tumor. (Chemodectoma). A 10 year old male Boxer presented with respiratory distress. The plain radiograph shows dorsal displacement of the trachea over the right heart. The terminal downward bend in the trachea is preserved. The barium study shows extrinsic pressure on the esophagus in the area of the tracheal displacement. At autopsy there was a heart base tumor, an adenoma of thyroid origin.

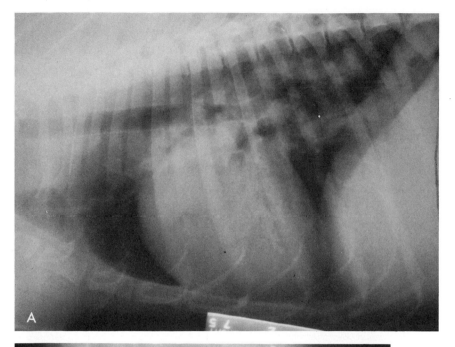

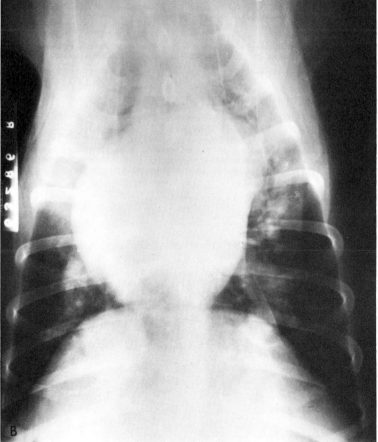

FIGURE 3-39. Dirofilaria immitis infestation. *A, B.* A 6 year old Afghan hound had a history of coughing. On the lateral view there is some enlargement of the right ventricle. The pulmonary vasculature is abnormal with distended and tortuous vessels. The vasculature is obscured in places. On the dorsoventral view the pulmonary artery segment is prominent and a large abnormal vessel is seen in the right caudal thorax. There is a superimposed interstitial pattern.
(Illustration continued on opposite page.)

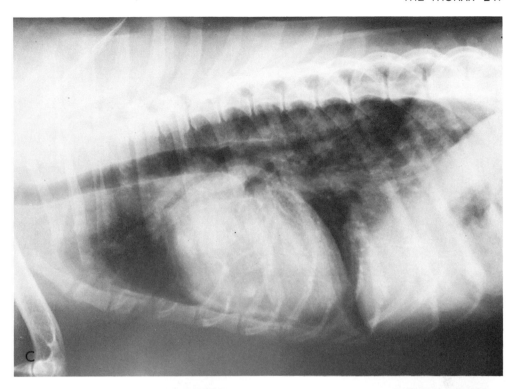

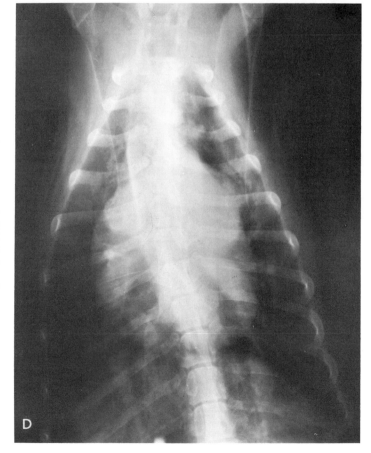

FIGURE 3-39 *Continued. C, D.* In this dog the right heart is enlarged and the pulmonary artery segment is prominent. Several abnormal vessels are seen in both lungs. An interlobar fissure is visible on the right side. Calcified bronchi, nonvascular linear marks and ill-defined irregular infiltrates can be seen on the lateral view. This is a mixed pattern indicating a pneumonia associated with the parasitic infestation. The dorsoventral view is rotated.

(*Illustration continued on following page.*)

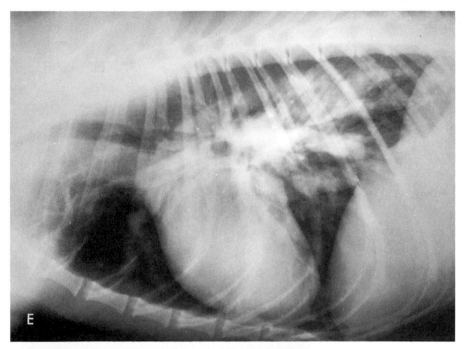

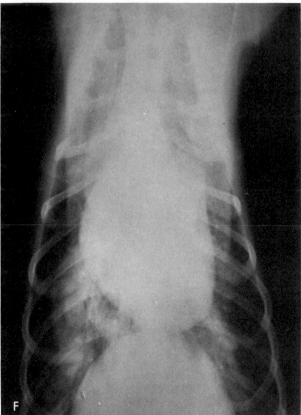

FIGURE 3–39 *Continued.* *E, F.* Another case in which both views show distended and tortuous pulmonary vessels. Some interstitial infiltration is present. The right ventricle is enlarged and the pulmonary artery segment is very prominent on the dorsoventral view.

(*Illustration continued on opposite page.*)

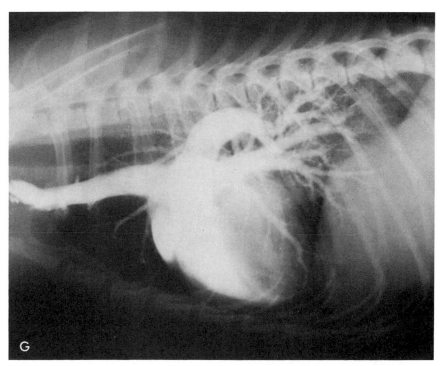

FIGURE 3–39 *Continued.*   G. A nonselective angiocardiogram through a jugular vein shows ballooning and distortion of the left pulmonary artery. Several large vessels are seen to be truncated (pruned) because of blockage by worms. Nonselective angiocardiography is very useful in the diagnosis of *Dirofilaria immitis* when the findings on plain radiographs are equivocal. (See Fig. 3–25 G).

The radiologic findings are very similar to those seen in *Dirofilariasis*. There is right ventricular enlargement, dilatation and pruning of the pulmonary arteries, and interstitial infiltration in the lungs. The changes seen are not as severe as those seen in *Dirofilariasis* and affect chiefly the branches of the pulmonary artery rather than the trunk. Nonselective angiocardiography is a simple method of demonstrating the vascular changes. (Fig. 3–40).

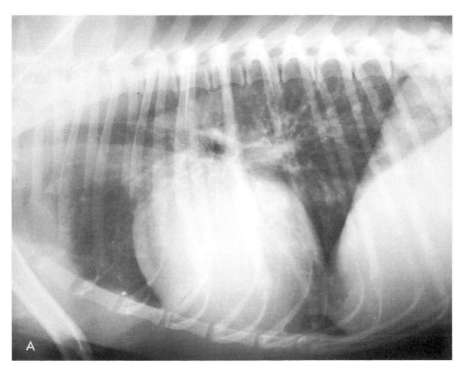

FIGURE 3–40. *A–C.* Angiostrongylus vasorum infestation. The right ventricle is enlarged on the lateral view. The pulmonary vasculature is abnormal. The larger vessels cannot be traced out to the periphery of the lung fields. In the ventrodorsal position the right ventricular enlargement is not so apparent, owing to the position of the heart. Interstitial changes are evident. A nonselective angiocardiogram via the jugular vein shows distortion of the pulmonary vessels with truncation of several large vessels. The changes seen are not as severe as those encountered with *Dirofilaria immitis.*

(*Illustration continued on opposite page.*)

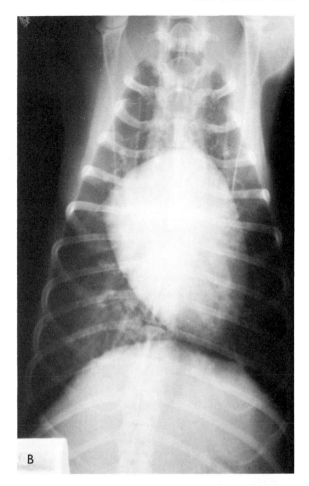

FIGURE 3–40. Continued.

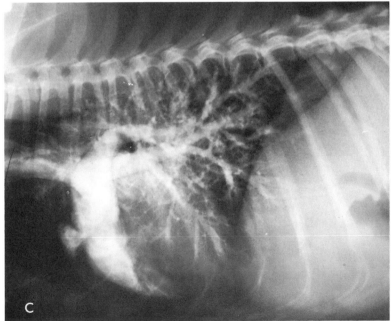

REFERENCES

Bhargava, A. K., Rudy, R. L., Diesem, C. D. (1969). Radiographic anatomy of the pleura in dogs as visualized by contrast pleurography. J.A.V.R.S. X. 61.

Bhargava, A. K., Burt, J. K., Rudy, R. L., Wilson, G. P. (1970). Diagnosis of mediastinal and heart base tumors in dogs using contrast pleurography. J.A.V.R.S. XI. 56.

Biery, D. N. (1974). Differentiation of lung diseases of inflammatory or neoplastic origin from lung disease in heart failure. Vet. Clinics of North America. (Nov., 1974). W. B. Saunders Co. Philadelphia.

Bohn, F. K., Rhodes, W. H. (1970). Angiograms and angiocardiograms in dogs and cats. Some unusual filling defects. J.A.V.R.S. XI. 21.

Brown, N. O., Zontine, W. J. (1976). Lung lobe torsion in a cat. J.A.V.R.S. XVII. 6. 219.

Buchanan, J. W. (1963). Persistent left cranial vena cava in dogs: angiocardiography, significance and coexisting anomalies. J.A.V.R.S. IV. 1.

Buchanan, J. W., Kelly, A. M. (1964). Endocardial splitting of the left atrium in the dog with hemorrhage and hemopericardium. J.A.V.R.S. V. 28.

Buchanan, J. W. (1965). Selective angiography and angiocardiography in dogs with acquired cardiovascular disease. J.A.V.R.S. VI. 5.

Buchanan, J. W., Patterson, D. F. (1965). Selective angiography and angiocardiography in dogs with congenital cardiovascular disease. J.A.V.R.S. VI. 21.

Burk, R. L. (1976). Radiographic definition of the phrenico-pericardial ligament. J.A.V.R.S. XVII. 6. 216.

Carlson, W. D. (1977). Veterinary Radiology. Lea and Febiger. Philadelphia.

Dear, M. G. (1971). Mitral incompetence in dogs of 0–5 years of age. J. Sm. Anim. Pract. 12. 1.

Dodd, K., Kealy, J. K., Lucey, M., Mehigan, C. (1973). Angiostrongylus vasorum. An angiographic study of the pulmonary circulation following treatment for the removal of adult parasites. Irish Vet. J. 27. 105.

Donahoe, J. M., Kneller, S. K., Lewis, R. E. (1976). In vivo pulmonary arteriography in cats infected with Dirofilaria immitis. J.A.V.R.S. XVII. 4. 147.

Douglas, S. W. (1970). Radiology of the normal canine thorax. J. Sm. Anim. Pract. 11. 669.

Douglas, S. W., Williamson, H. D. (1970). Veterinary Radiological Interpretation. Lea and Febiger. Philadelphia.

Douglas, S. W., Williamson, H. D. (1972). Principles of Veterinary Radiography. 2nd ed. Williams and Wilkins Co. Baltimore.

Douglas, S. W. (1974). The interpretation of canine bronchograms. J.A.V.R.S. XV. 1. 18.

Ettinger, S. J., and Suter, P. F. (1970). Canine Cardiology. W. B. Saunders Co. Philadelphia.

Ettinger, S. J. (1975). Textbook of Veterinary Internal Medicine of the Dog and Cat. 2 Vols. W. B. Saunders Co. Philadelphia.

Felson, B. (1973). Chest Roentgenology. W. B. Saunders Co. Philadelphia.

Grandage, J. (1974). The radiology of the dog's diaphragm. J. Sm. Anim. Pract. 15. 1. 1.

Hall, L. W. (1964). The accident case. V. The diagnosis of thoracic injuries. J. Sm. Anim. Pract. 5. 35.

Hamlin, R. L. (1959). Angiocardiography for the clinical diagnosis of congenital heart disease in small animals. J.A.V.M.A. 135. 12.

Hamlin, R. L. (1960). Radiographic anatomy of the heart and great vessels in healthy living dogs. J.A.V.M.A. 136. 265.

Hamlin, R. L. (1960). Radiographic diagnosis of heart disease in dogs. J.A.V.M.A. 137. 458.

Hamlin, R. L. (1968). I. Prognostic value of changes in the cardiac silhouette in dogs with mitral insufficiency. II. Analysis of the cardiac silhouette in dorsoventral radiographs from dogs with heart disease. J.A.V.M.A. 153. 1436.

Hayward, A. H. S. (1968). Thoracic effusions in the cat. J. Sm. Anim. Pract. 9. 75.

Kirk, R. W. (Editor). (1974). Current Veterinary Therapy. V. W. B. Saunders Co. Philadelphia.

Lindsay, F. E. F. (1974). Chylothorax in the domestic cat. A review. J. Sm. Anim. Pract. 15. 241.

Liu, S. K. (1970). Acquired cardiac lesions leading to congestive heart failure in the cat. Am. J. Vet. Res. 31. 2071.

Lord, P. F., Suter, P. F., Chan, K. F., Appleford, M. (1972). Pleural, extrapleural and pulmonary lesions in small animals. A radiographic approach to differential diagnosis. J.A.V.R.S. XIII. 4.

Lord, P. F., Tilley, L. P., Wood, A., Liu, S. K. (1974). Radiography and angiocardiography of feline cardiomyopathy. An abstract. J.A.V.R.S. XV. 2. 56.

Lord, P. F., Schaer, M., Tilley, L. P. (1975). Pulmonary infiltrates with eosinophilia in the dog. J.A.V.R.S. XVI. 4. 115.

Lord, P. F. (1977). Quantitative left ventricular cineangiocardiography in the dog. Measurement and usefulness of left ventricular volume. J.A.V.R.S. XVIII. 2. 51.

Miller, M. E., Christensen, G. C., Evans, H. E. (1964). Anatomy of the Dog. W. B. Saunders Co. Philadelphia.

Morgan, J. P., Silverman, S., Zontine, W. J. (1975). Techniques of Veterinary Radiography. Veterinary Associates, Davis, California.

Myer, W. (1978). Radiography Review: Pleural Effusion. J.A.V.R.S. XIX. 3. 75.

Myer, W., and Burt, J. K. (1973). Bronchiectasis in the dog. Its radiographic appearance. J.A.V.R.S. XIV. 2. 3.

Olsson, S. E. (1973). The Radiological Diagnosis in Canine and Feline Emergencies. Lea and Febiger. Philadelphia.

O'Brien, J. A., Buchanan, J. W., Kelly, D. F. (1966). Tracheal collapse in the dog. J.A.V.R.S. VII. 12.

Patterson, D. F. (1961). Angiocardiography. J.A.V.R.S. 1. 26.

Patterson, D. F. (1965). Congenital heart disease in the dog. Ann. N.Y. Acad. Sc. 127. 541.

Pechman, R. D. (1976). The radiographic features of pulmonary paragonimiasis in the dog and cat. J.A.V.R.S. XVII. 5. 182.

Rawlings, C. A., Lebel, J. L., Mitchum, G. (1970). Torsion of the left apical and cardiac pulmonary lobes in a dog. J.A.V.M.A. 156. 726.

Reif, J. S., and Rhodes, W. H. (1966). The lungs of aged dogs. A radiographic-morphologic correlation. J.A.V.R.S. VII. 5.

Reif, J. S. and Rhodes, W. H. (1968). Linear opacities in canine thoracic radiographs. J.A.V.R.S. IX. 57.

Reif, J. S., Snider, W. R., Kelly, D. F., Brodey, R. (1969). Cavitating pulmonary metastases in a dog. Case report. J.A.V.R.S. X. 12.

Rhodes, W. H., Patterson, D. F., Detweiler, D. K. (1960). Radiographic anatomy of the canine heart. Part I. J.A.V.M.A. 137. 283.

Rhodes, W. H., Patterson, D. F., Detweiler, D. K. (1963). Radiographic anatomy of the canine heart. Part II. J.A.V.M.A. 143. 137.

Schebitz, H. and Wilkens, H. (1977). Atlas of radiographic anatomy of the dog and cat. Paul Parey. Berlin and Hamburg.

Silverman, S., Poulos, P. W., Suter, P. F. (1976). Cavitary pulmonary lesions in animals. J.A.V.R.S. XVII. 4. 134.

Simon, G. (1971). Principles of Chest X-Ray Diagnosis. New York. Appleton-Century-Crofts.

Suter, P. F., and Chan, K. F. (1968). Disseminated pulmonary diseases in small animals. A radiographic approach to diagnosis. J.A.V.R.S. IX. 67.

Suter, P. F., Colgrove, D., Ewing, G. (1972). Congenital hypoplasia of the canine trachea. J.A.A.H.A. 8. 120.

Suter, P. F., Carrig, C. B., O'Brien, T. R., Koller, D. (1974). Radiographic recognition of primary and metastatic pulmonary neoplasms of dogs and cats. J.A.V.R.S. XV. 2. 3.

Suter, P. F. and Lord, P. F. (1974). Radiographic differentiation of disseminated pulmonary parenchymal diseases in dogs and cats. Veterinary Clinics of North America. (Nov., 1974). W. B. Saunders Co. Philadelphia.

Tashjian, R. J. and Albanese, N. M. (1960). A technique of canine angiocardiography. J.A.V.M.A. 136. 359.

Taylor, D. H., and Sittnikow, K. L. (1968). The diagnosis of canine cardiac disease. J. Sm. Anim. Pract. 9. 589.

Ticer, J. W. (1975). Radiographic Technique in Small Animal Practice. W. B. Saunders Co. Philadelphia.

Wyburn, R. S. and Lawson, D. D. (1967). Simple radiography as an aid to the diagnosis of heart disease in the dog. J. Sm. Anim. Pract. 8. 163.

4

BONES AND JOINTS

Bone lends itself very well to radiographic examination. It is relatively dense and contrasts well with the surrounding soft tissues. As living tissue it frequently reflects changes in general metabolism.

Structure

During development each long bone consists of a shaft, or diaphysis, and two extremities, or epiphyses. The diaphysis is composed of dense compact bone that surrounds the medullary cavity. The epiphysis is composed of spongy bone, and it supports the articular cartilage. Between the epiphysis and the diaphysis are the epiphyseal, or growth, plate and the metaphysis. The epiphyseal plate is often referred to as the epiphyseal line when seen on radiographs. It is also called the physis. The metaphysis is an area of spongy bone between the epiphyseal plate and the diaphysis. Both the epiphysis and the metaphysis show marked trabeculation on radiographs. Apophyses are accessory centers of ossification that do not contribute to the growth in length of a bone. They are sites of attachment for muscles and ligaments, for example the great trochanter of the femur. When the bone matures, the epiphysis fuses with the metaphysis and the physis disappears. (Figs. 4–1 and 4–2).

The periosteum is a connective tissue layer that covers bone except at articular surfaces. The articular surfaces are covered by articular cartilage. The periosteum has an outer fibrous layer, which serves for muscle and ligament attachments, and an inner, or cambium, layer capable of elaborating osteoblasts. The endosteum is a single layer membrane lining the medullary cavity. Both periosteum and endosteum elaborate the cells necessary for bone repair.

Development

Bone develops in one of two ways, by endochondral or by intramembranous ossification. In endochondral ossification bone develops on a preformed cartilaginous matrix. Most bones are formed in this way. The long bones increase in length by endochondral ossification. Intramembranous ossification takes place in bands of connective tissue. Flat bones are formed in this way and long bones increase in width in a similar manner. The increase in width of long bones by intramembranous ossification is initiated by the inner, or cambium, layer of the periosteum.

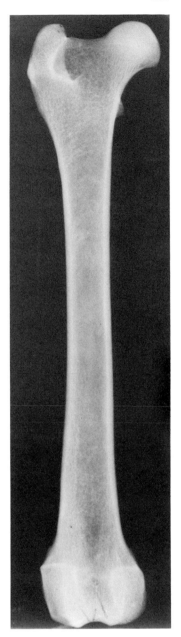

FIGURE 4–1. A marked trabecular pattern can be seen toward each end of the bone.

Living bone is constantly undergoing remodeling. The bone-forming cells are the osteoblasts that elaborate alkaline phosphatase, an indicator of bone activity. Osteoclasts are responsible for bone resorption. Osteocytes form from osteoblasts in mature bone. By means of cytoplasmic processes they help to keep the bone provided with the necessary metabolites. The normal functioning of bone, therefore, depends on a balance being maintained between the activities of these various cells.

Cartilage is radiolucent, and the first radiographic evidence of bone formation in a long bone is the appearance of a collar of mineralized matrix around the shaft. Later, other ossification centers appear.

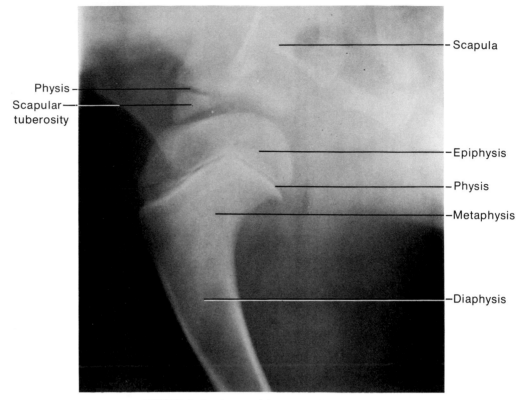

FIGURE 4–2. A normal immature shoulder joint.

Short bones, which develop by endochondral ossification, are found in the carpus and tarsus.

Flat bones, which develop by intramembranous ossification, are found in the head, the thorax (ribs), the pelvis, and in the proximal parts of the limbs, for example, the scapula.

Irregularly shaped bones are found in the skull, the vertebral column, and the pelvis.

Sesamoid bones form in tendons or in ligamentous tissue over which tendons pass. They are usually formed where the direction of a tendon changes or where friction may develop. They have an articular surface that is opposed to a long bone. The term fabella is used to describe a sesamoid bone in the gastrocnemius or popliteus muscles.

Radiography

At least two views taken at right angles to one another are usually required for proper evaluation of the status of a bone. In some instances oblique views may give additional information. It is important that the studies of the skeleton be made in standard positions; the reader is referred to textbooks of radiographic techniques for details of proper positioning.

Normal Appearance

In the young animal the physes appear as radiolucent bands separating the epiphyses from the metaphyses. When growth ceases the epiphyses and the metaphyses fuse and the physes are no longer seen. For some time a band of increased bone density is seen at the junction of the epiphysis and the metaphysis. This is sometimes referred to as an epiphyseal scar. (Fig. 4–3).

It is important to know the positions of the various centers of ossification in the young animal and the times at which they close. Subsidiary centers of ossification may be mistaken for abnormalities. Young animals appear to have very wide joint spaces because the cartilaginous models on which the epiphyses and the small bones of the carpus and tarsus are developing are radiolucent. Growth is completed in dogs and cats by about the tenth to the twelfth month of age. However, considerable variation may occur in the times of epiphyseal closure, even in animals of the same breed. In the long bones, the proximal humeral epiphysis is the last to fuse. The pelvic symphysis may not fuse for several years. The epiphyses of the cat tend to close somewhat later than those of the dog. (See table on pp. 258, 259).

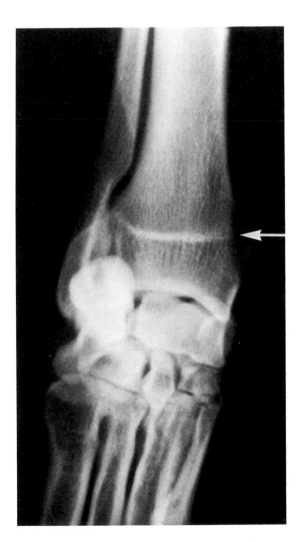

FIGURE 4–3. An epiphyseal scar (arrow) at the lower extremity of a radius.

Age at Appearance of Ossification Centers and of Bony Fusion in the Immature Canine

Anatomic Site	Age at Appearance of Ossification Center	Age When Fusion Occurs	Anatomic Site	Age at Appearance of Ossification Center	Age When Fusion Occurs
Scapula			Accessory		
Body	Birth		Body	2 wk	
Tuber scapulae	7 wk	4–7 mo	Epiphysis	7 wk	4 mo
			First	3 wk	
Humerus			Second	4 wk	
Diaphysis	Birth	—	Third	4 wk	
Proximal epiphysis	1–2 wk	10–13 mo	Fourth	3 wk	
Distal epiphysis		6–8 mo to shaft	Sesamoid bone	4 mo	
Medial condyle	2–3 wk	6 wk to lateral condyle	*Metacarpus*		
			Diaphysis	Birth	
			Distal epiphysis (2–5)*	4 wk	6 mo
Lateral condyle	2–3 wk		**Proximal epiphysis (1)***	5 wk	6 mo
Medial epicondyle	6–8 wk	6 mo to condyles	*Phalanges*		
			First phalanx		
Radius			Diaphysis (1–5)*	Birth	
Diaphysis	Birth	—	Distal epiphysis (2–5)*	4 wk	6 mo
Proximal epiphysis	3–5 wk	6–11 mo	Distal epiphysis (1)*	6 wk	6 mo
Distal epiphysis	2–4 wk	8–12 mo	*Second phalanx*		
			Diaphysis (2–5)*	Birth	
Ulna			Proximal epiphysis (2–5)*	5 wk	6 mo
Diaphysis	Birth		Second phalanx absent or fused with first in first digit.		
Olecranon	8 wk	6–10 mo			
Distal epiphysis	8 wk	8–12 mo	*Third phalanx*		
			Diaphysis	Birth	
Carpus			Volar sesamoids	2 mo	
Ulnar	4 wk		Dorsal sesamoids	4 mo	
Radial	3–4 wk				
Central	4–5 wk				
Intermediate	3–4 wk				

RESPONSE OF BONE TO INJURY OR DISEASE

Bone may respond to injury or disease in a number of ways.

DECREASED DENSITY. Bone may be resorbed as a result of trauma, disuse, metabolic disease, inflammation, or neoplasia. When resorption takes place, the bone loses its radiographic density at the site of resorption. The trabecular pattern becomes hazy or is lost. Decreased density may be localized in one bone, or in part of a bone, or it may be generalized throughout the skeleton in metabolic disturbances.

INCREASED DENSITY. Increased bone density is associated with increased mineralization. It may result from disease processes within the bone or be a response to trauma or stress. Continued abnormal stress on a bone may result in cortical thickening along the line of stress. The term sclerosis is often used to describe increased radiographic density in bone. Sclerotic margins frequently surround areas of infection. Sclerosis of the subchondral bone may be seen associated with arthritic changes in a joint.

Disease or trauma may, therefore, cause either an increase or a decrease

Age at Appearance of Ossification Centers and of Bony Fusion in the Immature Canine
(Continued)

Anatomic Site	Age at Appearance of Ossification Center	Age When Fusion Occurs	Anatomic Site	Age at Appearance of Ossification Center	Age When Fusion Occurs
Pelvis			Tuberosity	8 wk	6–8 mo to condyles
Pubis	Birth	4–6 mo			6–12 mo to shaft
Ilium	Birth	4–6 mo			
Ischium	Birth	4–6 mo	Distal epiphysis	3 wk	8–11 mo
Os acetabulum	7 wk	5 mo	Medial malleolus	3 mo	5 mo
Iliac crest	4 mo	1–2 yr			
Tuber ischii	3 mo	8–10 mo	*Fibula*		
Ischial arch	6 mo	12 mo	Diaphysis	Birth	
Caudal symphysis pubis	7 mo	5 yr	Proximal epiphysis	9 wk	8–12 mo
Symphysis pubis		5 yr	Distal epiphysis	2–7 wk	7–11 mo
Femur			*Tarsus*		
Diaphysis	Birth		Tibial	Birth–1 wk	
Proximal epiphysis (head)	2 wk	7–11 mo	Fibular	Birth–1 wk	
Trochanter major	8 wk	6–10 mo	Tuber calcis	6 wk	3–8 mo
Trochanter minor	8 wk	8–13 mo	Central	3 wk	
Distal epiphysis		8–11 mo to shaft	First	4 wk	
			Second	4 wk	
Trochlea	2 wk	3 mo condyles to trochlea	Third	3 wk	
			Fourth	2 wk	
Medial condyle	3 wk		Metatarsus and pelvic limb phalanges are approximately the same as the metacarpus and pectoral limb phalanges.		
Lateral condyle	3 wk				
Patella	9 wk				
Tibia			*Sesamoids*		
Diaphysis	Birth		Fabellar	3 mo	
Condyles			Popliteal	3 mo	
Medial	3 wk	6 wk to lateral	Plantar phalangeal	2 mo	
Lateral	3 wk	6–12 mo to shaft	Dorsal phalangeal	5 mo	

*Digit numbers
(From Ticer, J. W., 1975, Radiographic Technique in Small Animal Practice, p. 101. W. B. Saunders Co. Philadelphia).

in bone density. Areas of both increased and decreased density may be seen in the one bone. This is most commonly seen associated with infection or neoplasia.

PERIOSTEAL REACTION. The periosteum may react to irritation in a number of ways. If the periosteum is elevated from the underlying cortex, new bone formation occurs beneath the elevated periosteum. Periosteal reaction may be laminated ("onion skin"), smooth, palisade-like, or radiating ("sunburst" appearance). In destructive lesions in which a portion of the cortex is destroyed, a solid triangle of bone is often formed between the elevated periosteum, the intact cortex, and the lesion. This is referred to as "Codman's triangle." A smooth and intact periosteal reaction generally indicates a benign lesion, while a broken or interrupted pattern of response often indicates malignancy. (Fig. 4–4).

CHANGE IN SIZE OR CONTOUR. Bones may change in size or contour as a

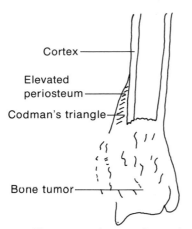

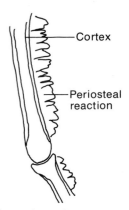

Cortex

Elevated periosteum

Codman's triangle

Bone tumor

The tumor elevates the periosteum, resulting in subperiosteal new bone formation.

Cortex

Periosteal reaction

This palisade-like periosteal reaction is seen in hypertrophic pulmonary osteopathy and sometimes in osteomyelitis.

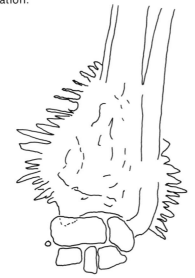

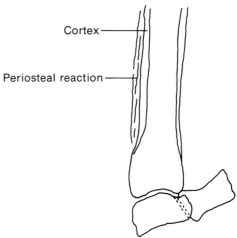

A "sunburst" type of periosteal reaction is sometimes, but not always, seen associated with osteosarcoma or chondrosarcoma.

Cortex

Periosteal reaction

A linear type of periosteal reaction may be seen with callus formation or it may result from metabolic disease or irritation of the bone from a variety of causes.

FIGURE 4–4. Four kinds of periosteal reaction.

result of disease or trauma during the growth period. Premature closure of a physis will cause a bone to be shorter than normal. The shortened bone may affect the growth of bones in its immediate neighborhood. Bone may remain thickened over the site of a healed fracture. (Fig. 4–5).

CHANGE IN TRABECULAR PATTERN.   Trabecular patterns are clearly seen in normal bones in the epiphyses and metaphyses. They tend to fade out in the diaphyses. Changes in trabecular pattern may be the first indication of a disease process. (Fig. 4–1).

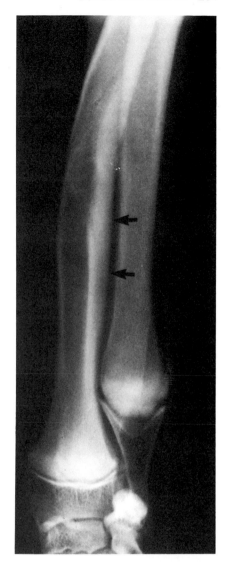

FIGURE 4–5. Thickening of the cortex at the site of a healed fracture in a young dog (arrows).

BONE ABNORMALITIES

Developmental

UNUNITED ANCONEAL PROCESS

Nonunion of the anconeal process of the ulna is the commonest form of elbow dysplasia. Nonunion of the ulnar coronoid process has also been described, though it is difficult to demonstrate radiographically. Nonunion of the anconeal process is seen most frequently in the German Shepherd (Alsatian) breed but it also occurs in other large breeds. In these animals there is usually a separate center of ossification for the anconeal process. This fuses with the diaphysis of the ulna between the fourth and the sixth month of age. Persistence of the physis beyond this time is abnormal. If fusion does not take place at the usual time, the anconeal process may become partially or completely detached from the ulnar diaphysis. The resulting intra-articular bone fragment precipitates secondary degenerative changes in the elbow joint. It has been suggested that this form of elbow dysplasia may be due to trauma rather than to a simple failure of the physis to close.

RADIOLOGIC SIGNS

a. A mediolateral view of the elbow joint taken with the joint in extreme flexion will show the ununited anconeal process.

b. If the condition has been present for some time secondary degenerative changes associated with osteoarthritis may be seen. (Fig. 4–6).

HIP DYSPLASIA

Hip dysplasia is a hereditary disease that affects the larger breeds of dogs, that is, dogs in the region of 30 pounds in weight and over. The breeds most commonly affected are the German Shepherd (Alsatian), the Labrador retriever, and the Rottweiler. The racing greyhound is rarely, if ever, affected. Much remains to be explained about hip dysplasia, and the reader is referred to the copious literature on the subject.

Since treatment of the condition is unsatisfactory, efforts are made to limit its occurrence by controlled breeding programs in which breeding is carried out only from normal or minimally affected animals. Radiography is the only method available for demonstrating conclusively the changes associated with the disease in the living animal.

In the United States, the Orthopedic Foundation for Animals (OFA), 817 Virginia Avenue, Columbia, Missouri, 65201, issues certificates of freedom from hip dysplasia. This is done following examination of radiographs by a

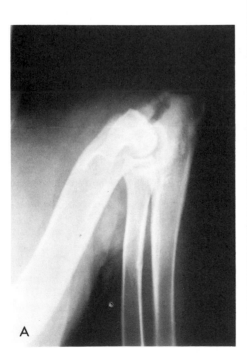
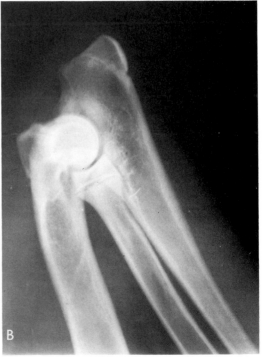

FIGURE 4–6. *A* shows nonunion of the processus anconeus of the ulna. This is best demonstrated with the elbow in extreme flexion. *B* shows a normal elbow, flexed.

panel of veterinary radiologists. A similar certification program is operated in Great Britain by the British Veterinary Association, 7 Mansfield Street, London, W1M OAT. If certification of an animal is required application should be made to the appropriate body for details of the required procedure.

It is advisable to wait until an animal is at least one year old before evaluating it radiographically for hip dysplasia. Earlier examination may be useful if the disease is suspected from clinical signs. Animals found to be free of hip dysplasia should be reexamined after one year. This is because some animals, apparently free from disease at one year of age, later develop secondary degenerative changes in the hip joints.

Radiography

a. Deep sedation or general anesthesia is advisable to facilitate proper positioning.

b. The animal is placed on its back with the hindlimbs drawn out behind. The extended hindlimbs are grasped in the region of the hocks and rotated inward so that the patellas overlie the femoral trochleas. Alternatively the limbs may be strapped to the table in this position. Inward rotation of the limbs enables the femoral necks to be clearly seen.

c. The pelvis should be parallel to the table top. The tail should not be allowed to tilt upward. The pelvis must not be rotated. This can be checked by feeling the distances between the wings of the ilia and the table top. The wings should be equidistant from the table.

d. The use of sand bags or a V tray can assist in maintaining the required position.

e. The legs should be retained as nearly parallel to one another as possible. This will result in the medial cortex of each femur overlying the corresponding ischial tuberosity. Holding the limbs actually parallel to one another is not usually possible in dogs with well-developed thigh muscles.

f. A grid should be used.

A "frog-leg" position is sometimes used. For this view the animal is placed on its back and the hips and stifles are fully flexed. This view may show changes in the femoral neck not seen on the more conventional ventrodorsal study.

If the film has been correctly made the following features can be noted:

a. The wings of the ilia appear symmetric.

b. The obturator foramina appear equal in size and symmetric in outline. If the obturator foramina are different in size, then the pelvis was rotated when the exposure was made. As a result of the rotation, the hip joint on the side of the smaller-appearing foramen will seem shallower than it really is and, conversely, the opposite hip will appear deeper than it actually is.

c. The dorsal acetabular edges should be visible through the femoral heads.

d. The patellas should overlie the femoral trochleas. (Fig. 4–7).

Normal Appearance

The normal hip joint has the following radiographic features:

a. The acetabulum is deep.

b. The femoral head is round and even, except at the fovea capitis where it is slightly flattened.

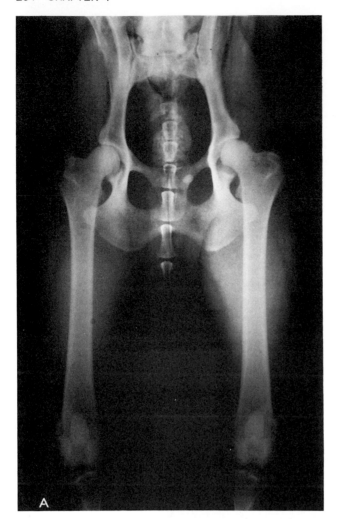

FIGURE 4–7.   *A.* Good position of a pelvis.

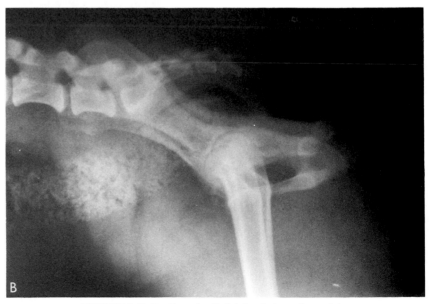

FIGURE 4–7 *Continued.*   *B.* A lateral view of a pelvis.

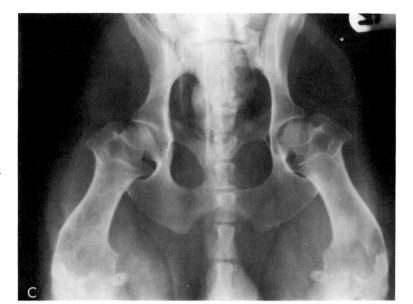

FIGURE 4–7 *Continued.* C. Pelvis of a Bassett hound.

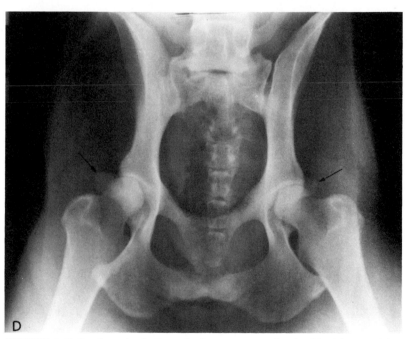

FIGURE 4–7 *Continued.* D. Teat shadows may overlie the hip joints and be mistaken for abnormalities (arrows).

c. The outline of the femoral head parallels the outline of the cranial acetabular edge from the cranial effective acetabular rim to the fovea capitis.

d. The femoral head fits snugly into the acetabulum and at least half of the head should be within the acetabulum. The center of the femoral head should lie to the inner side of the dorsal acetabular edge.

e. The joint space is even and regular and not increased in width.

f. There is no evidence of secondary degenerative joint changes. (Figs. 4–8 and 4–9).

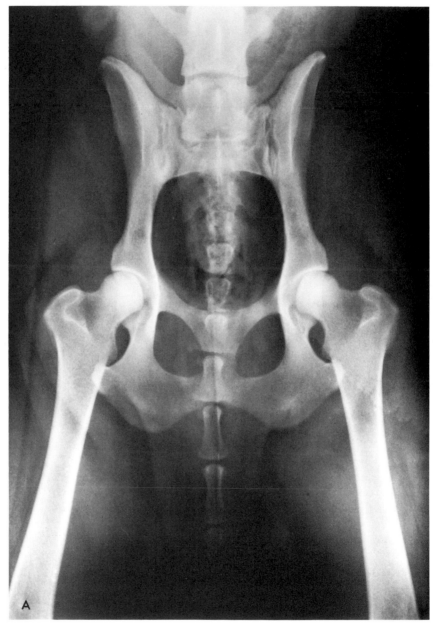

FIGURE 4–8. *A.* A normal pelvis.

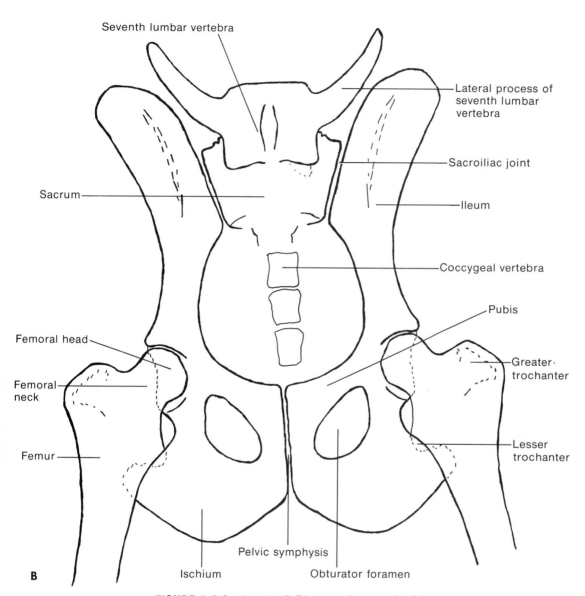

Seventh lumbar vertebra

Lateral process of seventh lumbar vertebra

Sacroiliac joint

Sacrum

Ileum

Coccygeal vertebra

Pubis

Femoral head

Greater trochanter

Femoral neck

Femur

Lesser trochanter

Ischium

Pelvic symphysis

Obturator foramen

B

FIGURE 4–8 *Continued.* *B*. Diagram of a normal pelvis.

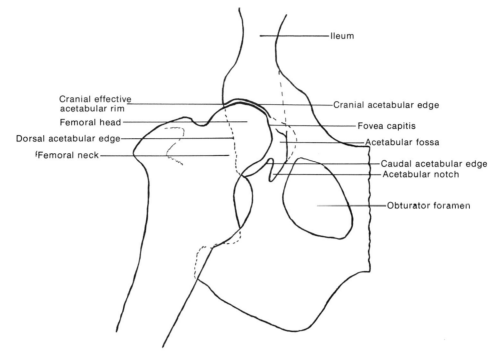

FIGURE 4–9.   Detailed diagram of the hip joint.

Signs of Hip Dysplasia

Many radiographic changes may be associated with hip dysplasia, depending on the severity of the condition when the examination is carried out. Not all possible changes are necessarily seen in one animal. Care, judgment, and experience are required in the interpretation of radiographs. The changes commonly seen associated with hip dysplasia are as follows:

a. The femoral head fits poorly in the acetabulum. The head may appear to be too small for the acetabulum.

b. The outline of the femoral head deviates from the outline of the acetabulum along the cranial and caudal acetabular edges. Some care is necessary in assessing this sign.

c. Subluxation or luxation of the femoral head is present. Subluxation is present if less than fifty per cent of the head is within the acetabulum. In cases of doubt, subluxation can be assessed by Norberg's method. This consists of measuring the angle formed between a line joining the centers of the femoral heads and a line joining the center of the head under examination with the cranial effective acetabular rim on the same side. This angle should be not less than 105°. (Fig. 4–10).

d. As a result of poor relationship between the femoral head and the acetabulum, secondary degenerative changes occur. These include the following:

    1. Irregular wear occurs on the femoral head, causing it to become misshapen and to lose its rounded appearance.

    2. The acetabulum becomes flattened or shallow and irregular in outline.

    3. New bone is produced around the acetabulum and on the femoral head and neck.

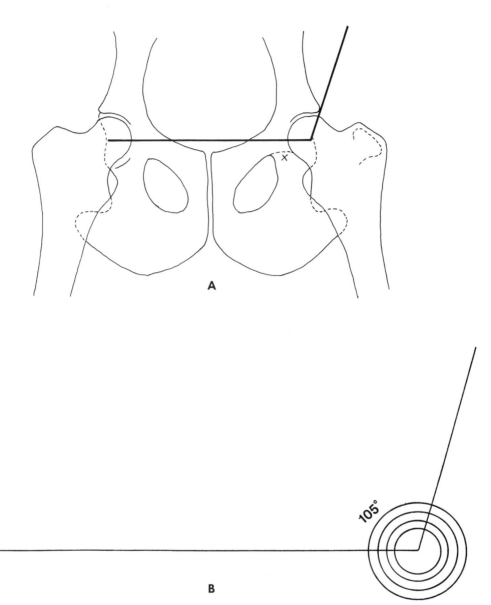

FIGURE 4–10. Norberg's Index. *A.* A line is drawn joining the centers of the femoral heads. From the center of the head under examination a second line is drawn through the cranial effective acetabular rim. The angle formed by these two lines should be not less than 105°. *B.* A transparent sheet of plastic material is prepared as follows. A series of concentric circles are drawn on the material and a small hole is punched at the center of the circles. Two lines originating at the center of the circles are drawn to form an angle of 105°. To examine a femoral head, the center of the head is found by placing the circles over the head and moving them about until a circle is found to conform to the outline of the head under examination. The center of the head is then marked with a pin or a pen through the hole at the center of the circles. The center of the other head is found in the same way. The predrawn lines can then be used to determine the angle. As the plastic is transparent, by turning it over the angles on both sides can be determined. Shenton's line: The curve on the inner aspect of the femoral neck, when projected, should be continuous with the cranial edge of the obturator foramen (dotted line at X in Fig. A.). If the hip joint is luxated or subluxated, the projected line will not be continuous with the edge of the foramen.

4. A line of increased density appears on the femoral neck along the line of attachment of the joint capsule. This is indicative of stress on the joint capsule. (Fig. 4–11).

5. The angle formed at the cranial effective acetabular rim is worn away, producing a flattened area at that point. This is referred to as "bilabiation."

6. There is an increase in density (sclerosis) of the subchondral bone along the cranial acetabular edge.

Osteoarthrosis is a common sequel to hip dysplasia and many of the changes seen are associated with degeneration of the joint.

The changes seen in hip dysplasia are sometimes graded according to their severity:

Grade I.   Minimal deviation from normal with minor subluxation and remodeling changes.

Grade II.   Marked lateral subluxation of the femoral head, which is one-fourth to one-half of the way out of the acetabulum.

Grade III.   The femoral head is one-half to three-quarters of the way out of the acetabulum and there are marked remodeling changes. Exostoses may be present on the femoral head and on the acetabulum.

Grade IV.   Luxation of the femoral head is present with flattening of the acetabular edge and the femoral head. Varying degrees of osteoarthrosis and osteosclerosis are seen. (Fig. 4–12).

Hip dysplasia is usually bilateral but occasional unilateral cases are seen. If only one hip is affected, trauma should be considered as a possible cause of any abnormalities seen.

Minor deviations from normal can be very difficult to assess and expressions such as "near normal" or "less than ideal, but within normal limits for the breed and age" are sometimes used to describe borderline cases. A more lenient view should be taken in interpreting radiographs of animals over two years of age in the absence of evidence of degenerative joint disease.

CONGENITAL LUXATION OF THE PATELLA

This may result from malformation of the femoral trochlea, poor alignment between the distal femur and the proximal tibia, rotation of the proximal extremity of the tibia, which displaces the tibial tuberosity medially, or a combination of all these. There may be an associated abnormal angulation of the distal femoral extremity. These abnormalities result in the patellar straight ligament being out of line with the trochlear groove.

RADIOLOGIC SIGNS

a. The patella is seen to lie to the medial side of the femur in the craniocaudal view. The displaced patella may be difficult to demonstrate in young animals before it has become fully mineralized. Lateral displacement is much less common.

b. In the lateral view the patella is not seen in its usual position.

c. The associated bone abnormalities are frequently evident. A skyline view of the trochlear groove may be helpful. (Fig. 4–13).

Text continued on page 276

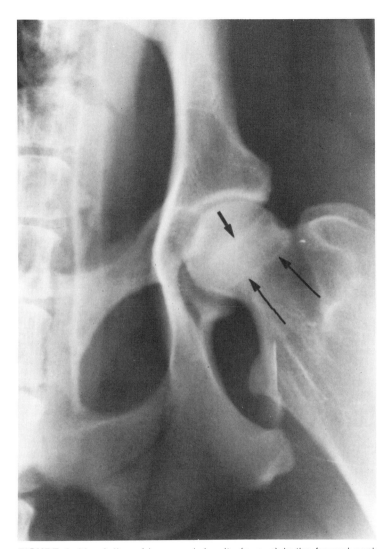

FIGURE 4–11. A line of increased density (arrows) in the femoral neck indicative of stress along the line of attachment of the joint capsule. This should not be confused with the epiphyseal scar, which can also be seen (small arrow). There is sclerosis of the subchondral bone along the cranial acetabular edge.

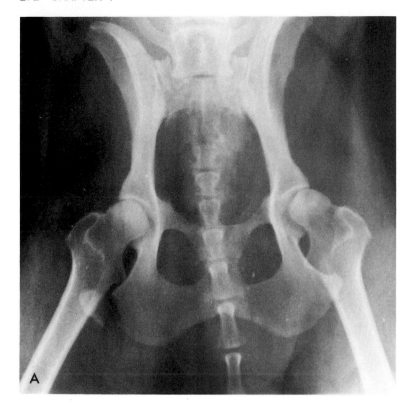

FIGURE 4–12. Four degrees of hip dysplasia. *A.* Minimal dysplastic changes are evident, particularly in the left hip. There is loss of parallelism between the femoral head and the cranial acetabular edge. There is a minor degree of subluxation in the left hip. (Grade I dysplasia). There is a fracture of the right ischium.

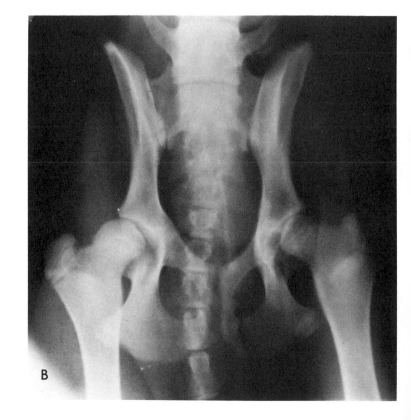

FIGURE 4–12 *Continued. B.* Marked remodeling changes are present in both acetabula. The left femoral head is about one-half the way out of the acetabulum. The femoral necks appear thickened because of the small femoral heads (Grade II dysplasia).

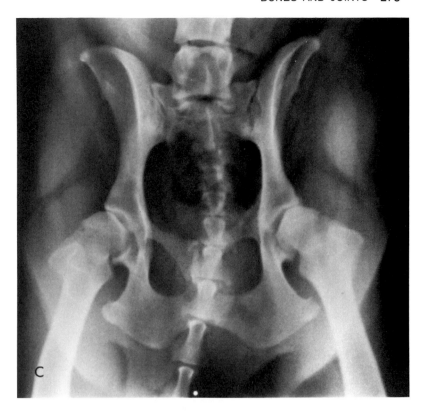

FIGURE 4–12 *Continued. C.* Severe remodeling changes are seen in the acetabula and the femoral heads. The femoral necks are grossly thickened. The right femoral head is over 50 per cent luxated. (Grade III dysplasia).

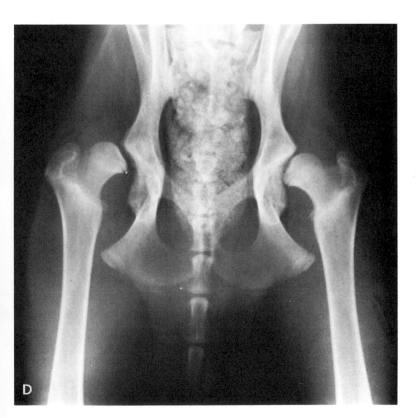

FIGURE 4–12 *Continued. D.* The acetabula are flattened. The heads of the femurs are no longer within the acetabula. Inflammatory new bone formation is present particularly in the acetabula and less obviously on the femoral necks. (Grade IV dysplasia).

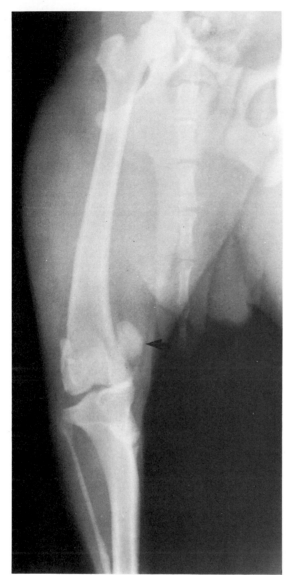

A

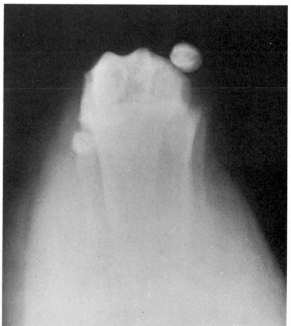

B

FIGURE 4–13. *A.* Luxation of the patella. The displaced patella can be seen on the medial aspect of the stifle (arrow). The stifle joint is deformed. *B.* A skyline view of a displaced patella.

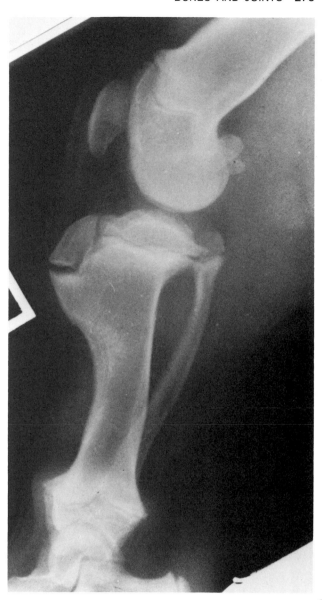

FIGURE 4–14. Bones of a young Bassett hound.

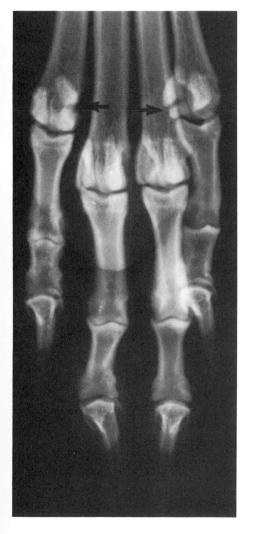

FIGURE 4–15. Bipartite sesamoids (arrows). The second and seventh sesamoids are most commonly affected by this anomaly.

ACHONDROPLASIA

The features of this condition are seen in the chondrodystrophic breeds such as the dachshund and the Bassett hound. The bones are short, thickened, and bent, with prominent tuberosities. (Fig. 4–14).

Dwarfism has been reported in the Alaskan malamute.

BIPARTITE SESAMOIDS

Two sesamoid bones are present above the palmar aspect of each metacarpophalangeal and metatarsophalangeal articulation. They are numbered from 1 to 8 from the medial to the lateral side. The second and the seventh are frequently bipartite. This developmental anomaly should not be mistaken for a fracture. (Fig. 4–15).

RETAINED CARTILAGE CORE IN THE ULNA

Retained hypertrophied enchondral cartilage is occasionally seen in the distal ulnar metaphysis in some large dogs. It may retard growth of the ulna.

RADIOLOGIC SIGNS

a. A wedge of radiolucent cartilage is seen in the distal ulnar metaphysis.

b. The cartilaginous wedge is often surrounded by a zone of sclerosis.

c. Interference with growth of the ulna may cause the radius to bend cranially.

d. The lower radial epiphysis becomes distorted as a result of the growth disturbance in the ulna. (Fig. 4–16).

CONGENITAL MALFORMATIONS

Various congenital anomalies, such as polydactylism or absence of one or more phalanges, are occasionally encountered. (Fig. 4–17).

MULTIPLE EPIPHYSEAL DYSPLASIA

This has been described in beagle puppies. Punctate lesions are seen in the epiphyses; they have a stippled appearance and there is failure of ossification at the epiphyseal centers. Affected pups show a swaying hindleg gait, sagging hocks, and forelimb lameness. Adults show periodic lameness.

Fractures

A fracture may be defined as a solution or break in the continuity of a bone. It may be the result of trauma or it may occur because the bone has been weakened by disease (pathologic fracture).

For descriptive purposes fractures may be classified as follows:

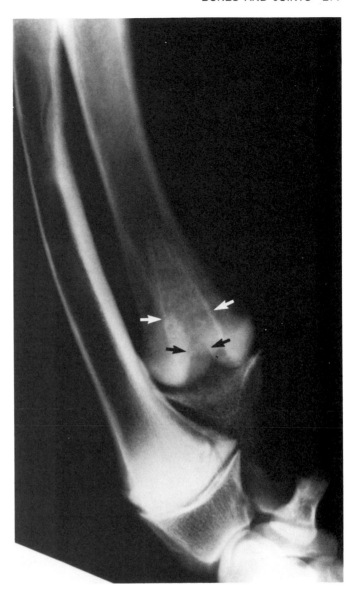

FIGURE 4–16. A retained cartilaginous core in the ulna (black arrows). Interference with ulnar growth has caused the radius to bend cranially. The core has a sclerotic margin (white arrows).

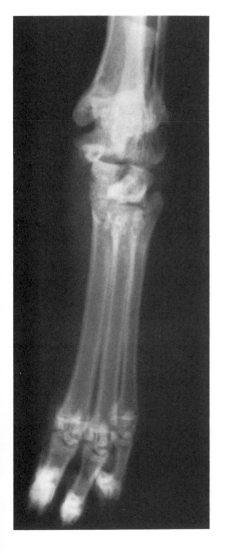

FIGURE 4–17. Congenital anomalies of digits.

COMPLETE OR INCOMPLETE. In a complete fracture there is a break through the entire substance of the bone. An incomplete fracture retains some degree of continuity between the fractured ends, such as occurs in a fissure fracture or a greenstick fracture. In a fissure or hairline fracture there is a thin fracture line without any separation of the fractured ends. It does not involve the full depth of the bone. A greenstick fracture is a fracture through the cortex on one side of a bone, while the opposite cortex remains intact.

CLOSED OR OPEN (COMPOUND). A closed fracture has no communication with the exterior. An open, or compound, fracture is associated with a wound in the skin. On radiographs, air shadows can usually be seen in the soft tissues at the site of a compound fracture.

SIMPLE OR COMMINUTED. A simple fracture has only two fracture fragments, while a comminuted fracture has three or more associated fragments.

TRANSVERSE, OBLIQUE, OR SPIRAL. In a transverse fracture the fracture line is at right angles to the long axis of the bone. An oblique fracture has the fracture line obliquely directed relative to the long axis of the bone. In a spiral fracture the fracture line winds along the long axis of the bone.

AVULSION OR CHIP. In an avulsion fracture a bone fragment is pulled away from a bone at the point of attachment of a tendon, muscle, or ligament. A chip fracture is a separation of a small piece of bone without disruption of its general continuity. Chip fractures usually occur at or near joint margins.

EPIPHYSEAL OR DIAPHYSEAL. An epiphyseal fracture, or perhaps more correctly an epiphyseal separation or slip, occurs when the epiphysis of a bone is displaced from its normal position. The movement takes place at the physis. An epiphysis may be the site of a fracture without a concomitant epiphyseal separation. A diaphyseal fracture is a fracture of the shaft of a bone.

IMPACTED OR OVERRIDING. An impacted fracture has the fracture fragments embedded in one another. In an overriding fracture one of the fracture fragments lies partially alongside the other.

Most fractures are readily recognized on radiographs, as there is usually some separation of the fractured ends. The fracture line appears as an area of radiolucency between the fracture fragments. It is essential to have at least two views of any bone under examination, made at right angles to one another. In fractures with little or no displacement an oblique view may also be required to demonstrate the fracture line. A fracture line can be missed if one relies on one view alone. Two views are also required to relate the positions of the fracture fragments to one another. Physes must not be confused with fracture lines.

When describing a fracture it is usual to consider the proximal fragment as fixed and to describe the distal fragment as displaced relative to the proximal. A selection of fractures is shown in Figure 4–18.

In the study of fractures radiography may be required for one or more of the following reasons:

a. To confirm a clinical diagnosis.

b. To demonstrate the positions, relationships, and nature of fractured bone fragments with a view to deciding on the best method of treatment.

c. To determine the age of a fracture.

d. To assess the degree of repair.

e. To visualize a suspected fracture not demonstrable clinically.

Text continued on page 291

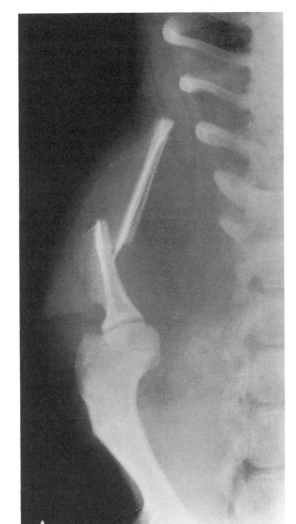

FIGURE 4–18. A selection of fractures. *A.* Fracture of the scapula.

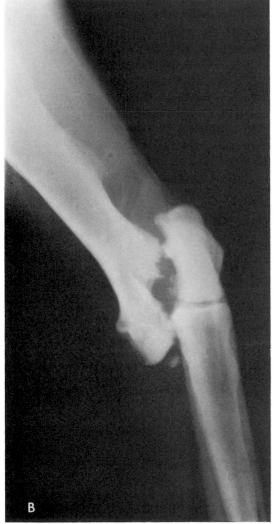

FIGURE 4–18 *Continued.* *B.* Fracture of the lateral epicondyle of the humerus.

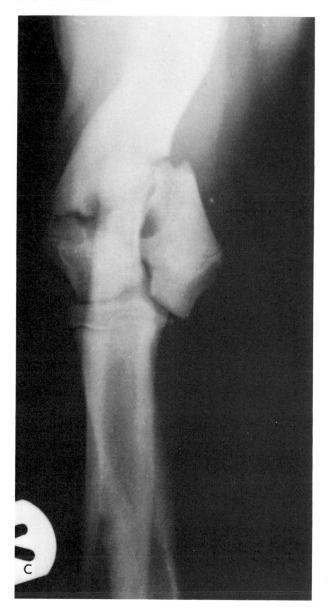

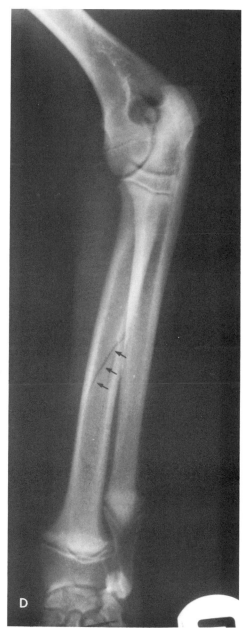

FIGURE 4–18 *Continued.   C.* Fractures of both medial and lateral humeral epicondyles. (Y fracture).

FIGURE 4–18 *Continued.   D.* A fissure fracture in a radius (arrows).

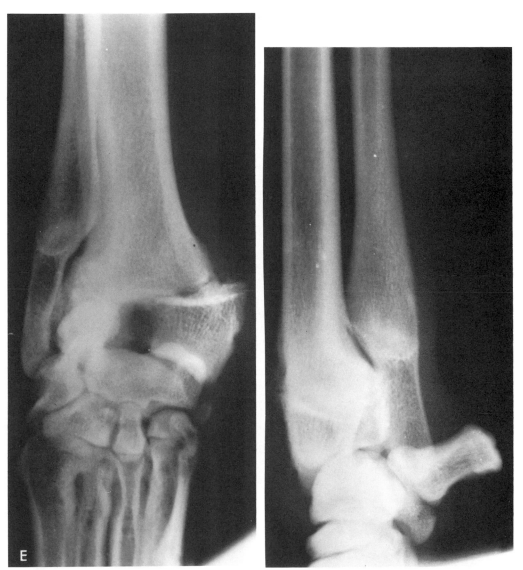

FIGURE 4–18 *Continued. E.* Separation and fracture of the lower epiphysis of a radius. The separation is not readily seen on the lateral view. This illustrates the necessity for two views. This is not a recent injury, as a periosteal reaction can be seen on the cranial aspect of the distal radius.

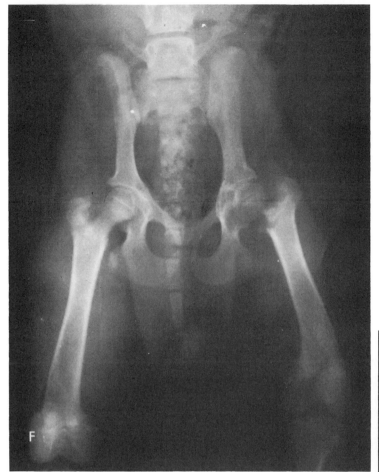

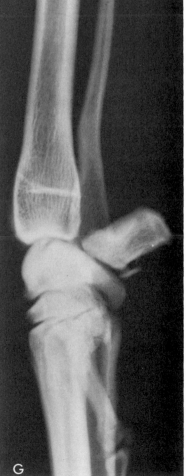

FIGURE 4–18 Continued. F. A fracture of the left femoral neck. The femoral head and neck have lost their normal density because of resorption of bone. This is common with intracapsular fractures, as they usually interfere with the blood supply.

FIGURE 4–18 Continued.   G. Fracture of the accessory carpal bone. This is a common injury in the racing greyhound. The commonest site of fracture is the one illustrated, though fracture may occur at any of the angles of the bone.

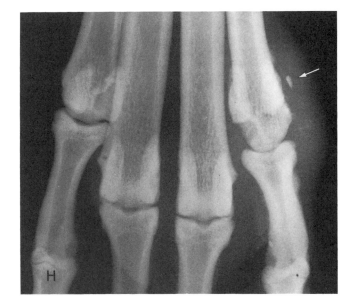

FIGURE 4–18 *Continued.* *H.* An avulsion fracture (arrow) at the distal extremity of a large metacarpal bone. This is seen, particularly in racing greyhounds, as a result of stretching or rupture of the collateral ligament of the adjacent joint. There is an associated soft tissue swelling.

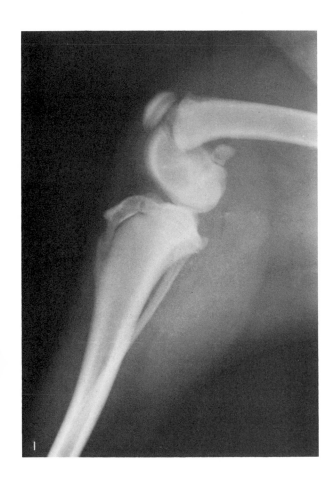

FIGURE 4–18 *Continued.* *I.* An epiphyseal separation at the distal end of a femur. Note the smooth appearance of the end of the femoral shaft. A true fracture would have a more irregular appearance.

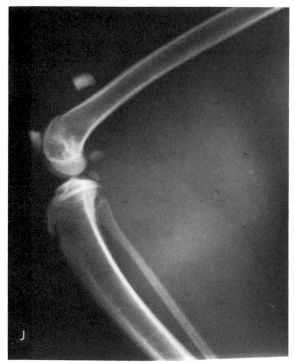

FIGURE 4–18 *Continued.* *J.* Fracture of the patella in a cat.

FIGURE 4–18 *Continued.* *K.* Separation of the proximal epiphysis and crest of a tibia.

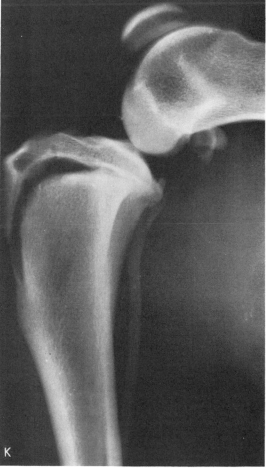

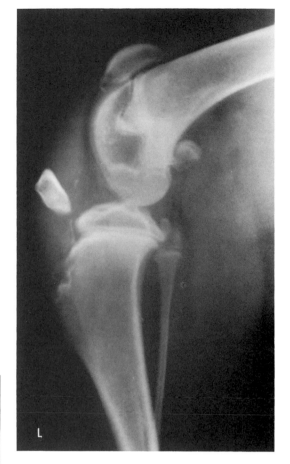

FIGURE 4–18 *Continued.   L.* Separation of the tibial tuberosity.

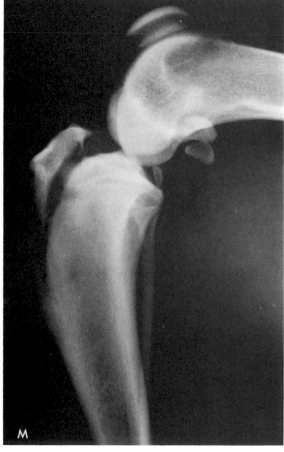

FIGURE 4–18 *Continued.   M.* Separation of the tibial tuberosity and crest.

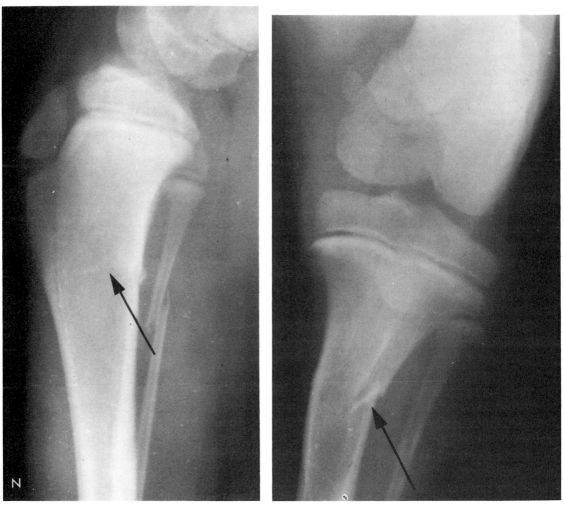

FIGURE 4–18 *Continued.* *N.* A greenstick (folding) fracture. Such fractures may appear as lines of increased density within the bone (arrows).

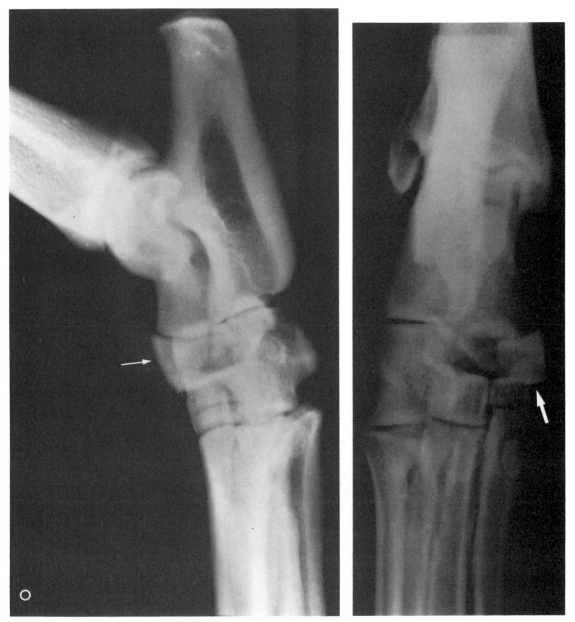

FIGURE 4–18 *Continued.*   *O.* Fracture of the central tarsal bone. This is a common injury in the racing greyhound. The right leg is most commonly affected in dogs racing on left-hand tracks. The fractured fragment is displaced medially and dorsally (arrows). Note that the hock has not collapsed. (See Fig. 4–18 *P*).

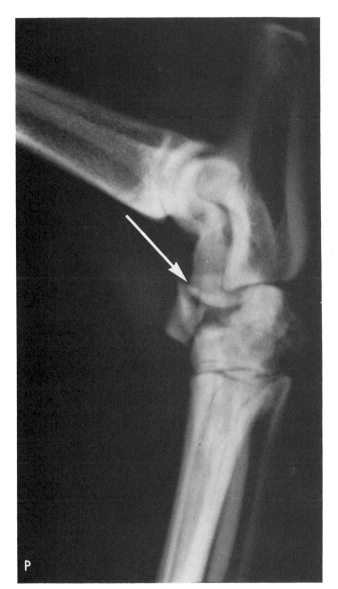

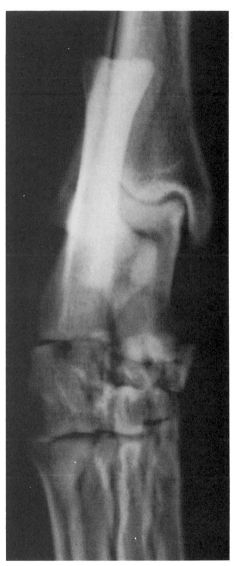

FIGURE 4–18 *Continued.* *P.* Fracture of the central tarsal bone with collapse of the hock. The fracture is comminuted and the tibial tarsal bone is displaced distally (arrow). Such fractures carry a poorer prognosis than the type illustrated in Figure 4–18 *O.* The fourth tarsal bone is also fractured.

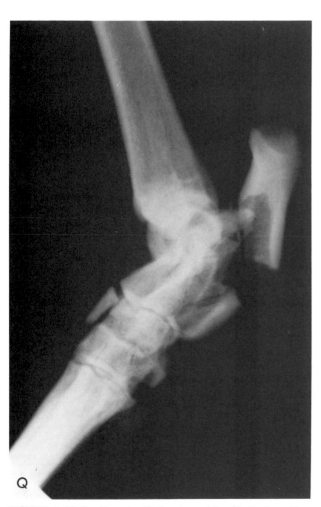

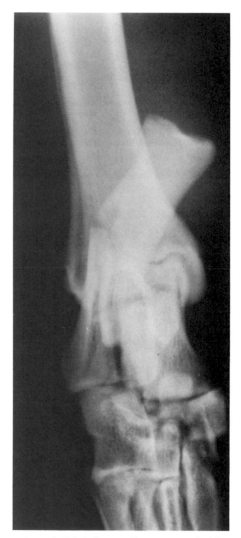

FIGURE 4–18 *Continued.* Q. Fracture of the fibular tarsal bone. In greyhounds this is frequently accompanied by a fracture of the central tarsal bone, as in this case.

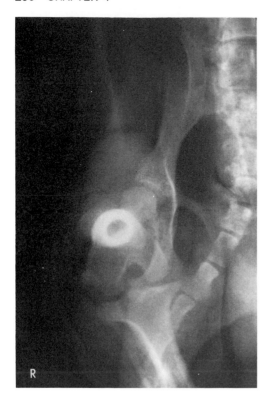

FIGURE 4–18 *Continued.* *R.* Fracture of the femur. If the fractured shaft lies end-on to the x-ray beam a peculiar "ring" effect is sometimes produced. This might be mistaken for a foreign body.

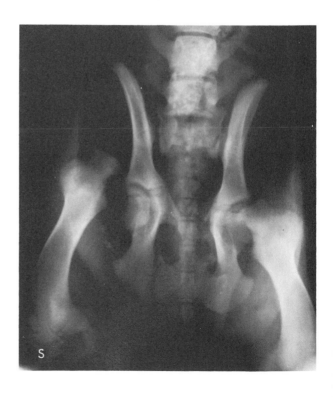

FIGURE 4–18 *Continued.* *S.* Epiphysiolysis. The term "epiphysiolysis" is used to denote separation of an epiphysis, particularly the femoral capital epiphysis. This pelvis has sustained multiple injuries.

Fracture Repair

After a fracture occurs the increased vascularity associated with vasodilation, changes in the pH of the tissue fluid, and osteoclastic activity result in a resorption of bone along the fractured ends. The hematoma that is present at the fracture site becomes organized and the resulting primitive repair tissue eventually becomes mineralized. This results in a bony callus. At first the callus is large and irregular in outline. Later, remodeling takes place and the callus is incorporated into the general bone structure.

In cases in which apposition of the fractured ends has been accurately achieved and maintained by surgical methods, for example in compression plating, repair takes place, for the most part, by periosteal and endosteal extension rather than by organization of a hematoma. Little, if any, callus is then seen.

Radiology of Fracture Repair

From a knowledge of repair processes one can deduce what the radiographic appearance will be at various stages of bone repair. It must be emphasized that not all bones heal in exactly the same way or to the same time scale. The bones of young animals heal more rapidly than do those of older animals. Disease processes, local or metabolic, may retard bone healing. The following time scale may be used as a general indicator of the changing radiographic appearance of a healing fracture.

RECENT FRACTURE The fracture lines are sharp and well defined. There is an associated soft tissue swelling.

ONE WEEK TO TEN DAYS. The fracture lines are no longer sharp because of the resorption of bone along the fractured ends. The soft tissue swelling has subsided. Hairline fractures may be more clearly seen at this time than immediately after their occurrence.

TWO TO THREE WEEKS. There is evidence of periosteal reaction and some mineralization of the callus. The fracture line is being bridged.

FOUR TO EIGHT WEEKS. The fracture line becomes filled-in with bony callus and there is advanced bridging of the fracture area with new bone. A large callus is still present.

EIGHT TO TWELVE WEEKS. The callus is being remodeled and organized and is being incorporated into the general bone structure. The amount of visible callus is decreasing. (Fig. 4–19).

The process of reorganization and remodeling may take several months. The time factor at this stage of repair is very variable and depends on the amount of displacement and distortion originally present.

In assessing whether or not a fracture line has been bridged by callus, care must be taken not to confuse overlapping tongues of callus for actual union. Oblique views may be required to accurately evaluate the degree of repair. Little or no callus may be visible following compression plating. (Fig. 4–20).

RADIOLOGIC SIGNS OF UNION

a. Bridging of the fracture area with new bone.

b. Obliteration of the fracture line. This should be demonstrated on more than one view.

Text continued on page 295

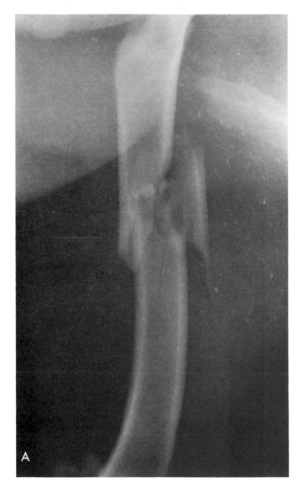

FIGURE 4–19. Three stages in the repair of an untreated fracture. *A.* Recent fracture.

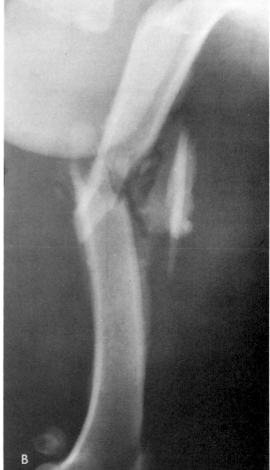

FIGURE 4–19 *Continued.* *B.* Three weeks after occurrence callus formation is evident.

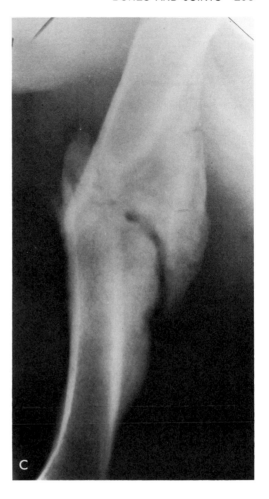

FIGURE 4–19 *Continued.* *C.* Ten weeks after occurrence there is excessive callus formation incorporating the fragments. The fracture line is not yet completely bridged. The delayed union is probably due to the comminution.

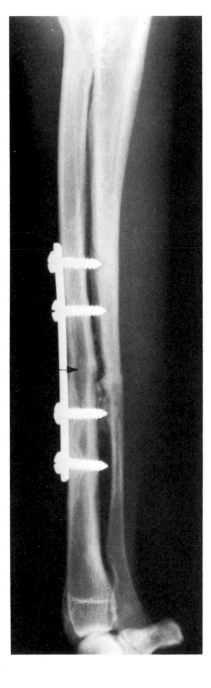

FIGURE 4–20. No callus formation is visible at the site of injury in this healed fracture of the radius (arrow). There is some callus associated with the ulnar fracture.

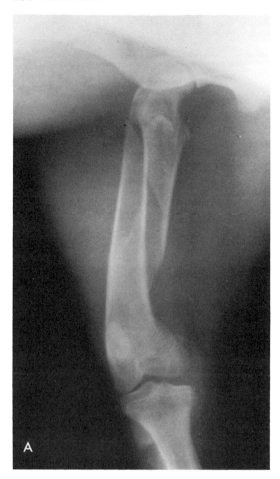

FIGURE 4–21.   *A.* An oblique overriding fracture of the femur. *B.* Five weeks later remodeling is evident.

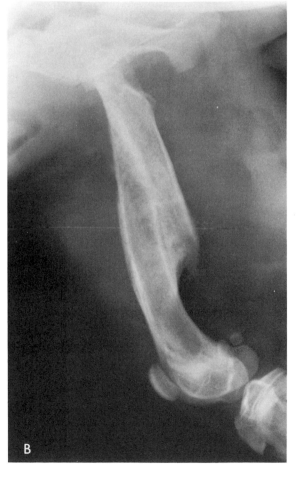

c. Remodeling of the callus with restoration of the continuity of the cortex and medullary cavity.

d. Restoration of the normal trabecular pattern. (Fig. 4–21).

Nonunion Fracture

Occasionally, the fractured ends of a bone fail to unite. This is most commonly seen in the smaller breeds of dogs. The radius and ulna and the tibia and fibula are most commonly affected, though nonunion is encountered in other bones. The cause remains obscure. Movement of the fractured ends is probably a primary factor.

RADIOLOGIC SIGNS

a. A clearly visible fracture line long after the fracture was sustained.

b. Poor callus formation and the callus does not bridge the fracture line efficiently.

c. Rounding off of the fractured ends, which become sclerotic with thickened cortices and bone formation within the medullary cavity. This is sometimes called an "elephant foot" callus.

d. Generalized decreased density in the bones of the affected limb distal to the fracture due to atrophy of disuse.

Judgment must be exercised in correlating clinical and radiographic findings. There may be good clinical union with restoration of a considerable amount of function, although radiographically a fracture line has not been completely bridged. (Fig. 4–22).

Malunion

Malunion is present when a fracture has healed with the fracture fragments in an abnormal position, resulting in distortion of the bone. Its significance depends on its severity and on the site. Remodeling processes may minimize its effects. Malunion may be the cause of secondary arthritic changes in joints above and below the fracture because of abnormal stresses being placed on them as a result of the bone distortion. (Fig. 4–23).

Premature Closure of Physes

Trauma may precipitate premature closure of a physis. It is not very common. The radius and ulna are the bones commonly affected.

Following premature closure of the distal ulnar physis, the radius continues to grow in length though ulnar growth has ceased or has been considerably retarded. This results in cranial bowing of the radius with outward deviation of the lower limb (valgus deformity). The cortex along the caudal concave side of the radius increases in thickness and the distance between the radius and ulna increases. The bowing of the radius causes changes in the elbow and radiocarpal joints. The elbow may become subluxated and the radiocarpal joint distorted. (Fig. 4–24).

Text continued on page 301

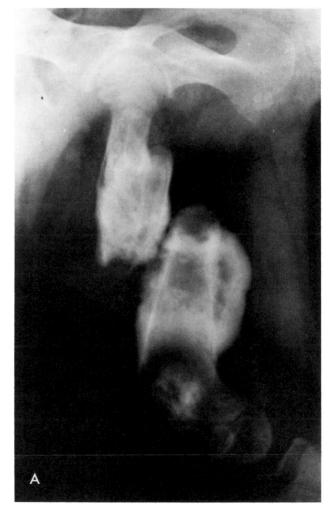

FIGURE 4–22. Examples of nonunion fracture. *A.* An old femoral fracture. Although there is considerable callus formation the fracture line has not been bridged. The fractured ends have become rounded off.

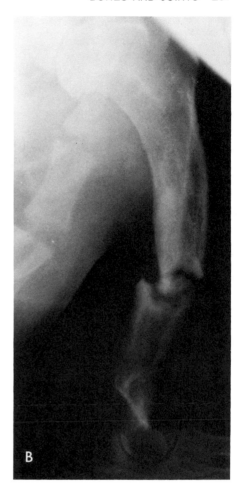

FIGURE 4–22 *Continued.*   *B.* An eight month old fracture of the humerus. The fracture line is still obvious and there is no callus formation. The fractured ends are sclerotic.

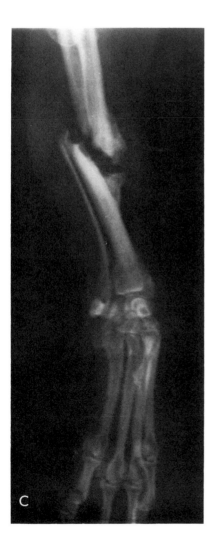

FIGURE 4–22 *Continued.*   *C.* A nonunion fracture in the radius and ulna. The proximal fractured end of the radius shows the so-called "elephant foot" appearance. Disuse osteoporisis is evident distal to all three fractures.

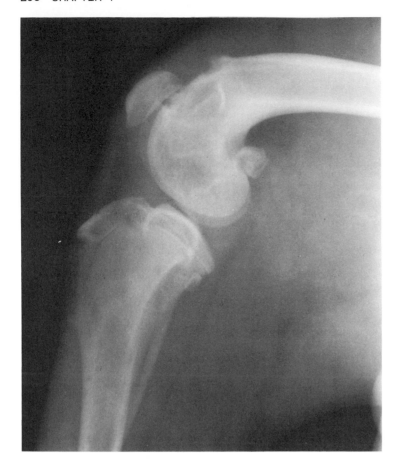

FIGURE 4-23. Malunion of a fracture. This femoral fracture has healed with a distorted angle between the femoral shaft and the condyles.

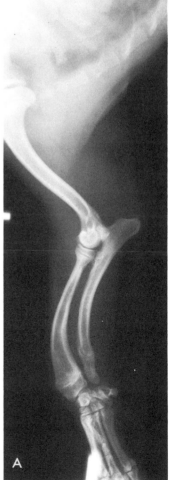

FIGURE 4-24. *A.* Premature closure of the distal ulnar physis. There is marked bowing of the radius and the humero-ulnar joint is subluxated.

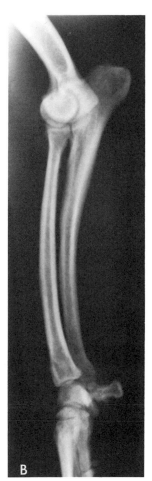

FIGURE 4–24 *Continued.* B. Radiograph of a normal limb for comparison.

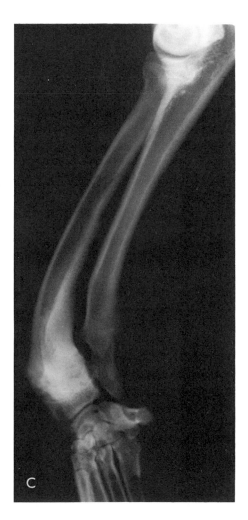

FIGURE 4–24 *Continued.* C. Premature closure of the distal ulnar physis showing bowing of the radius and marked thickening of the cortex of the radius on its concave side.

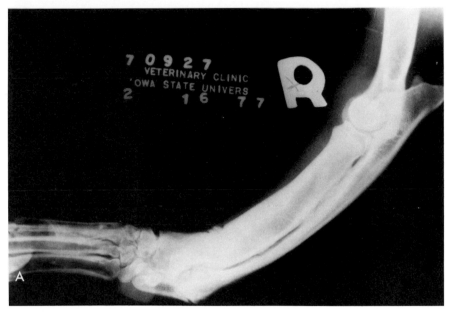

FIGURE 4–25*A.* Premature closure of the distal radial physis. This film was made with the animal bearing weight on the limb.

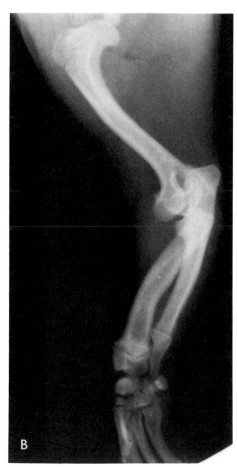

FIGURE 4–25*B.* Premature closure of the proximal radial physis has resulted in shortening of the radius, bowing of the ulna, subluxation of the humero-radial joint and of the radio-carpal joint.

Premature closure of the distal radial physis is not as common as premature closure of the distal ulnar physis. If it occurs the ulna increases in length relative to the radius and subluxation of the radiocarpal joint may ensue. Premature closure of the proximal radial physis is also occasionally seen. (Fig. 4–25).

Infection in Bone

OSTEOMYELITIS

This is not common in the dog or cat. It is, perhaps, more frequently seen in cats. It may arise as a direct result of infection in a wound, traumatic or surgical, or it may be blood borne. Infection in bone results in death of the bone tissue. The dead bone is resorbed and replaced by fibrous connective tissue. Healthy bone in the neighborhood of the infection tends to proliferate in an attempt to confine the infection.

RADIOLOGIC SIGNS

Osteomyelitis will exhibit some or all of the following radiographic features:

a. Loss of normal trabecular pattern. This is often seen in the metaphysis of the bone, which is the most common site of infection.

b. Lysis, or destruction, of bone. This appears as an area of radiolucency within the bone. It is sometimes seen as an area of decreased density around a bone screw if infection follows fracture repair.

c. Sclerosis. Around the area of lysis there is an area of increased density. This represents an apparent attempt by the body to confine the area of infection. This is called the involucrum.

d. Periostitis. The periosteum becomes elevated and there is subperiosteal new bone formation. This may extend for a considerable distance on either side of the area of infection. The periosteal reaction tends to develop parallel to the cortex.

e. Cortical destruction. The cortex becomes thinned or even eroded at the site of infection.

f. Sequestrum formation. This is an area of dead bone that appears radiographically denser than the surrounding bone from which it is separated by a radiolucent zone of osteolysis. Sequestrum formation is rare in dogs and cats.

g. The infection spreads readily to adjacent bones and joints.

If serial radiographs are made during the course of treatment the condition may be seen to be resolving. The normal bone structure begins to reappear in cases that are responding satisfactorily. The radiographic appearance of osteomyelitis is very variable. It is often difficult, if not impossible, to distinguish with certainty between it and neoplasia. (Fig. 4–26).

One cannot distinguish between living and dead bone radiographically unless there has been collapse of the bone trabeculae. Following collapse of bone trabeculae, dead bone appears denser than normal bone.

Fungal infections usually provoke a multifocal type of osteomyelitis that may give a mottled appearance to the affected bone. Coccidioidomycosis, seen in the southwestern United States, causes a reaction in bone that is, for the most part, sclerotic in nature. Adjacent bones may become involved. In blastomycosis there may be involvement of bone from a soft tissue focus of infection. Osteolysis is the principal feature. (Fig. 4–26).

Text continued on page 306

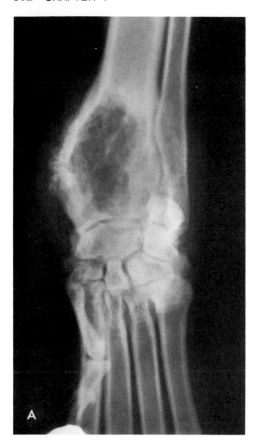

FIGURE 4–26. Some examples of osteomyelitis. *A. B.* These craniocaudal and lateral views of the distal radius show a classic case of osteomyelitis. There is a central area of bone destruction surrounded by a well-defined sclerotic border. There is a palisade-type of periosteal reaction and the lesion is sharply demarcated. Because of the site and degree of bone lysis, this might be interpreted as an osteosarcoma.

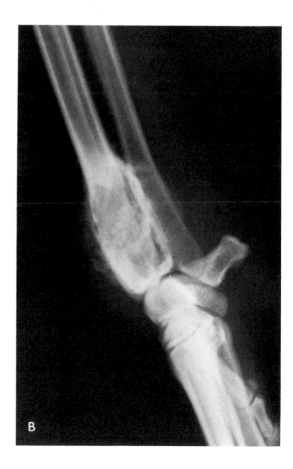

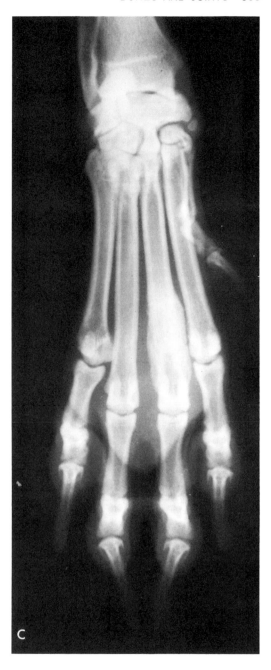

FIGURE 4–26 *Continued. C, D.* Osteomyelitis, due to coccidioidomycosis, in a large metacarpal bone. The lesion is primarily sclerotic in nature.

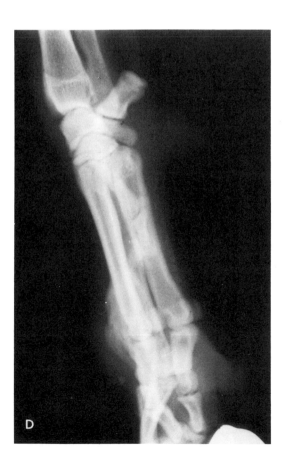

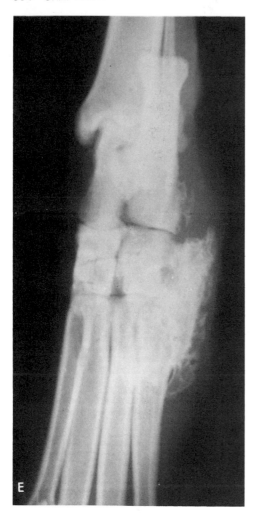

FIGURE 4–26 *Continued. E.* Osteomyelitis provoking a profuse periosteal reaction.

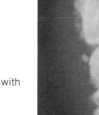

FIGURE 4–26 *Continued. F.* Periostitis associated with osteomyelitis.

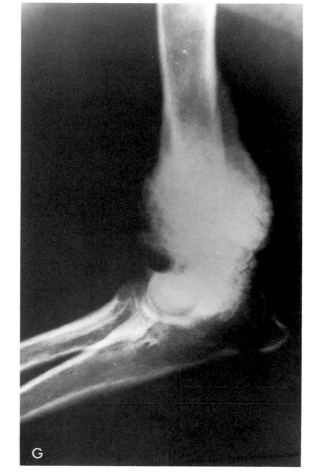

FIGURE 4–26 *Continued.* *G.* Coccidioidomycosis in a humerus.

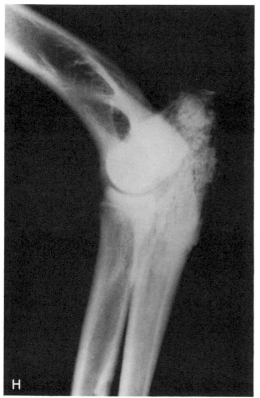

FIGURE 4–26 *Continued.* *H.* Blastomycosis in an ulna.

NEOPLASIA OF BONE

Bone neoplasia, while not common in dogs and cats, is nonetheless seen regularly, particularly in dogs. Diagnosis may present some difficulty. It is often quite impossible to diagnose the type of tumor present from a radiograph. Usually, however, a reasoned opinion can be given as to whether a neoplasm is malignant or benign.

Malignant Bone Tumors

RADIOLOGIC SIGNS OF MALIGNANCY

a. Bone destruction. Osteolysis is practically a consistent feature of malignancy. Loss of the normal trabecular pattern may be the first sign of disease. The cortex at the site of the tumor may be destroyed or at least expanded and thinned due to the growing neoplasm.

b. New bone formation. Accompanying bone destruction there is often disorganized new bone formation. The new bone may extend into and invade the surrounding soft tissues.

c. Indefinite outline. There is no clearly demarcated division between affected and normal bone. The lesion fades imperceptibly into normal bone.

d. Periosteal reaction. The periosteum becomes elevated at the site of the lesion and subperiosteal new bone formation occurs. A triangle of new bone is formed between the elevated periosteum, the shaft of the bone, and the lesion. This is Codman's triangle. (Fig. 4–4). It may also be seen in other conditions occasionally, for example in osteomyelitis.

e. Soft tissue swelling. There is usually an associated large soft tissue swelling that may be invaded by the tumor.

f. Poor reaction. There is failure of the tissue defenses to confine the lesion. The term "aggressive" is sometimes used to describe a lesion that is defeating the tissue defenses. Sclerosis, if present, is disorganized in distribution.

g. Pathologic fracture. Neoplastic bone breaks easily. A pathologic fracture may be the first clinical evidence of disease.

h. Metastases. Metastatic lesions may be found elsewhere in the body.

All the above signs are not always seen in any individual case. Some cases of osteomyelitis show many of the features of malignancy. (Fig. 4–27).

OSTEOSARCOMA (OSTEOGENIC SARCOMA)

This is the most common malignant bone tumor of dogs and cats. It is seen more commonly in the dog. Over 80 per cent of all bone malignancies in dogs are osteosarcomas. Most cases occur between the fifth and the ninth year of age. The large breeds are much more susceptible than the small breeds. It is rarely seen in dogs under 25 pounds in weight.

Three types of osteosarcoma can be distinguished:

1. Lytic type. (Osteoclastic). This is characterized by lysis or destruction of bone with little or no defensive response. There is early destruction of the cortex with extension into the surrounding soft tissues. Early metastatic spread is usual.

2. Sclerotic type. (Osteoblastic). The principal feature of this type is new bone formation with increased radiographic density of the affected bone.

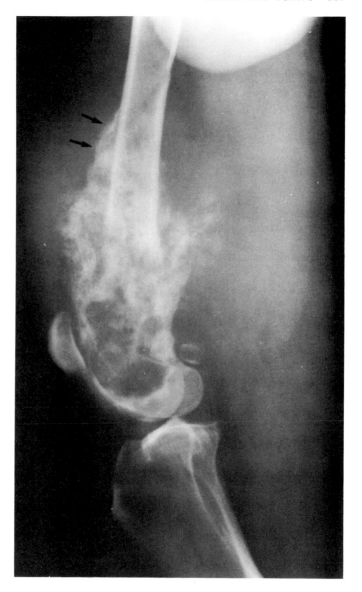

FIGURE 4–27. A characteristic malignant bone tumor. There are areas of lysis and areas of sclerosis. The cortex has been eroded and extension is occurring into the surrounding soft tissues. There is a large soft tissue swelling. A Codman's triangle is present (arrows). The lesion fades imperceptibly into the normal bone proximally without any line of demarcation. This was an osteosarcoma.

3. Mixed type. Areas of bone destruction and bone production are intermixed with one another. The bone has a disorganized appearance. This is the commonest type seen.

FEATURES OF OSTEOSARCOMA

a. Osteosarcoma will have many or all of the radiographic features of a malignant bone tumor. It usually arises in the medullary cavity.

b. Osteosarcoma occurs most commonly at predilection sites. These are the distal extremities of the radius, tibia, and femur and the proximal extremity of the humerus. Less commonly involved are the proximal femur and tibia, the skull, the vertebrae, the ribs, and the pelvis.

c. The lesion begins in the metaphysis but rarely crosses a joint space. The subchondral bone is usually spared.

d. About fifty per cent of cases show a so-called "sunburst" type of periosteal reaction. Spicules of periosteal new bone radiate outward from the cortex. (Fig.

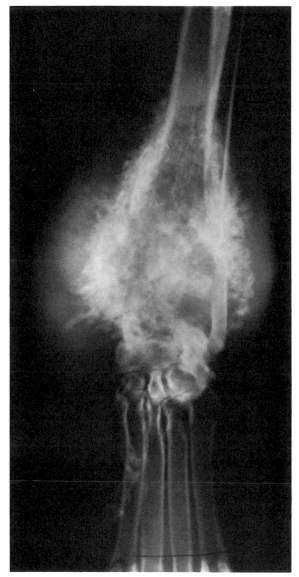

FIGURE 4–28. The classic "sunburst" appearance of an osteosarcoma. This appearance is not seen in all cases of osteosarcoma.

4–28). Periosteal reaction, without invasion, is often seen on adjacent bones, for example on the ulna if the radius is affected.

e. Osteosarcomas usually metastasize to the lungs. The tumor foci appear as rounded, discrete densities ("cannonball" metastases). Metastatic foci under about 1 cm in diameter may not be visible radiographically. Hence, failure to demonstrate metastases on chest radiographs does not mean that the lungs are free of the disease. Metastases to other bones are rare.

Multicentric osteosarcoma, that is, osteosarcoma arising in more than one bone at the same time, has been reported. Osteosarcoma may arise in soft tissue. This is occasionally seen in degeneration of mixed mammary tumors in the bitch. It may arise following esophageal infestation with *Spirocerca lupi*.

Parosteal osteosarcoma arises in the periosteum or parosteal connective tissue. It is uncommon. Masses of periosteal new bone surround the site. It is a slow-growing tumor. The cortex remains intact until late in the disease and metastatic spread is slow. An affected animal may survive for up to two years. (Fig. 4–29).

FIBROSARCOMA

This tumor is primarily lytic in nature and results in widespread bone destruction. It is slow growing and frequently invades an adjacent joint space.

CHONDROSARCOMA

Chondrosarcoma is a neoplasm of cartilage that primarily affects the flat bones, such as the ribs, the scapula, or the pelvis. Lysis of bone is a marked feature. Periosteal reaction is not prolific. Metastases develop slowly and less frequently than with osteosarcoma.

MULTIPLE MYELOMA

Myeloma is a tumor of cells of the type normally found in the bone marrow. It may affect bone. Lesions are seen at several sites and appear as sharply defined "punched-out" areas of lysis without any surrounding reaction.

METASTATIC LESIONS

It would appear that metastasis of neoplasms to bone is much rarer in the dog and cat than in man. Metastatic disease should be considered in the differential diagnosis of solitary destructive lesions especially if they occur at unusual sites. It is impossible, however, to differentiate a metastatic lesion from a primary bone tumor.

Other bone neoplasms, for example, reticulum cell sarcoma, hemangiosarcoma, and malignant synovioma, are occasionally seen. Attempts to differentiate one type of bone malignancy from another on radiographic evidence alone are not likely to be successful. The primary problem remains one of differentiating bone malignancy from osteomyelitis. (Fig. 4–30).

Text continued on page 316

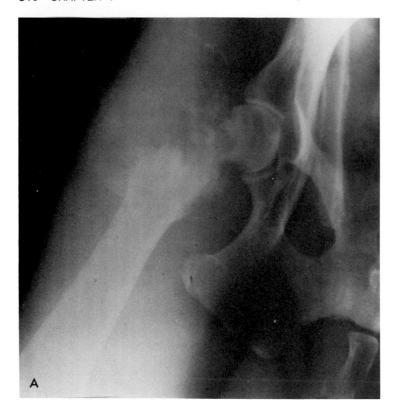

FIGURE 4–29. Some examples of osteosarcoma. *A.* A primarily lytic lesion in the proximal femur. There is gross cortical destruction and invasion of the surrounding soft tissues.

FIGURE 4–29 *Continued. B.* A sclerosing type of tumor. No lysis is evident and the lesion is fairly well demarcated.

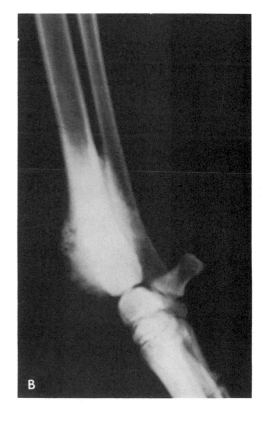

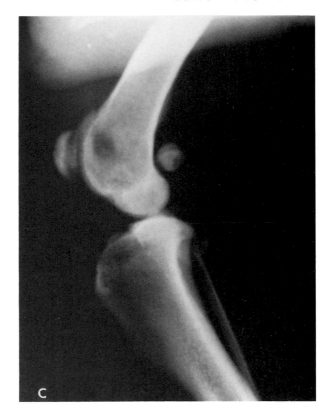

FIGURE 4-29 *Continued.* *C.* A small lytic lesion in the distal femur. There is no surrounding reaction.

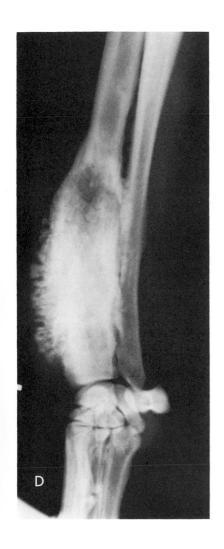

FIGURE 4-29 *Continued.* *D.* A mixed type of osteosarcoma. Areas of lysis and areas of sclerosis are intermixed. There is a palisade-type of periosteal reaction and a well marked Codman's triangle.

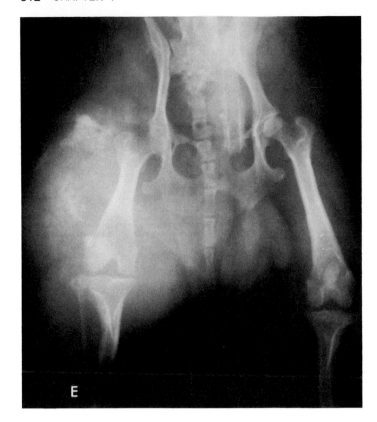

FIGURE 4–29 *Continued.* *E.* An osteosarcoma arising in the soft tissues of the thigh.

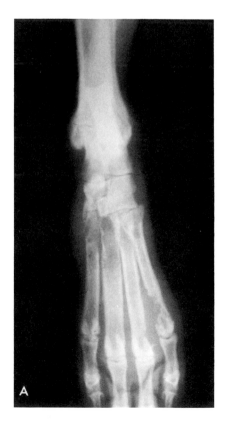

FIGURE 4–30. *A.* An undifferentiated sarcoma affecting the metatarsal bones.

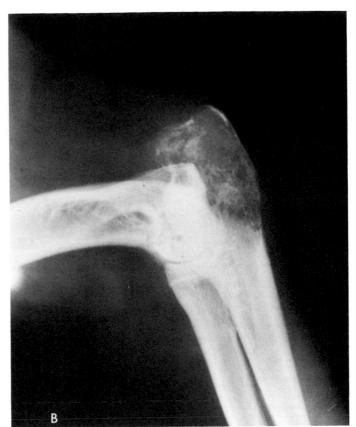

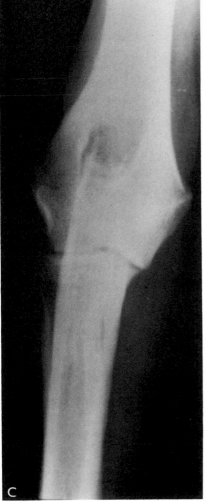

FIGURE 4–30 *Continued.   B, C.* A reticulum cell sarcoma affecting the ulna. There is loss of bone density in the olecranon on the craniocaudal view also.

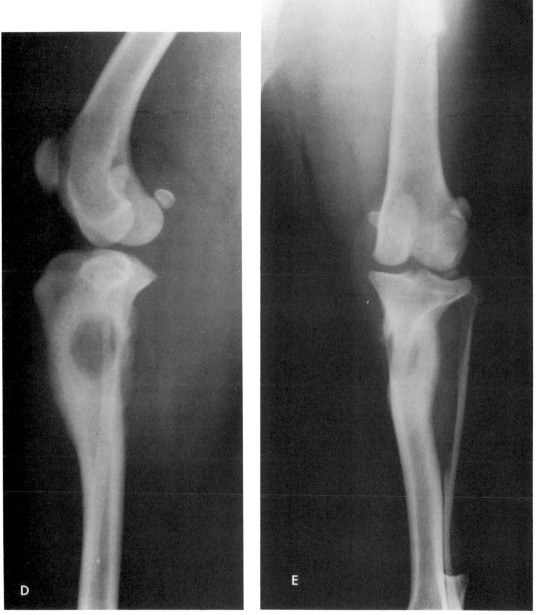

FIGURE 4–30 *Continued.   D, E.*   A fibrosarcoma in a tibia. A "window" effect is produced by bone lysis. The periosteal reaction is relatively mild.

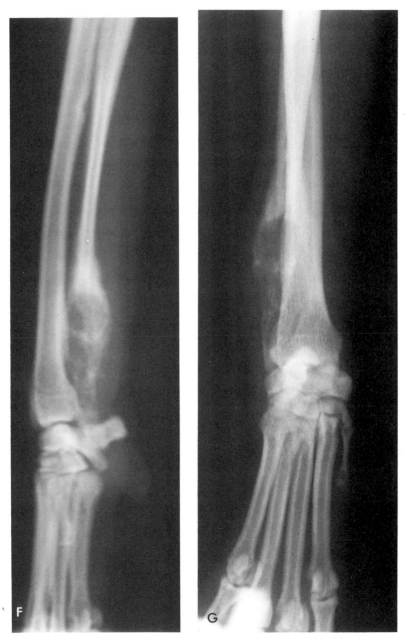

FIGURE 4–30 *Continued. F, G.* Hemangiosarcoma in an ulna. The lesion is primarily destructive. The radius is not involved.

Benign Bone Tumors

Benign bone tumors are rare in the dog and cat. The features of a benign tumor are as follows:

  a. It has well-demarcated edges.
  b. It provokes no periosteal reaction.
  c. It does not invade the surrounding soft tissues, though it may displace them.

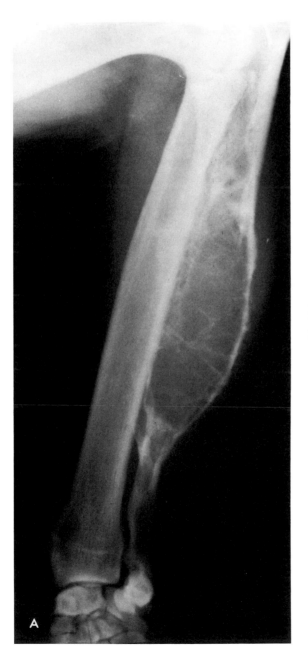

FIGURE 4–31. *A.* A large cystic lesion in the ulna. The lesion is expansile and has caused marked thinning of the cortex.

Bone cysts are rare. They may cause expansion of bone with loss of the normal trabecular pattern and a central area of radiolucency. They are sharply demarcated from the surrounding bone. The cortex is thinned and there is no accompanying bone reaction.

Multiple cartilaginous exostoses (osteochondroma) have been seen in dogs. They appear as protrusions in the metaphyses of bones and they grow with the developing skeleton. The cortex and medullary cavity of the affected bone are continuous with the tumor. Pressure on surrounding structures may cause symptoms. They cease to grow when the skeleton matures. (Fig. 4–31).

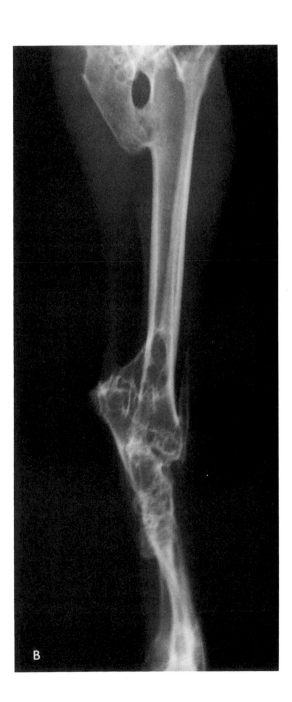

FIGURE 4–31 *Continued. B.* Multiple cartilaginous exostoses. The medullary cavity and cortex of the bone is continuous with that of the exostoses. In this case there were deformities of the adjacent joints.

Metabolic Bone Diseases

Bone is affected by changes in the composition of the circulating blood. Abnormalities of the body's metabolic processes may cause disease in bone. Changes in bone usually reflect severe, rather than mild, metabolic disturbances. It is said that the calcium content of bone must be reduced by about 50 per cent before radiographic changes become evident. Metabolic disease should be suspected when changes are seen in several bones. Solitary bone lesions are not likely to be due to metabolic causes.

JUVENILE OSTEODYSTROPHY

(Juvenile Osteoporosis. Osteodystrophia Fibrosa. Nutritional Osteodystrophy. Nutritional Secondary Hyperparathyroidism. Nutritional Osteoporosis.)

This condition is regularly seen in young dogs and cats. It affects animals fed exclusively, or almost exclusively, on meat. It is due to a deficiency of calcium, which may be aggravated by a high vitamin D intake. Excess intake of phosphorus will produce the same condition even in the presence of a sufficiency of calcium. Affected animals may appear to be well nourished but they often present with symptoms associated with locomotor impairment. This is usually due to pathologic fractures. Affected animals may be reluctant to stand or move. If capable of movement they do so gingerly and with difficulty. The term "osteogenesis imperfecta" for this condition is a misnomer, as the problem is dietary. Feeding a

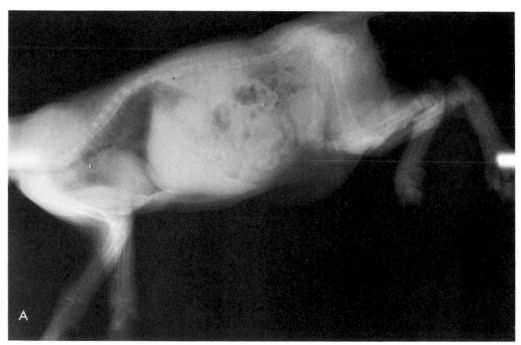

FIGURE 4–32. Juvenile Osteodystrophy. *A.* This radiograph of the skeleton of a three month old domestic cat shows the bones to be poorly mineralized. There is little contrast between the bones and the soft tissues. The spine is deformed in the lumbar region. There was splaying of the legs and hindquarter pain.

balanced diet results in rapid remineralization of the bones. Deformities due to fractures, however, may persist.

RADIOLOGIC SIGNS

a. Generalized skeletal demineralization (osteoporosis), in which the bones appear to have almost the same density as the soft tissues.

b. The cortices of the bones are extremely thin and "shell-like."

c. There is a thin line of increased density along the epiphyseal edge of the metaphysis.

d. The physes are normal in width.

e. Pathologic fractures are regularly seen. They are generally of the folding type; that is, there is practically no separation of the fractured ends, but the bone is bent in the manner of a greenstick fracture, one cortex often remaining intact. Old fractures appear as lines of increased density in the shaft of the bone.

f. Some long bones may have an abnormal shape due to malunion of earlier healed fractures.

g. The spine is often abnormal in shape particularly in the lumbar area. Compression fractures of vertebrae may occur. (Fig. 4–32).

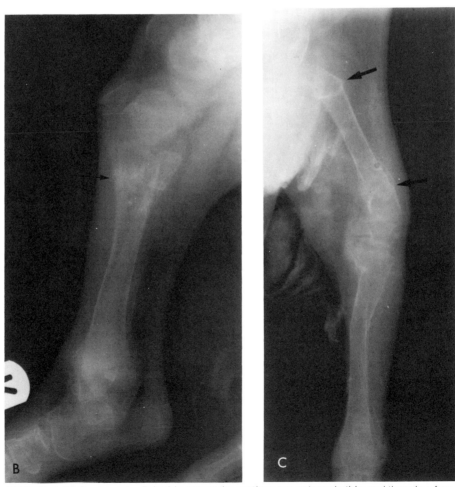

FIGURE 4–32 *Continued. B.* In this puppy the cortices are extremely thin and there is a fracture in the upper third of the tibia (arrow). *C.* This cat shows bowing of the tibia and the femur is fractured in two places (arrows).

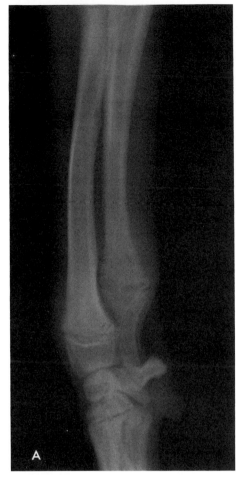

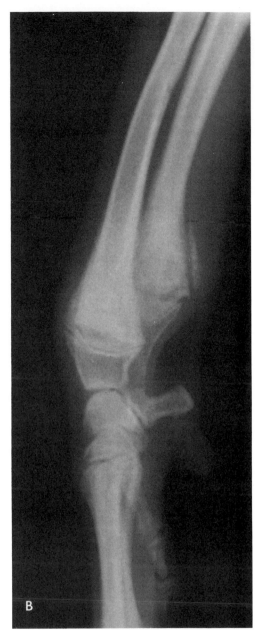

FIGURE 4-33. Hypertrophic Osteodystro-phy. *A.* Radiolucent bands are seen in the radial and ulnar metaphyses. There is some soft tissue swelling.

FIGURE 4-33 *Continued. B, C.* The same case eight days later. The radiolucent zones have become more marked, particularly in the radius. The metaphyses have a dense appearance. A cuff of ossified tissue is developing outside the ulnar cortex.

HYPERTROPHIC OSTEODYSTROPHY (JUVENILE SCURVY)

This is a disease of bone seen in young rapidly growing dogs of the larger breeds. Affected animals develop hot, painful swellings at the ends of the long bones, notably at the carpus and tarsus. There is accompanying anorexia and fever. Various opinions have been expressed as to the etiology. As vitamin C deficiency has been postulated as a cause, the term "juvenile scurvy" is sometimes applied to the condition.

RADIOLOGIC SIGNS

a. A radiolucent band appears in the metaphysis of an affected bone. (Trummel-feldzone).

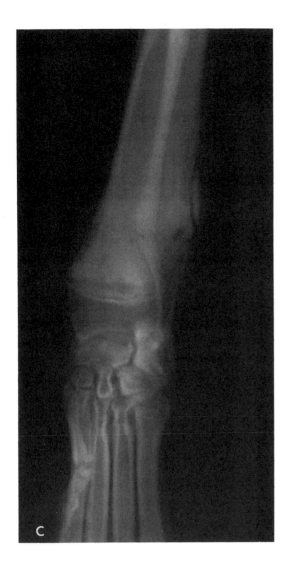

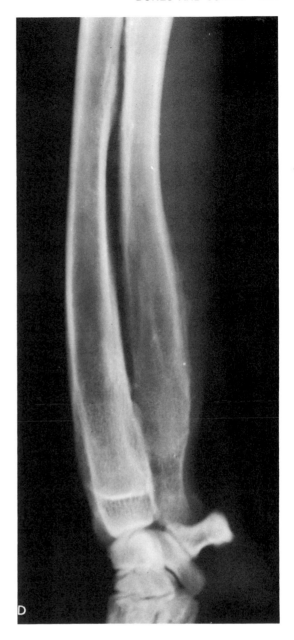

FIGURE 4–33 *Continued. D.* The healing phase. The cuffs are being incorporated into the bones, resulting in widening of the metaphyses.

 b. Within a week or ten days an irregular collar of bone forms around the metaphysis outside the cortex.

 c. As the disease progresses, the metaphysis becomes denser than normal and the trabecular pattern is lost.

 d. The physes remain normal in width.

 e. As the changes progress the collar of bone surrounding the metaphysis fuses with the shaft. The metaphysis appears widened as a result.

 f. Over a period of months remodeling of the bone occurs and the abnormalities gradually disappear. There may be some residual thickening of the shaft of the bone in the metaphyseal area.

  The disease is apparently self-limiting and eventual recovery is usual. (Fig. 4–33).

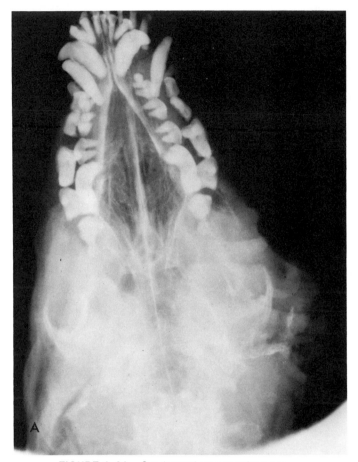

FIGURE 4–34. *See legend on opposite page.*

RENAL OSTEODYSTROPHY

(Rubber Jaw. Renal Rickets. Renal Osteitis Fibrosa. Renal Secondary Hyperparathyroidism).

A secondary hyperparathyroidism may result from renal insufficiency, causing phosphate retention. Increased parathormone secretion causes mineral withdrawal from the bones. The skull is usually affected first.

RADIOLOGIC SIGNS

a. There is a marked decrease in density of the bones of the skull. The teeth stand out very prominently because of loss of density in the skull bones. This gives an

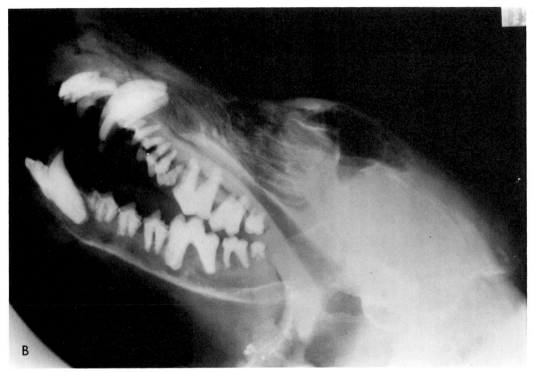

B

FIGURE 4–34. *A, B.* Gross demineralization of the skull due to renal osteodystrophy. The zygomatic arches have virtually disappeared and the mandibles are thinned. The teeth stand out prominently because of lack of bone density in the skull.

appearance of "floating teeth." Loss of the lamina dura, the dense bone outside the peridontal membrane, is first noted in early cases.

b. The mandibles appear to be grossly thinned and in places may be radiographically absent. The zygomatic arches are similarly affected.

c. The normal trabecular patterns of the skull bones are lost.

d. Elsewhere some demineralization of bone may be noted, subperiosteal bone resorption in particular. This gives a flat, reticulated, or lace-like, appearance to bone in that area. This sign is not always seen.

e. Dystrophic calcification in the soft tissues is occasionally seen. (Fig. 4–34).

HYPERTROPHIC PULMONARY OSTEOARTHROPATHY

(Hypertrophic Osteoarthropathy. Hypertrophic Osteopathy).

This is a response in bone to chronic disease in an intrathoracic structure. It has also been described associated with carcinoma of the bladder. It may be seen associated with neoplasia of the lungs whether primary or secondary, with chronic infectious diseases, or with lung abscess. The exact causal mechanism is obscure. It may be associated with circulatory disturbances.

RADIOLOGIC SIGNS

a. Periosteal new bone formation is seen along the shafts of the long bones and the phalanges. The earliest changes are seen in the phalanges. The small bones of the carpus and tarsus are less severely affected.

b. The new bone is laid down at right angles to the long axis of the bone in so-called "palisade" fashion. This gives the bone an irregular appearance. Individual areas of a bone may be more severely affected than others.

c. As the disease progresses the new bone tends to become smooth.

d. If the pulmonary disease is successfully treated the bony lesions rapidly regress. Vagotomy on the side of the thoracic lesion results in regression of the bone changes (Fig. 4–35).

HYPERVITAMINOSIS A

Cats fed excess amounts of liver may suffer from hypervitaminosis A and a mineral imbalance characterized by a gross calcium deficiency and excess phosphorus. The presenting symptoms depend on the location of the lesions. They include stiffness, reluctance to move, abnormal posture, foreleg or hindleg lameness, and constipation. Cats between two and four years of age are most commonly affected.

RADIOLOGIC SIGNS

a. New bone formation is seen on the vertebrae, especially in the cervical area. The lumbar and thoracic vertebrae may also be involved. The rest of the skeleton may exhibit varying degrees of demineralization.

b. The new bone formation is most clearly seen on the ventral aspects of the vertebral bodies. This should not be confused with the spondylosis sometimes seen in older cats. Generally, the lesions associated with hypervitaminosis A are larger and more extensive than they are in spondylosis.

c. New bone formation may occur at other sites, such as around the shoulder, elbow, and stifle joints, and on the pelvis.

d. Periarticular ankylosis of the vertebral joints develops as the disease progresses.

e. Disuse osteoporosis may be evident, particularly in the bones of the forelimb.

f. Isolated skeletal lesions may be confused with neoplasms. (Fig. 4–36).

RICKETS

It is now generally believed that rickets is rarely seen clinically in the dog and cat. The disease is characterized by a failure of mineralization of the cartilaginous matrix at the epiphyseal plate. It may be due to a deficiency of calcium, phosphorus, or vitamin D.

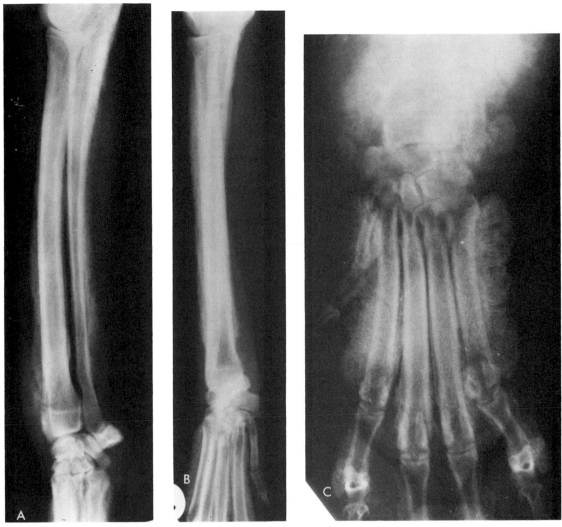

FIGURE 4–35. Hypertrophic Pulmonary Osteoarthropathy. *A, B.* Periosteal new bone formation can be seen along the lengths of the radius and ulna. A palisade-type of periosteal reaction is seen on the metacarpal bones. *C.* A gross example.

RADIOLOGIC SIGNS

a. Widening of the physes is usually seen. Normally it is but a few millimeters in width. The plate appears to be irregular in outline.

b. The metaphyseal edge of the bone at the physis becomes wider than usual, irregular in outline, and concave, giving a mushroom effect to the bone in that area.

c. Long bones may show some degree of demineralization and bending or bowing may be present. (Fig. 4–37).

"IDIOPATHIC OSTEODYSTROPHY"

Normal variations in the metaphyses of young dogs have been called "Idiopathic Osteodystrophy." Some dogs, particularly of the larger breeds, show a wide

Text continued on page 329

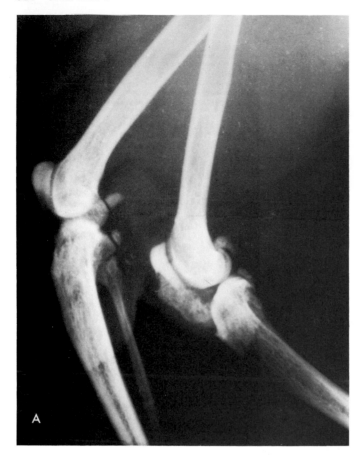

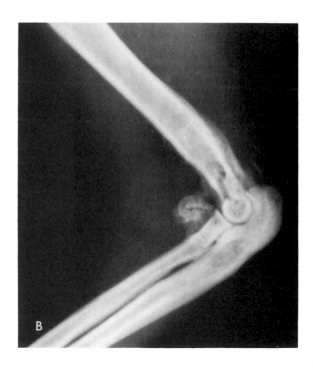

FIGURE 4-36. *A. B.* Hypervitaminosis A. Radiographs of an adult cat fed almost exclusively on liver and heart. It became progressively lame on all limbs. The trabecular patterns are coarse, the cortices are thickened, and there is calcification in the soft tissues around the stifle and the elbow. (Courtesy of Dr. Wayne Riser).

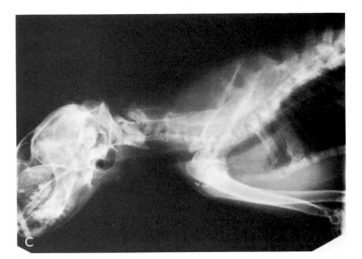

FIGURE 4–36 *Continued.* C. Hypervitaminosis A. New bone formation on the cervical and thoracic vertebrae of a cat being fed exclusively on liver.

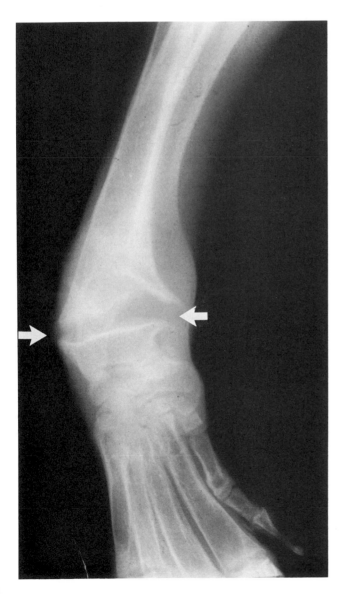

FIGURE 4–37. Rickets in a dog. The distal radial physis is widened (arrows) and the metaphysis has an irregular, flared and concave edge. The bones appear osteoporotic. (Courtesy of Dr. Wayne Riser).

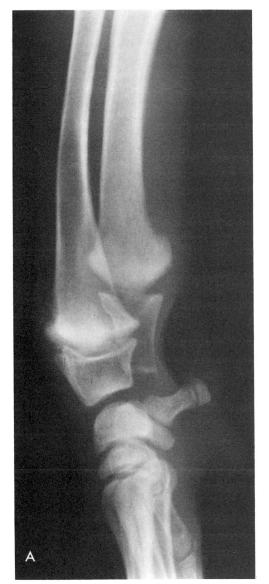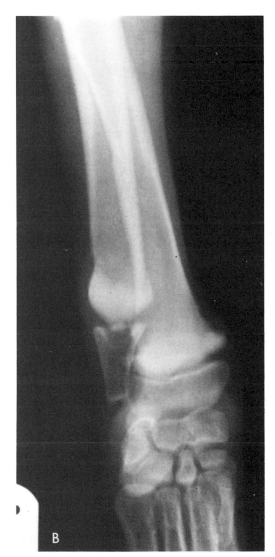

FIGURE 4–38 *A, B.* Idiopathic osteodystrophy.

metaphyseal edge at the physis. The metaphysis is increased in density. The bone edge adjacent to the metaphysis may be irregular in outline on the diaphyseal side. The epiphysis and the physis appear to be normal. In normal dogs there may be considerable variation in the density of the metaphysis adjacent to the physis. (Fig. 4–38).

The significance of these changes is not apparent and it is probable that they do not constitute a clinical entity. They are frequently misdiagnosed as rickets.

Specific Bone Diseases

AVASCULAR NECROSIS OF THE FEMORAL HEAD

(Legg-Perthes Disease. Legg-Calvé-Perthes Disease. Osteochondritis Deformans Juvenilis. Osteochondrosis. Coxa Plana).

Young dogs under one year of age, of the smaller breeds, may be affected by this disease. The etiology is uncertain. There is a local ischemia of bone in the femoral head. The presenting sign is lameness, often intermittent, with frequently some degree of atrophy of the muscles about the hip. It is usually unilateral but bilateral involvement is not uncommon.

RADIOLOGIC SIGNS

a. Areas of decreased bone density are seen in the femoral head and, in some cases, in the femoral neck. Early cases may show areas of increased density due to trabecular collapse.

b. The joint space of the hip becomes wider than normal.

c. The femoral head loses its rounded contour and becomes flattened, particularly cranially. The areas of decreased density become more marked as the disease progresses.

d. The acetabulum becomes shallow and its cranial edge becomes flattened to accommodate the changing shape of the femoral head. Sclerosis of the acetabular subchondral bone may occur.

e. Fragmentation of the femoral head may appear with discontinuity of the articular surface.

f. The femoral neck becomes thicker and secondary degenerative joint changes develop with new bone formation.

g. A varus deformity may develop; that is, the angle between the femoral neck and the shaft of the femur becomes smaller.

All the above changes are not necessarily seen in any one individual case. (Fig. 4–39).

OSTEOCHONDRITIS DISSECANS (OSTEOCHONDROSIS)

Osteochondritis dissecans may affect the shoulder joint in large dogs. It usually occurs between the fourth and the ninth month of age. It is characterized by shoulder lameness. Not infrequently it is bilateral; both shoulders should be examined if the condition is suspected.

A small defect appears in the subchondral bone at the caudal third of the humeral head. It may be covered, or partially covered, by a piece of dead articular cartilage. The distal humerus and the femoral condyles are less commonly affected.

Three views of the shoulder joint are advisable to demonstrate the caudal third

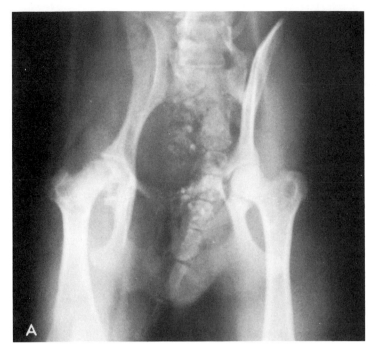

FIGURE 4–39. Legg-Perthes disease. *A.* Areas of decreased density are seen in the right femoral head and neck. The femoral head is misshapen and compensatory changes are occurring in the acetabulum

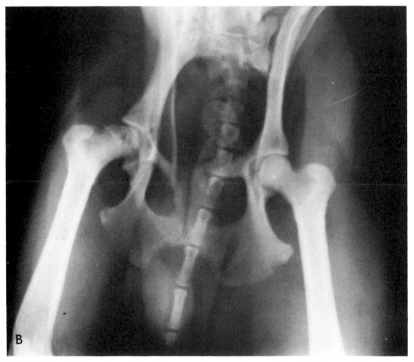

FIGURE 4–39 *Continued. B.* A more advanced case. The right femoral head has lost its rounded contour. The neck is thickened. The cranial acetabular edge is flattened. The joint space is widened and the head does not sit well into the acetabulum.

of the humeral head adequately: a mediolateral view, a mediolateral view with the limb rotated cranially, and a mediolateral view with the limb rotated caudally. Sedation is advisable, as these movements may be resented. Both shoulders should be examined. Arthrography may be useful, especially in the demonstration of a flap of cartilage over the bone defect. (See page 372).

RADIOLOGIC SIGNS

a. A defect is seen in the subchondral bone in the caudal third of the humeral head.

b. The defect frequently has a sclerotic margin.

c. A loose flap of calcified cartilage may be identified over the defect. This is not always seen.

d. Radiopaque fragments of calcified cartilage may be seen lying free within the joint capsule, usually in the caudal recess. Such bodies are termed "joint mice." They may increase in size over a period of time even though they have no attachments within the joint.

e. Advanced cases show degenerative changes in and about the joint. (Fig. 4–40).

CRANIOMANDIBULAR OSTEOARTHROPATHY

(Craniomandibular Osteopathy. Mandibular Periostitis. Craniomandibular Osteodystrophy).

This disease, of unknown etiology, is seen in young West Highland white terriers. Less frequently affected are Boston, Scottish, and Cairn terriers and more rarely other small breeds. There have been isolated reports of its occurrence in large breeds. Affected animals are usually under two years of age. The presenting signs are difficulty and pain in opening the mouth and in chewing food. The pain may be intense. Affected animals may recover after a period of several months, while some animals have to be euthanized because of inability to feed. The condition has to be distinguished from eosinophilic myositis.

RADIOLOGIC SIGNS

a. Periosteal new bone formation and sclerosis are seen affecting both mandibles, which are thickened and irregular in appearance.

b. Masses of new bone formation are seen in the area of the tympanic bullae of the petrous temporal bone. The occipital bones are similarly affected. (Fig. 4–41).

c. Some cases may show changes in the limbs similar to those seen in hypertrophic osteodystrophy. (See page 320).

PANOSTEITIS

(Canine Panosteitis. Enostosis. Eosinophilic Panosteitis. Juvenile Osteomyelitis.).

This is a disease of the long bones that affects the larger breeds of dogs, notably the German Shepherd (Alsatian). Most cases occur between the fifth and the twenty-fourth month of age, though animals up to five years old may be affected. Males are more commonly affected than are females. The etiology is unknown and the disease is self-limiting.

The presenting sign is usually a "shifting-leg" lameness, the lameness occurring first in one limb and then in another. Affected bones are painful to deep palpation. The humerus, radius and ulna, and the femur are most commonly affected.

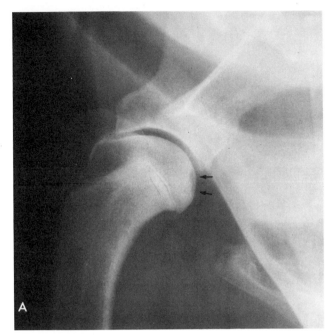

FIGURE 4–40. Osteochondritis dissecans in the humeral head. *A.* A radiolucent defect is seen in the caudal third of the humeral head (arrows).

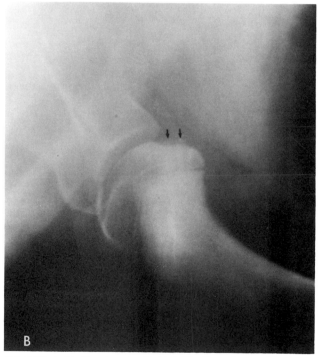

FIGURE 4–40 *Continued.* *B.* Calcification of a cartilaginous flap (arrows). The flap covers a large defect in the subchondral bone.

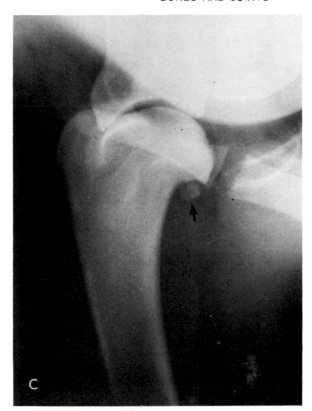

FIGURE 4–40 *Continued. C.* A cartilaginous flap is free in the caudal pouch of the joint capsule (arrow).

RADIOLOGIC SIGNS

a. Areas of increased bone density appear within the medullary cavity of an affected bone, particularly in the region of the nutrient foramen.

b. Loss of the normal trabecular pattern and accentuation of the areas of increased density tend to give a mottled or patchy appearance to the medullary cavity.

c. Coarse trabeculae arise from the endosteal surface of the cortex.

d. Bones that have been affected for some time may show a smooth type of periosteal reaction. The reaction is not very prolific and it is not seen in all cases.

e. As the disease progresses the abnormal densities gradually disappear but the endosteal face of the cortex remains irregular. As the patchy densities disappear the medullary cavity becomes more radiolucent than normal and coarse trabeculation may be noted.

f. There may be some slight residual cortical thickening. (Fig. 4–42).

ARTERIOVENOUS FISTULA

An arteriovenous fistula is a communication between an artery and a vein that bypasses the capillaries. It may be congenital or acquired due to trauma. It is rare in dogs and even rarer in cats. Arteriovenous fistula may affect bone, causing a mild periosteal reaction and some loss of bone density in the region of the fistula. A large fistula may cause pain in the limb, lameness, and ulceration. Pulsation may be felt in a peripheral vein. A small fistula may pass unnoticed. Angiography is required to demonstrate the lesion. (Fig. 4–43).

Text continued on page 338

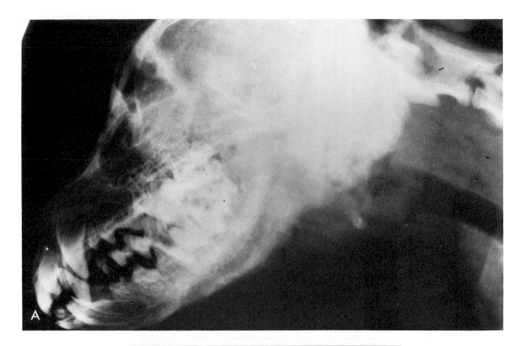

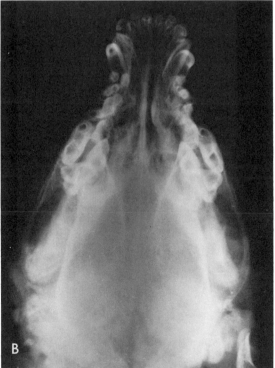

FIGURE 4–41 *A. B.* Craniomandibular osteopathy. Masses of new bone can be seen around the petrous temporal bone and along the rami of the mandibles.

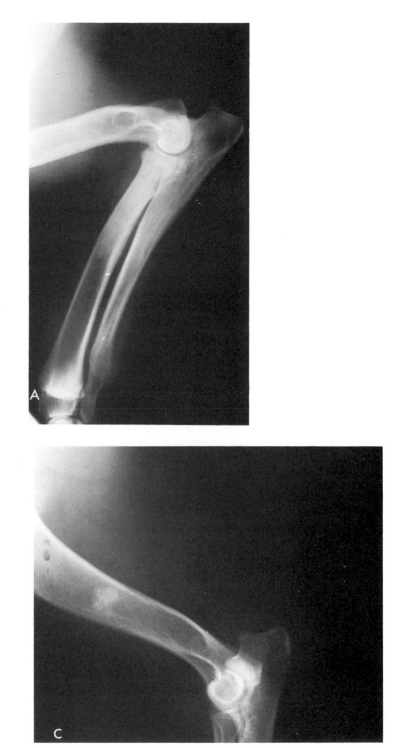

FIGURE 4–42. Canine panosteitis. *A.* Areas of increased density can be seen in the medullary cavities of both the radius and ulna. *B.* Lesions of panosteitis extending into the distal third of the tibia. *C.* A lesion in the mid-humerus that has almost healed. The trabecular pattern is coarse and the endosteum appears irregular.

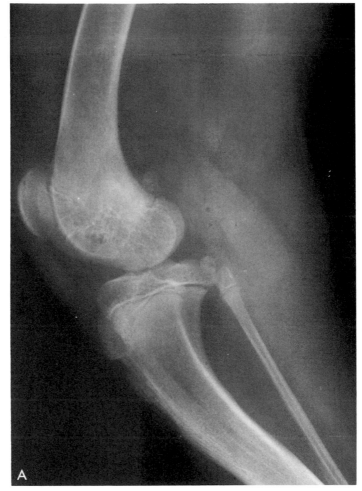

FIGURE 4–43. Arteriovenous fistula. *A.* The trabecular pattern in the epiphyses of the femur and tibia is coarse and there is loss of normal bone density.

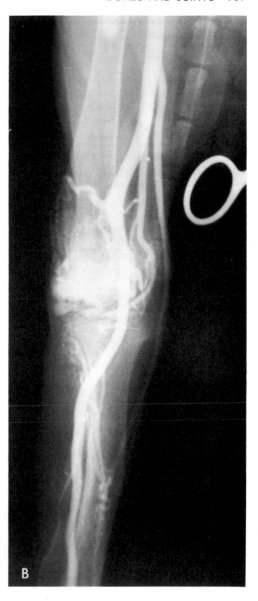

FIGURE 4–43 *Continued.*   *B.*   An angiogram shows a massive proliferation of vessels due to an arteriovenous fistula.

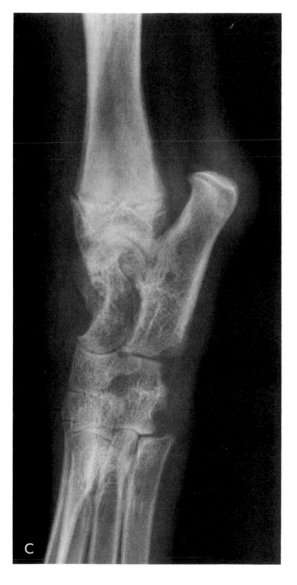

FIGURE 4–43 *Continued.*   *C.*   The hock of the same animal showing loss of bone density and coarse trabeculation. A second fistula was present at the hock. There was pulsation in the saphenous vein.

JOINTS

A synovial (diarthrodial) joint consists of two opposing bone surfaces each covered by articular cartilage and surrounded by a joint capsule. The inner layer of the joint capsule, or synovial membrane, secretes synovial fluid, a thin layer of which separates the opposing articular cartilages. Some synovial joints contain intra-articular ligaments, menisci, fat pads, or synovial projections.

The articular cartilages, the synovial fluid, and the joint capsule are not visible on radiographs. The subchondral bone, which is visible, merges smoothly with the cortex of the metaphysis. The joints in young animals appear to be much wider than those of the adult. This is because the immature, largely cartilaginous epiphysis is not fully visualized. The ossifying epiphysis often has an irregular outline that should not be mistaken for an abnormality.

Joint Abnormalities

LUXATIONS (DISLOCATIONS)

Luxations usually present no problems of diagnosis, provided adequate radiographic studies are available. The articular surfaces of the joint are seen to be displaced. Two views, at right angles to one another, are necessary for a proper evaluation of the degree and direction of the displacement. Luxations may easily be missed if only one view is relied on. A careful search should be made to detect small fracture fragments associated with a luxation, as they may interfere with attempts at reduction.

Anatomic abnormalities of joint surfaces would suggest that a luxation may be congenital. Comparison with the opposite limb, if it is normal, is advisable.

Subluxations are more difficult to evaluate than frank luxations. Views made with the animal bearing weight on the affected limb, if that is possible, may show a displacement not seen on a conventional radiograph. (Figs. 4–44 to 4–50; see also Fig. 4–8).

OSTEOARTHROSIS (OSTEOARTHRITIS)

Degenerative joint disease is more common than inflammatory disease and so the term osteoarthrosis should probably be preferred to osteoarthritis. Osteoarthrosis may result from many causes, including advancing age, injury, and any condition that puts excessive stress on a joint.

RADIOLOGIC SIGNS

a. Lipping of the joint margins with osteophyte formation.

b. Sclerosis of the subchondral bone. This results from wear of the articular cartilage and consequent increased stress on the subchondral bone.

c. Narrowing of the joint space may occur, though this is not a common finding in dogs and cats.

d. Cystic areas may develop in the subchondral bone. This is not common.

e. Subluxation may occur. This may be evident only on weight-bearing studies.

f. The disease may be secondary to a primary joint abnormality, for example osteoarthrosis associated with hip dysplasia.

g. Distention of the joint capsule may displace fascial planes in the neighborhood. This is most frequently noted around the stifle joint.

h. Remodeling of joint surfaces is frequently seen. (Fig. 4–51).

Text continued on page 369

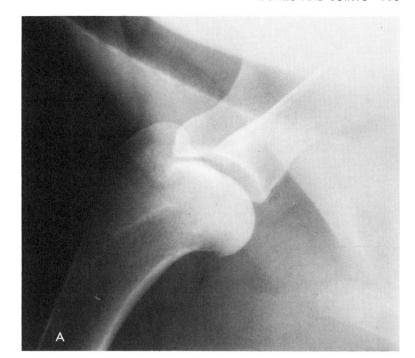

FIGURE 4–44. *A.* The shoulder joint.

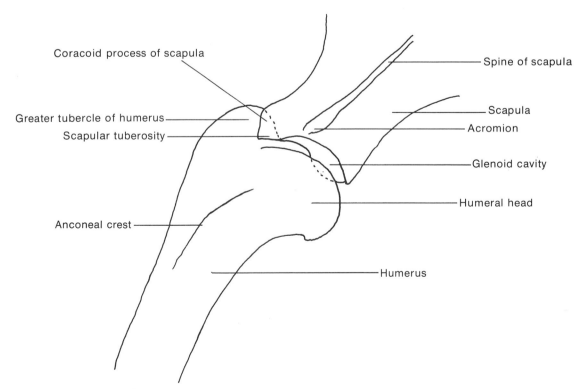

Coracoid process of scapula

Spine of scapula

Greater tubercle of humerus

Scapula

Scapular tuberosity

Acromion

Glenoid cavity

Humeral head

Anconeal crest

Humerus

FIGURE 4–44 *Continued.* *B.* Lateral view of a normal shoulder joint.

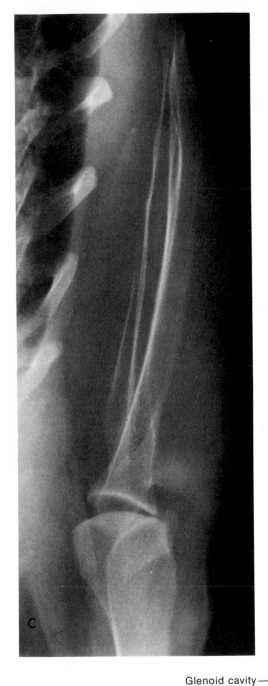

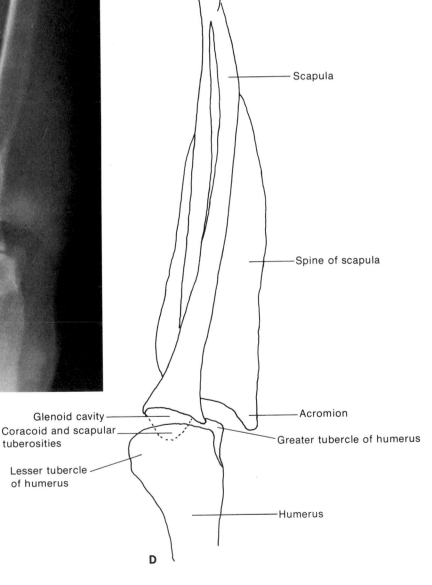

FIGURE 4–44 *Continued.* *C, D.* Craniocaudal view of a normal shoulder joint.

Scapula

Spine of scapula

Glenoid cavity

Coracoid and scapular tuberosities

Lesser tubercle of humerus

Acromion

Greater tubercle of humerus

Humerus

FIGURE 4–44 *Continued. E, F.* Lateral and craniocaudal views of the shoulder of a cat. A rudimentary clavicle is present (arrows).

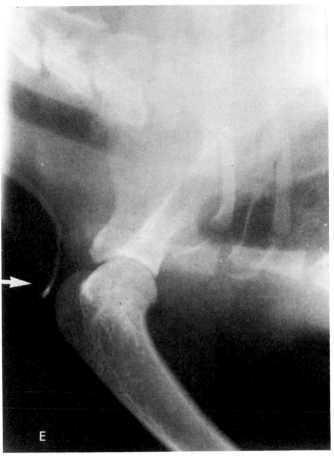

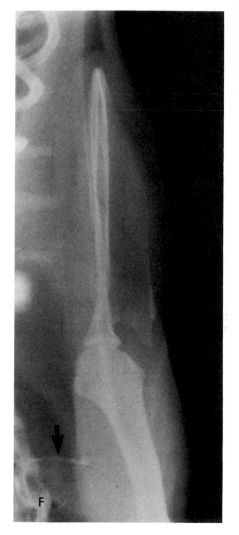

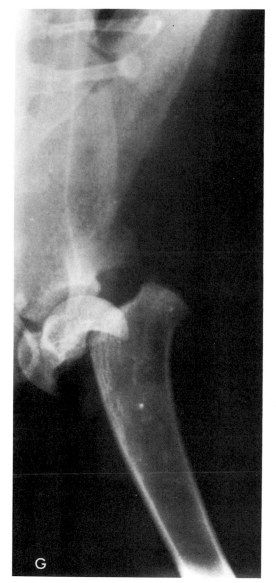

FIGURE 4–44 *Continued.* G. Separation of a fractured proximal humeral epiphysis in a cat.

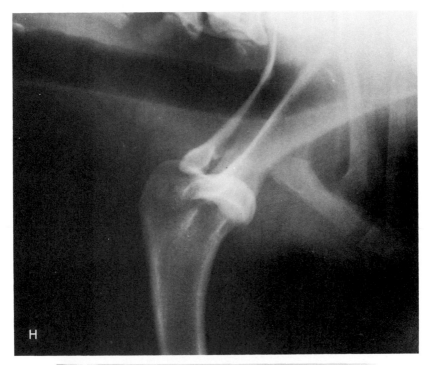

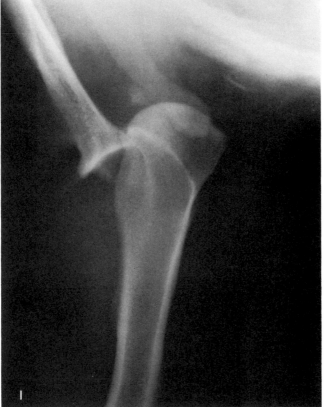

FIGURE 4–44 *Continued.* *H, I.* Luxation of the shoulder joint. The displacement can easily be missed on a lateral view.

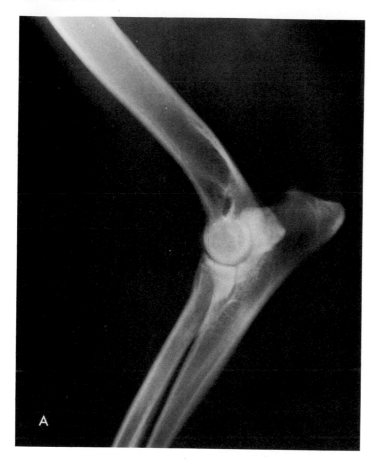

FIGURE 4–45 *A, B.* Lateral view of the elbow joint.

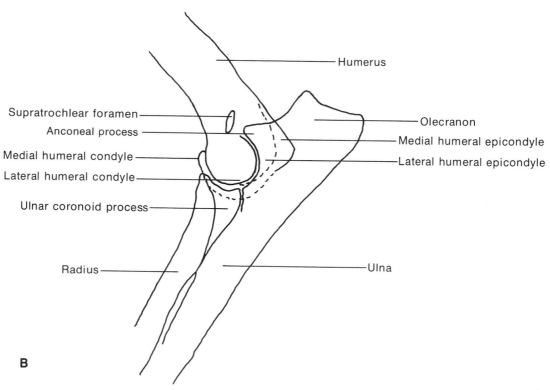

Humerus

Supratrochlear foramen

Olecranon

Anconeal process

Medial humeral epicondyle

Medial humeral condyle

Lateral humeral epicondyle

Lateral humeral condyle

Ulnar coronoid process

Radius

Ulna

B

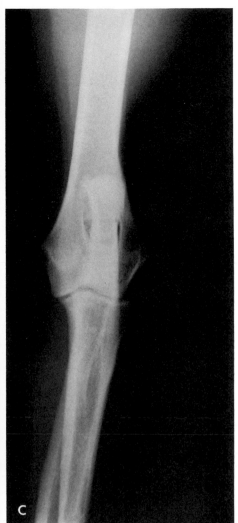

C

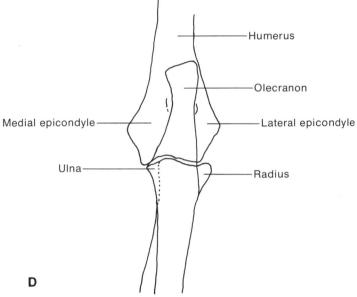

FIGURE 4–45 *Continued.* *C, D.* Craniocaudal view of the elbow joint.

Humerus

Olecranon

Medial epicondyle

Lateral epicondyle

Ulna

Radius

D

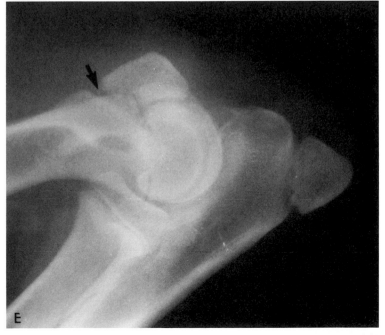

FIGURE 4–45 *Continued.* *E.* Elbow joint of an immature dog. Note the growth plate associated with the medial epicondyle of the humerus (arrow).

E

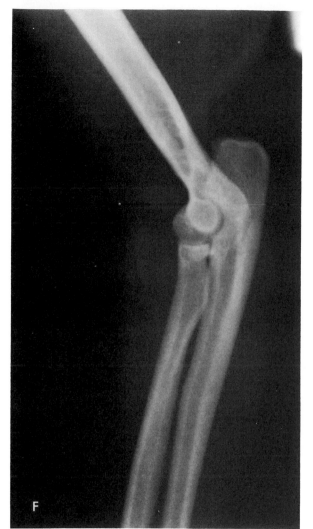

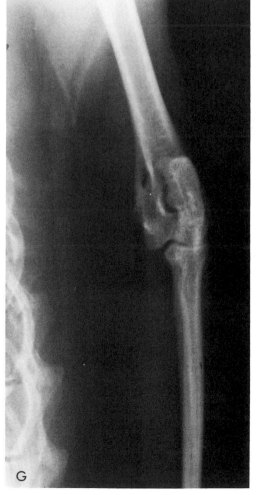

FIGURE 4–45 *Continued.* *F, G.* The elbow of a cat.

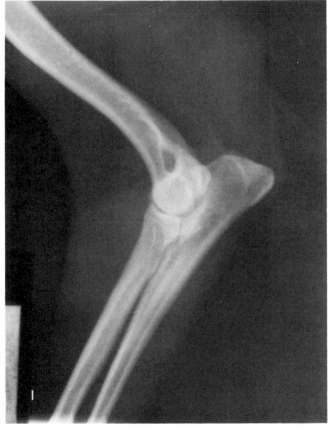

FIGURE 4–45 *Continued.* *H, I.* Subluxation of the elbow joint. The displacement is not visible on the lateral view.

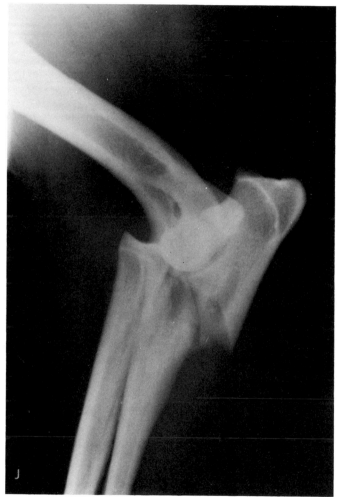

FIGURE 4-45 *Continued.* *J.* Dislocation of the elbow joint associated with a fracture of the ulna. (Monteggia's fracture).

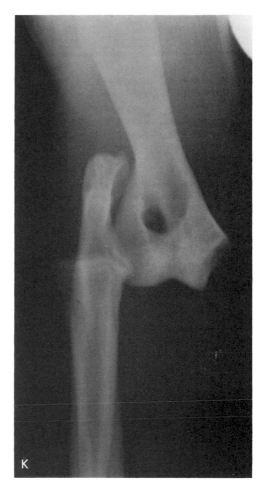

FIGURE 4–45 *Continued.* *K, L.* Luxation of the elbow joint without an associated fracture.

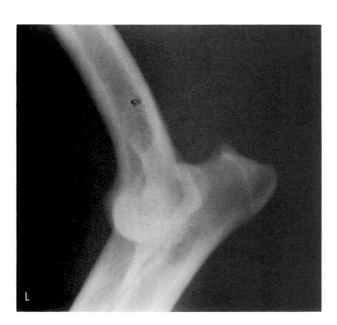

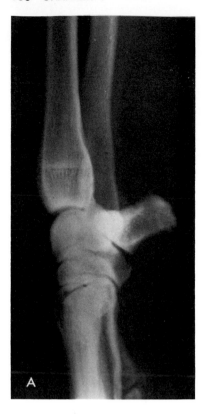

FIGURE 4–46 *A, B.* Lateral view of the carpus.

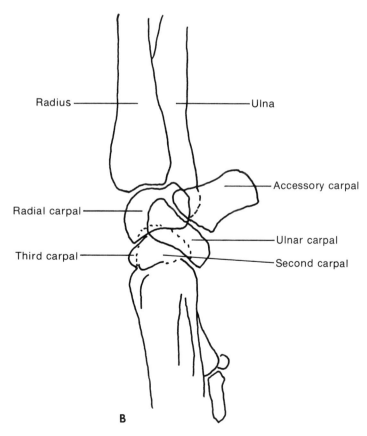

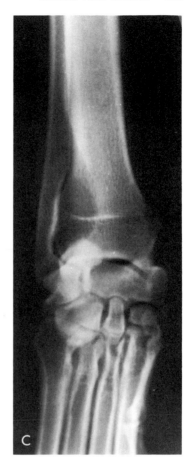

FIGURE 4–46 *Continued.   C, D.* Dorsopalmar view of the carpus.

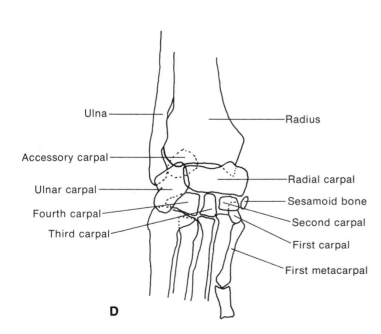

Ulna

Accessory carpal

Ulnar carpal

Fourth carpal

Third carpal

Radius

Radial carpal

Sesamoid bone

Second carpal

First carpal

First metacarpal

D

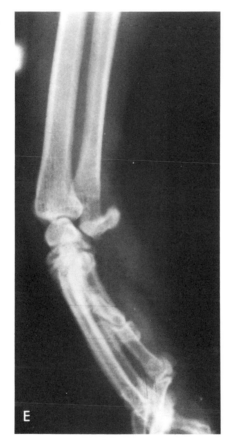

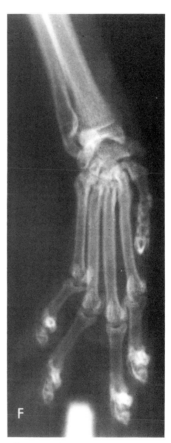

FIGURE 4–46 *Continued.* *E, F.* Carpus of a cat.

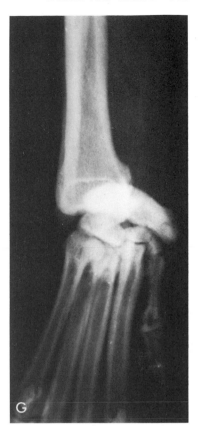

FIGURE 4–46 *Continued.* G. Luxation of the radiocarpal joint.

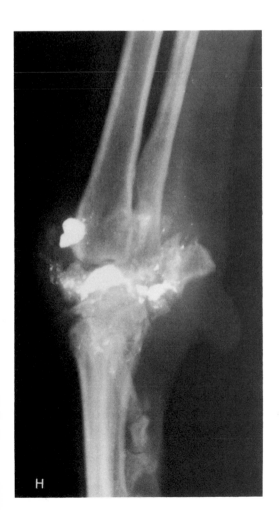

FIGURE 4–46 *Continued.* H. Severe damage to the carpus caused by a high velocity bullet.

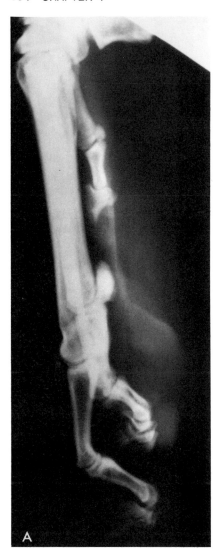

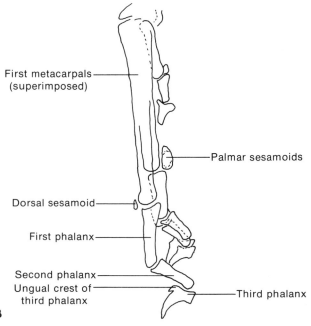

FIGURE 4–47 *A, B.* Lateral view of the metacarpus.

First metacarpals (superimposed)

Palmar sesamoids

Dorsal sesamoid

First phalanx

Second phalanx

Ungual crest of third phalanx

Third phalanx

B

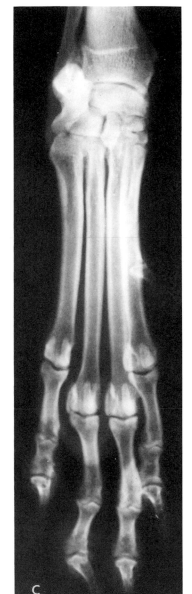

FIGURE 4–47 *Continued.* *C, D.* Dorsopalmar view of the metacarpus.

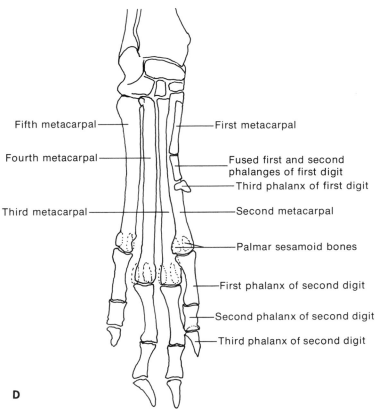

Fifth metacarpal————————————First metacarpal

Fourth metacarpal————————————Fused first and second
phalanges of first digit

——Third phalanx of first digit

Third metacarpal————————————Second metacarpal

——Palmar sesamoid bones

——First phalanx of second digit

——Second phalanx of second digit

——Third phalanx of second digit

C

D

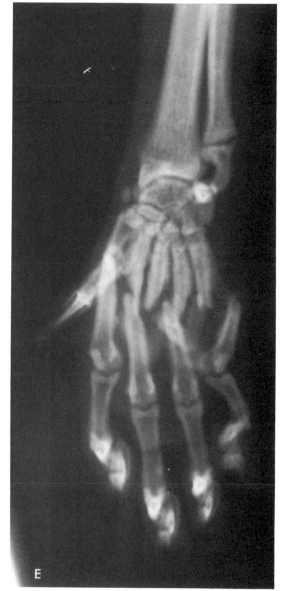

FIGURE 4–47 *Continued. E.* Multiple fractures of the metacarpal bones in a cat.

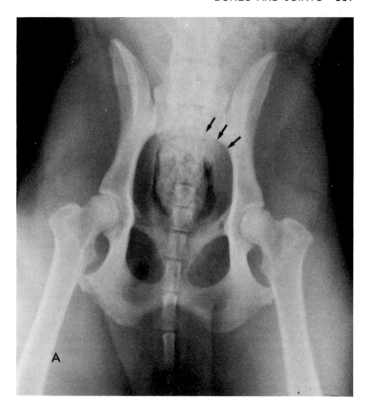

FIGURE 4–48A. A normal pelvis of a dog. Note how the line of the inner aspect of the shaft of the ilium blends smoothly with the line of the sacrum (arrows). The sacroiliac joint may disrupt the continuity of the line but not its direction.

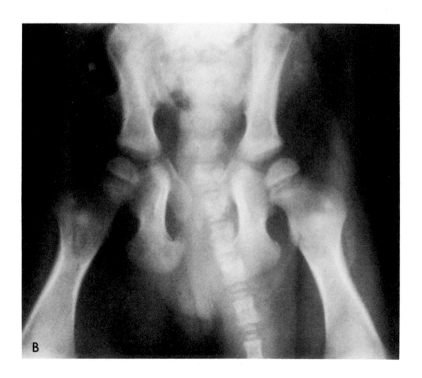

FIGURE 4–48 Continued. B. Pelvis of an immature dog. Note the wide joint spaces and the several physes. Cartilaginous ossification centers at the caudal aspect of the ischium and the cranial aspect of the ilium may not fuse with the pelvis until the dog is several years old. Closure of the pelvic symphysis may be likewise delayed.

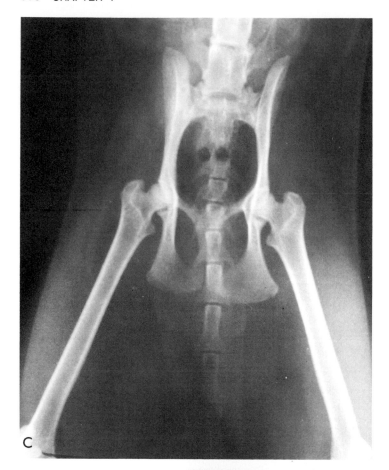

FIGURE 4–48 *Continued.* *C.* Normal pelvis of a cat. The pelvis is slightly rotated.

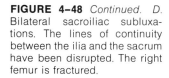

FIGURE 4–48 *Continued.* *D.* Bilateral sacroiliac subluxations. The lines of continuity between the ilia and the sacrum have been disrupted. The right femur is fractured.

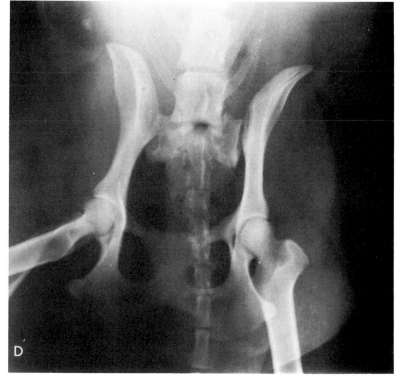

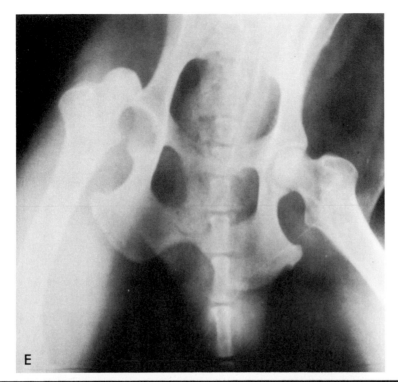

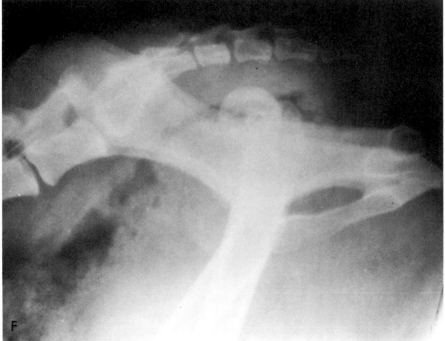

FIGURE 4–48 *Continued.* *E, F.* Luxation of the right hip joint of a dog. The lateral view is necessary to determine the direction and degree of displacement in the vertical plane.

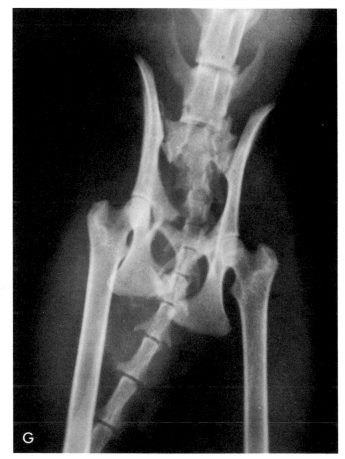

FIGURE 4–48 *Continued. G.* Severe damage to the pelvis of a cat. There are fractures of the pubis and ischium on the right side and the right sacroiliac joint is subluxated.

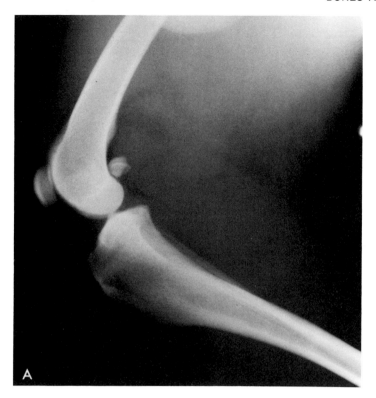

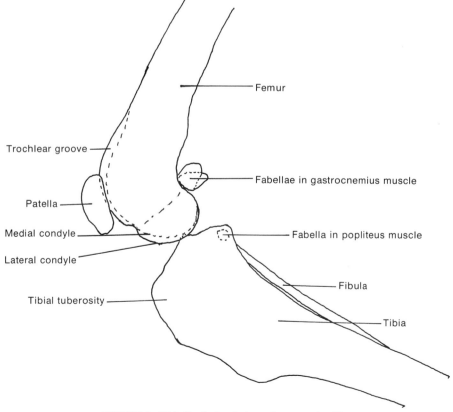

Femur

Trochlear groove

Fabellae in gastrocnemius muscle

Patella

Medial condyle

Fabella in popliteus muscle

Lateral condyle

Fibula

Tibial tuberosity

Tibia

FIGURE 4–49 *A, B.* Lateral view of a normal stifle.

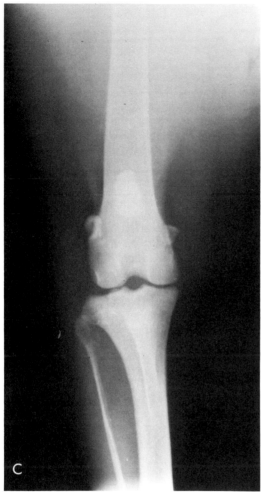

FIGURE 4–49 *Continued.   C, D.* Craniocaudal view of a normal stifle.

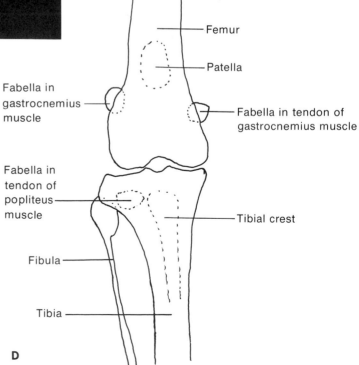

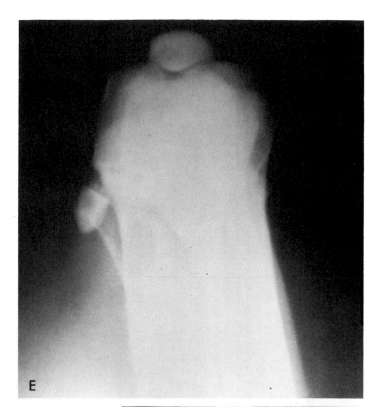

FIGURE **4–49** *Continued. E.* Skyline view of the patella and trochlear groove.

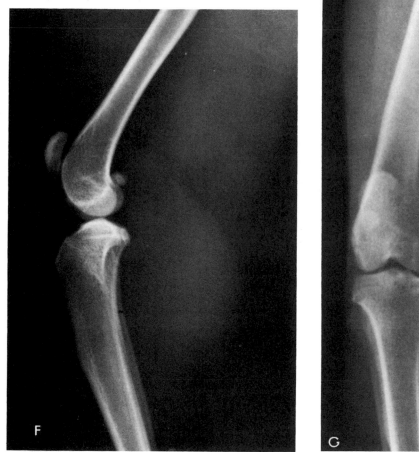

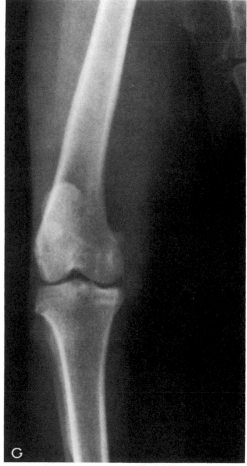

FIGURE **4–49** *Continued. F, G.* Stifle joint of a cat.

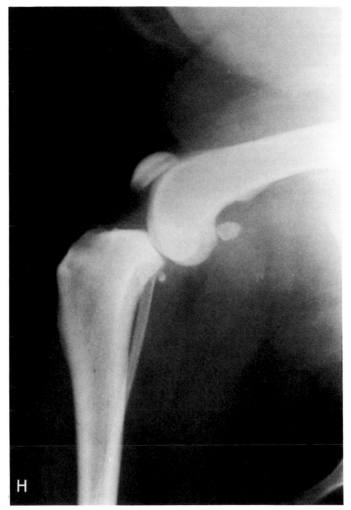

FIGURE 4–49 *Continued.* *H.* Subluxation of the stifle joint due to rupture of the cranial cruciate ligament. This injury does not usually produce a visible radiographic displacement.

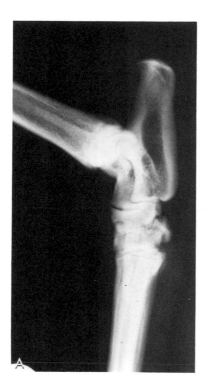

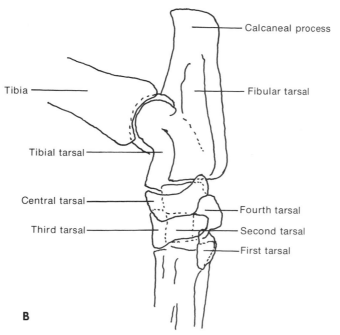

Calcaneal process

Fibular tarsal

Tibia

Tibial tarsal

Central tarsal

Third tarsal

Fourth tarsal

Second tarsal

First tarsal

B

FIGURE 4–50 *A, B.* Lateral view of the tarsus of a dog.

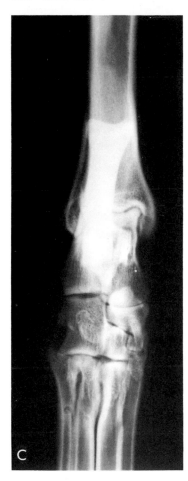

FIGURE 4–50 *Continued.* *C, D.* Dorsopalmar view of the tarsus of a dog.

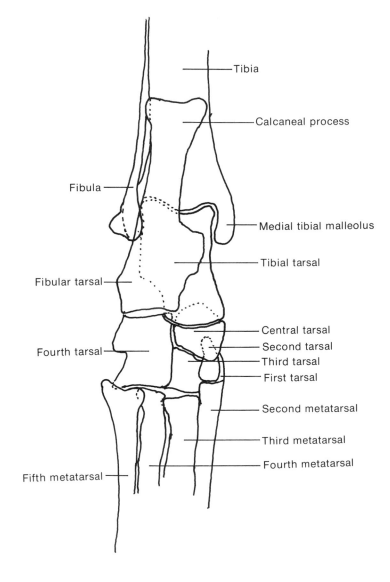

Tibia

Calcaneal process

Fibula

Medial tibial malleolus

Tibial tarsal

Fibular tarsal

Central tarsal

Second tarsal

Third tarsal

First tarsal

Fourth tarsal

Second metatarsal

Third metatarsal

Fourth metatarsal

Fifth metatarsal

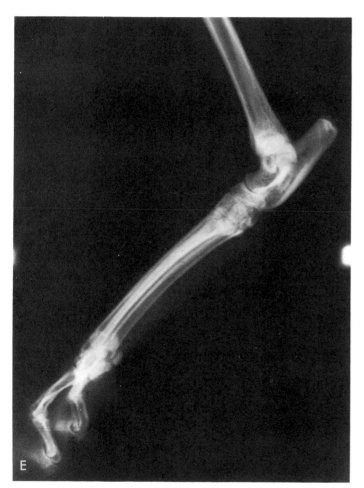

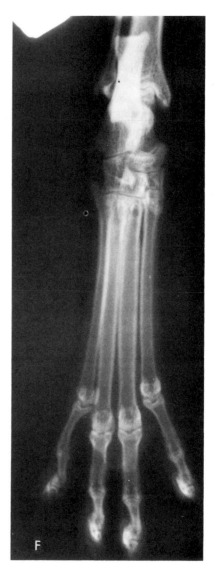

FIGURE 4–50 *Continued.* *E, F.* Tarsus and digits of a cat.

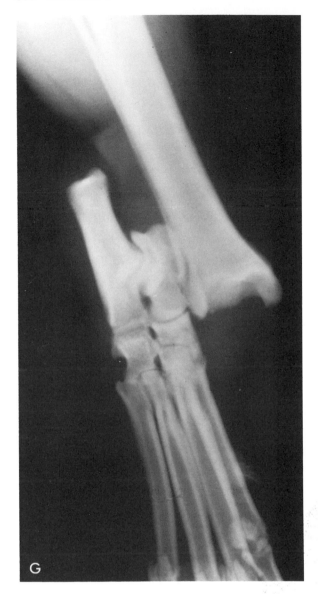

G

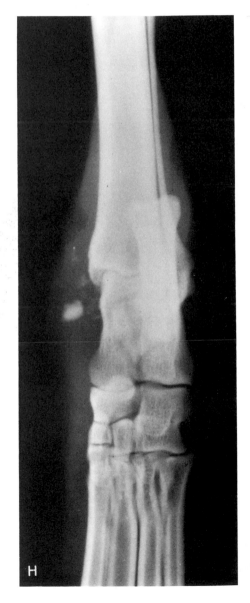

H

FIGURE 4–50 *Continued.* *G.* Luxation of the tibiotarsal joint.

FIGURE 4–50 *Continued.* *H.* Fracture of the medial malleolus of the tibia.

SEPTIC ARTHRITIS

This is not common in dogs and cats. It is usually a sequel to a wound. Rarely is it blood borne in origin.

RADIOLOGIC SIGNS

a. Erosion of the subchondral bone occurs, making the joint space appear wider than normal.

b. Bone destruction causes the opposing bone edges to appear irregular in outline.

c. There is usually marked periosteal reaction on the bones immediately above and below the affected joint.

d. Changes associated with osteomyelitis will be seen in the affected bones. (See page 301).

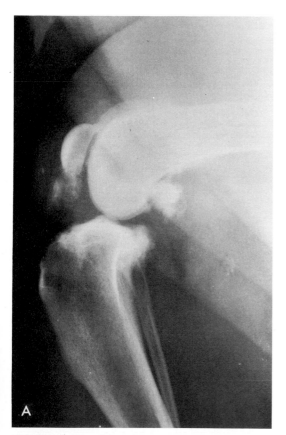
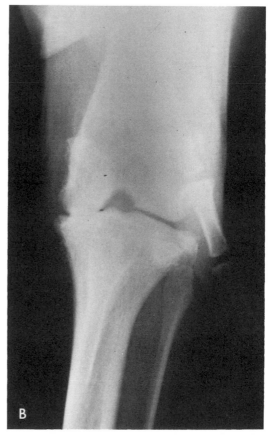

FIGURE 4–51. Joint disease. *A.* Degenerative changes in the stifle joint of a dog. There is intra-articular calcification below the patella, inflammatory new bone formation around the fabellae and on the caudal aspect of the tibia. There is sclerosis of the subchondral bone of the tibia. *B.* Narrowing of the joint space and inflammatory changes on the medial aspects of the femur and tibia indicate osteoarthrosis.

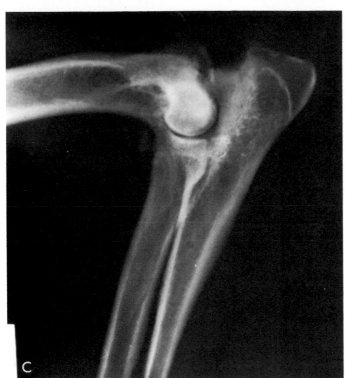

FIGURE 4–51 *Continued. C, D.* Osteoarthrosis of the elbow joint.

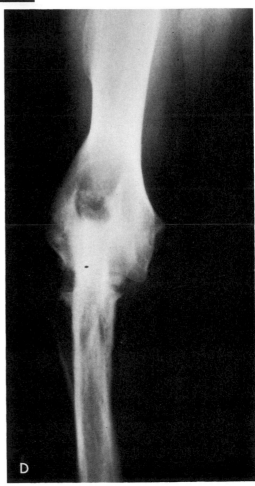

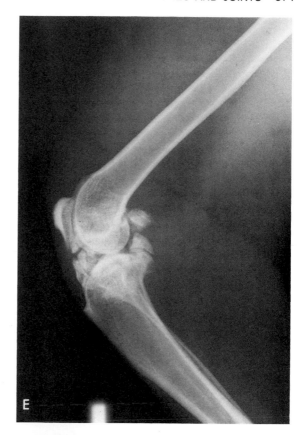

FIGURE 4-51 *Continued. E, F.* Chondromatosis (Osteochondromatosis) in a cat. This condition may, or may not, be associated with arthritis. Parts of the synovial membrane become cartilaginous and later they may calcify or ossify. The etiology is unknown. This cat was "getting stiff" for about one year but was not disabled.

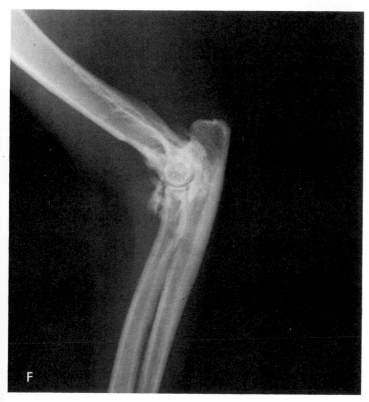

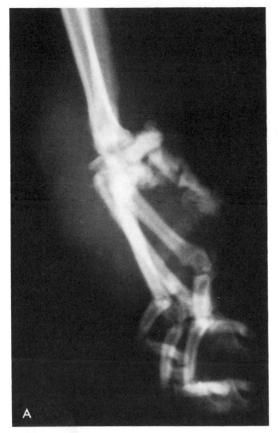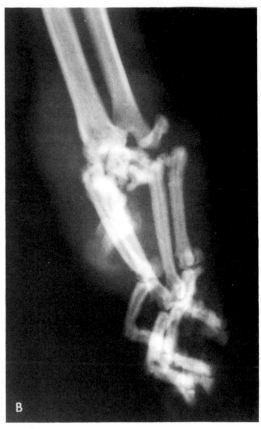

FIGURE 4–52*A, B.* Gross destruction of a carpal joint of a cat due to septic arthritis. There is a large associated soft tissue swelling.

e. In some cases swelling of the joint capsule and thickening of the synovial membrane may displace fascial planes in the neighborhood. This may be seen because of the fat within the fascial planes. The joint space may be widened owing to accumulation of exudate within the joint. (Fig. 4–52).

RHEUMATOID ARTHRITIS

Rheumatoid arthritis has been described in the dog. It is apparently very rare. Radiographic changes include periarticular soft tissue swelling, rarefaction, and, later, destruction of subchondral bone. Areas of bone lysis may occur at the points of ligamentous attachment and luxation may follow.

LUPUS ERYTHEMATOSUS ARTHRITIS

Systemic lupus erythematosus may affect young adult bitches. Joint changes, including thickening of the joint capsule and bone resorption, may occur.

Arthrography

Arthrography is not, as yet, widely practiced in veterinary radiology. Its use has been almost entirely confined to the shoulder joint. A positive contrast medium

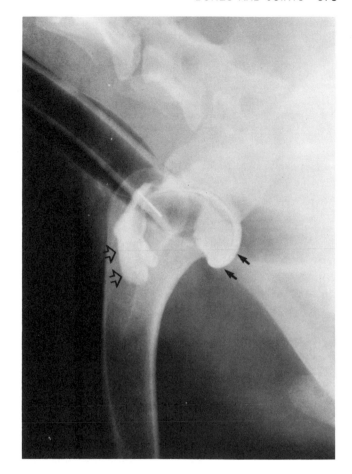

FIGURE 4–53. Positive contrast arthrogram of a shoulder joint of a dog. The articular cartilages are clearly outlined as radiolucent lines between the contrast material and the subchondral bone. Contrast material is seen in the tendon sheath of the biceps muscle cranially (open arrows) and in the caudal recess of the shoulder joint (closed arrows). The metallic density is a marker in an endotracheal tube.

is preferred. Sodium diatrizoate solution (Hypaque 50%, Winthrop Laboratories) or meglumine diatrizoate solution (Renografin 60%, E. R. Squibb & Sons) may be used. Synovial fluid is first aspirated from the joint and the contrast material is then injected. From 4 to 9 ml of contrast solution are used, depending on the size of the animal. The joint is entered about 1 cm below the acromion process using a 20 gauge needle. The needle is directed distally and caudally. (Fig. 4–53).

REFERENCES

Ackerman, N., Halliwell, W. H., Renze, L. G. and Corley, E. A. (1973). Solitary osteochondroma in a dog. J.A.V.R.S. XIV, 2, 13.

Archibald, J. (1974). Canine Surgery. 2nd Archibald edition. American Veterinary Publications, Inc. Santa Barbara, California.

Banks, W. C. (1971). Parosteal osteosarcoma in a dog and a cat. J.A.V.M.A. 158. 1412.

Barrett, R. B., Schall, W. D. and Lewis, R. E. (1968). Clinical and radiographic features of canine eosinophilic panosteitis. J. Amer. Anim. Hosp. Ass. 4. 94.

Bingel, S. A., Brodey, R. S., Allen, H. L. and Riser, W. H. (1975). Haemangiosarcoma of bone in the dog. J. Sm. Anim. Pract. 15. 303.

Böhning, R. H., Suter, R. P., Hohn, R. B. and Marshall, J. (1970). Clinical and radiologic survey of canine panosteitis. J.A.V.MA. 156. 870.

Brodey, R. S. (1970). Canine and feline neoplasia. Adv. Vet. Sc. and Comp. Med. 14. 309.

Brodey, R. D., Medway, W. and Marshak, R. R. (1971). Renal osteodystrophy in the dog. J.A.V.M.A. 139. 329.

Brodey, R. S., Sauer, R. M. and Medway, W. (1963). Canine bone neoplasms. J.A.V.M.A. 143. 471.

Brodey, R. S., Reid, C. F. and Sauer, R. M. (1966). Metastatic bone neoplasms in the dog. J.A.V.M.A. 148. 29.

Brodey, R. S., Riser, W. H. and Allen, H. (1973). Hypertrophic pulmonary osteoarthropathy in a dog with carcinoma of the urinary bladder. J.A.V.M.A. 162. 357.

Brown, S. G. (1975). Joint diseases; skeletal diseases. In Textbook of Veterinary Internal Medicine of the Dog and Cat. Stephen J. Ettinger, Editor. W. B. Saunders Co. Philadelphia.

Campbell, J. R. (1964). Metabolic bone dystrophies. J. Sm. Anim. Pract. 5. 229.

Campbell, J. R. (1968). Radiology of the epiphysis. J.A.V.R.S. IX. 11.

Carlson, W. J. (1977). Veterinary Radiology, Gillette, E., Thrall, D. E. and Lebel, J. H., Editors. 3rd Ed. Lea & Febiger, Philadelphia.

Carrig, C. B. and Morgan, J. P. (1975). Asynchronous growth of the canine radius and ulna — early radiographic changes following experimental retardation of longitudinal growth of the ulna. J.A.V.R.S. XVI. 4. 121.

Cawley, A. J. and Archibald, J. (1959). Ununited anconeal processes of the dog. J.A.V.M.A. 134. 454.

Clayton-Jones, D. G. and Vaughan, L. C. (1970). Disturbance in the growth of the radius in dogs. J. Sm. Anim. Pract. 11. 453.

Craig, P. H. and Riser, W. H. (1965). Osteochondritis dissecans in the proximal humerus of the dog. J.A.V.R.S. VI. 40.

Douglas, S. W. and Williamson, H. D. (1972). Principles of Veterinary Radiography. 2nd ed. Williams and Wilkins Co. Baltimore.

Douglas, S. W. and Williamson, H. D. (1970). Veterinary Radiological Interpretation. Lea and Febiger. Philadelphia.

Ettinger, S., Campbell, L., Suter, P. F., DeAngelis, M. and Butler, H. C. (1968). Peripheral arteriovenous fistula in a dog. J.A.V.M.A. 153. 1055.

Ettinger, Stephen J., Editor. (1975). Textbook of Veterinary Internal Medicine of the Dog and Cat. 2 vols. W. B. Saunders Co. Philadelphia.

Fletch. S. M., Smart, M. E., Pennock, P. W. and Subden, R. E. (1973). Clinical and pathologic features of chondrodysplasia (dwarfism) in the Alaskan Malamute. J.A.V.M.A. 162. 357.

Henricson, B., Norberg, I. and Olsson, S. E. (1966). On the etiology and pathogenesis of hip dysplasia. A comparative review. J. Sm. Anim. Pract. 7. 673.

Huff, R. W. and Brodey, R. S. (1964). Multiple bone cysts in a dog—a case report. J.A.V.R.S. V. 40.

Larsen, J. S. and Corley, E. A. (1971). Radiographic evaluations in a canine hip dysplasia control program. J.A.V.M.A. 159. 989.

Lawson, D. D. (1963). The radiographic diagnosis of hip dysplasia in the dog. Vet. Rec. 75. 445.

Lee, R. (1970). A study of the radiographic and histological changes occurring in Legg-Calvé-Perthe's disease (LCP) in the dog. J. Sm. Anim. Pract. 11. 621.

Lee, R. (1974). Legg-Perthe's disease in the dog. The histological and associated radiological changes. J.A.V.R.S. XV. 1. 24.

Lewis, R. M. and Hathaway, J. E. (1967). Canine systemic lupus erythematosus presenting with symmetrical polyarthritis. J. Sm. Anim. Pract. 8. 273.

Ling, G. V., Morgan, J. P. and Pool, R. R. (1974). Primary bone tumors in the dog. A combined clinical, radiographic, and histologic approach to early diagnosis. J.A.V.M.A. 165. 55.

Ljunggren, G. (1967). Legg-Perthe's disease in the dog. Acta Orthop. Scand. Suppl. 95.

Ljunggren, G. and Olsson, S. E. (1975). Osteoarthrosis of the shoulder and elbow joints in dogs. A pathologic and radiographic study of necropsy material. J.A.V.R.S. XVI. 2. 33.

Liu, S. K., Suter, P. F., Fischer, C. A. and Dorfman, H. D. (1969). Rheumatoid arthritis in a dog. J.A.V.M.A. 154. 495.

Meschan, I. (1966). Roentgen Signs in Clinical Practice. W. B. Saunders Co. Philadelphia.

Miller, M. E., Christensen, G. C. and Evans, H. E. (1964). Anatomy of the Dog. W. B. Saunders Co. Philadelphia.

Morgan, J. P. (1969). Radiological pathology and diagnosis of degenerative joint disease in the stifle joint of the dog. J. Sm. Anim. Pract. 10. 541.

Morgan, J. P. (1972). Radiology in Veterinary Orthopedics. Lea and Febiger. Philadelphia.

Morgan, J. P. (1974). Systematic radiographic interpretation of skeletal diseases in small animals. Vet. Clin. N. Amer. Radiology. W. B. Saunders Co. Philadelphia.

Morgan, J. P., Silverman, S. and Zontine, W. J. (1975). Techniques of Veterinary Radiography. Veterinary Associates. Davis, California.

Neher, G. M. and Carter, J. M. (1963). Understanding the pathology of your arthritic patient. J.A.V.R.S. V. 15.

Nunamaker, D. M., Biery, D. W. and Newton, C. D. (1973). Femoral neck anteversion in the dog. Its radiographic measurement. J.A.V.R.S. XIV. 1. 45.

O'Brien, T. R. (1971). Developmental deformities due to arrested epiphyseal growth. Vet. Clin. N. Amer. 1. 441. W. B. Saunders Co. Philadelphia.

O'Brien, T. R., Morgan, J. P. and Suter, P. F. (1971). Epiphyseal plate injury in the dog; a radiographic study of growth disturbance in the forelimb. J. Sm. Anim. Pract. 12. 19.

Oduye, O. O. and Losos, G. J. (1972). Multiple myeloma in a dog. J. Sm. Anim. Pract. 13. 257.

Olsson, S. E. (1971). Degenerative joint disease (osteoarthrosis). A review with special reference to the dog. J. Sm. Anim. Pract. 12. 333.

Olsson, S. E. (1975). Osteochondritis dissecans in the dog. Proc. Amer. An. Hosp. Ass. 42nd Ann. Meeting. Cincinnati, Ohio. Vol. I. 360.

Olsson, S. E. (1975). Lameness in the dog. A review of the lesions causing osteoarthrosis of the shoulder, elbow, hip, stifle and hock joint. Proc. Amer. Anim. Hosp. Ass. 42nd Ann. Meeting. Cincinnati, Ohio. Vol. I. 363.

Olsson, S. E. (1976). Osteochondrosis — a growing problem to dog breeders. Gaines Progress, Summer, 1976. Gaines Dog Research Center, White Plains, New York.

Owen, L. N. and Stevenson, D. E. (1961). Observations on canine osteosarcomata. Res. Vet. Sci. 2. 117.

Owen, L. N. (1969). Bone tumours in man and animals. Butterworths, London.

Paatsama, W., Rokkanen, P., Jussila, J. and Sittnikow, K. (1971). A study of osteochondritis dissecans of the canine humeral head using histological, OTC bone labelling, microradiographic and microangiographic methods. J. Sm. Anim. Pract. 12. 603.

Pennock, P. W. (1974). Radiographic diagnosis of joint diseases. Vet. Clin. N. Amer. Radiology. W. B. Saunders Co. Philadelphia.

Pennock, P., Jönsson, L. and Olsson, S. E. (1966). Multiple myeloma in a dog. J. Sm. Anim. Pract. 7. 343.

Priester, W. A. (1972). Sex, size, and breed as risk factors in canine patellar dislocation. J.A.V.M.A. 160. 740.

Rasmussen, P. G. (1972). Multiple epiphyseal dysplasia in Beagle puppies. Acta Radiologica. Suppl. 319, 251.

Riser, W. H. (1964). Radiographic differential diagnosis of skeletal diseases of young dogs. J.A.V.R.S. V. 15.

Riser, W. H. and Shirer, J. F. (1965). Normal and abnormal growth of the distal foreleg in large and giant dogs. J.A.V.R.S. VI. 50.

Riser, W. H., Parkes, L. J. and Shirer, J. F. (1967). Canine craniomandibular osteopathy. J.A.V.R.S. VIII. 23.

Riser, W. H. (1973). The dysplastic hip joint. Its radiographic and histologic development. J.A.V.R.S. XIV. 2. 35.

Riser, W. H. (1973). Growth and development of the normal canine pelvis, hip joints and femurs from birth to maturity. A radiographic study. J.A.V.R.S. XIV. 2. 24.

Schebitz, H. and Wilkens, H. (1968). Atlas of Radiographic Anatomy of the Dog and Horse. Paul Parey, Berlin and Hamburg.

Slocum, B., Colgrove, D. J., Carrig, C. B. and Suter, P. F. (1973). Acquired arteriovenous fistula in two cats. J.A.V.M.A. 162. 271.

Smith, R. N. (1963). The pelvis of the young dog. Vet. Rec. 76. 975.

Sumner-Smith, G. and Cawley, A. J. (1970). Nonunion fractures in the dog. J. Sm. Anim. Pract. 11. 311.

Suter, F. P. and Carb, A. V. (1969). Shoulder arthrography in dogs — radiographic anatomy and clinical application. J. Sm. Anim. Pract. 10. 407.

Ticer, J. W. (1975). Radiographic Technique in Small Animal Practice. W. B. Saunders Co. Philadelphia.

Tirgari, M. and Vaughan, L. C. (1973). Clinical-pathologic aspects of osteoarthritis in the shoulders of dogs. J. Sm. Anim. Pract. 14. 353.

Van Sickle, D. (1975). Selected orthopedic problems in the growing dog. Monograph. Amer. Anim. Hosp. Ass.

Vaughan, L. C. and Jones, D. G. C. (1968). Osteochondritis dissecans of the head of the humerus in dogs. J. Sm. Anim. Pract. 9. 283.

Walker, M. A., Lewis, R. E., Kneller, S. K., Thrall, D. E. and Losonsky, J. M. (1974). Radiographic signs of bone infection in small animals. J.A.V.M.A. 908.

Walton, G. S. and Gopinath C. (1972). Multiple myeloma in a dog with some unusual features. J. Sm. Anim. Pract. 13. 703.

Watson, A. D. J., Huxtable, C. R. R. and Farrow, B. R. H. (1975). Craniomandibular osteopathy in Doberman Pinschers. J. Sm. Anim. Pract. 16. 11.

Whittick, W. G. (1974). Canine Orthopedics. Lea and Febiger. Philadelphia.

Zontine, W. J. (1972). Bilateral stress pattern in the distal ulnar metaphyses of a Great Dane. J.A.V.R.S. XIII. 53.

5

THE SKULL, VERTEBRAL COLUMN, AND RIBS

THE SKULL

Radiography is commonly employed to study the bone structure of the skull. Contrast techniques are available to demonstrate associated soft tissue structures. Generalized or diffuse diseases of the central nervous system are usually diagnosed by methods other than radiography.

The skull is a difficult area to study radiologically. Its bone structure is very complex and its shape varies widely in different breeds of dogs. Superimposition of important structures makes detailed examination of individual parts difficult.

Anatomy

Three types of head shapes are recognized in dogs. The long, narrow type of head, as seen in collies, is called doliocephalic; mesaticephalic indicates a head of medium shape, such as that of the German Shepherd; brachycephalic indicates a short, wide head like that of the Pekingese or Boston terrier. The brachycephalic type presents most problems for the radiologist.

The skull is made up of some 50 bones and a detailed anatomic description of them is not helpful. Attention will be concentrated on the radiographic anatomy.

Radiography

Many different views are used to demonstrate individual structures within the skull. The basic views are the lateral, the dorsoventral or ventrodorsal, left and right lateral obliques, frontal, and open mouth. Anesthesia or sedation makes positioning easier and safer.

LATERAL VIEW.   The patient is placed in lateral recumbency. A foam rubber wedge is placed under the nose and mandible so that the sagittal plane of the skull lies parallel to the tabletop. The beam is centered midway between the ear and the eye dorsal to the zygomatic arch. (Fig. 5–1*A, B*).

VENTRODORSAL VIEW. The animal is placed in dorsal recumbency. A foam rubber block is placed under the neck behind the skull. The occipitoatlantal articulation is extended so that the hard palate lies parallel to the tabletop. It can be maintained in that position by a bandage or tape placed across the mandibles and fixed to the table. The beam is centered between the mandibles at a level midway between the eyes and the ears. This view is best to demonstrate the cranium, since the mandibles are projected laterally and the calvarium is closer to the film. The sinuses are more clearly seen than on the dorsoventral view, though it is more difficult to achieve bilateral symmetry on the ventrodorsal view. (Fig. 5–1*C, D*).

DORSOVENTRAL VIEW. The animal is placed in sternal recumbency. The head is pressed down to the table so that the hard palate lies parallel to the tabletop. It can be maintained in that position by a bandage passed across the neck, behind the skull, and fixed to the table. The x-ray beam is centered between the eyes and the ears on the midline. While it is easier to achieve bilateral symmetry in this view than in the ventrodorsal view, there is more distortion because the calvarium is farther from the film. (Fig. 5–1*E*).

OBLIQUE VIEW. The patient is placed in lateral recumbency. In most breeds, if the head lies flat on the table an oblique view will be achieved with a beam directed at right angles to the tabletop. If necessary, a wedge of foam rubber can be placed under the mandible to rotate the skull. Alternatively, the beam may be suitably angled relative to the tabletop.

Oblique views are used to study the temporomandibular joints, the osseous bullae, the frontal sinuses, the dorsal edge of the orbit, and, in the open mouth position, the maxillary and mandibular dental arcades. Oblique views enable some structures to be demonstrated without superimposition of the contralateral side. (Fig. 5–1*F*).

FRONTAL VIEW. The patient is placed in dorsal recumbency and the neck flexed so that the hard palate lies perpendicular to the tabletop. The head is held in position with a bandage or tape around the nose. The beam is directed at right angles to the tabletop along the line of the hard palate and centered between the eyes. The nasal passages and frontal sinuses can be demonstrated in this view. This frontal view, with the mouth open, can be modified to demonstrate the osseous bullae. Varying the angle of the hard palate to the tabletop, it may also be used to outline the calvarium. (Fig. 5–1*G, H*).

Normal Appearance

The appearance of the normal skull on these various views is best demonstrated by illustrations (Fig. 5–1). Figure 5–1*I, J* show the normal appearance of the skull of a cat.

Abnormalities

In an examination of the skull, because the bone structures are bilaterally symmetric, it is frequently possible to compare a unilateral abnormality with the corresponding normal structure on the opposite side.

Text continued on page 382

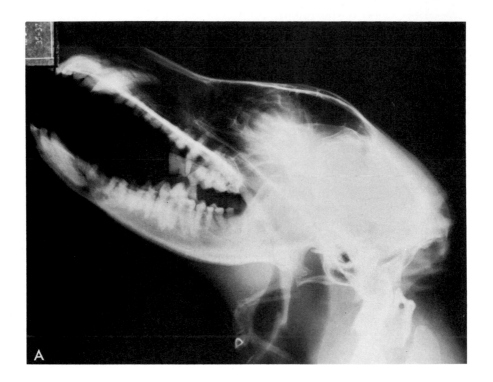

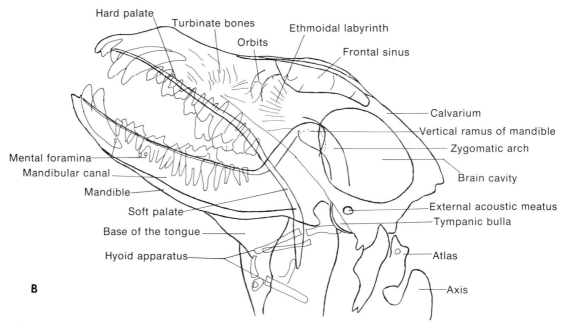

Hard palate · Turbinate bones · Ethmoidal labyrinth

Orbits · Frontal sinus

Calvarium

Vertical ramus of mandible

Zygomatic arch

Mental foramina

Brain cavity

Mandibular canal

Mandible

External acoustic meatus

Tympanic bulla

Soft palate

Base of the tongue

Atlas

Hyoid apparatus

Axis

B

FIGURE 5–1.   Normal skull. *A, B.*   Lateral view.

(Illustration continued on the opposite page.)

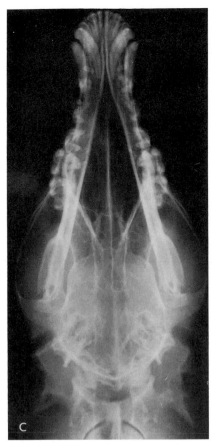

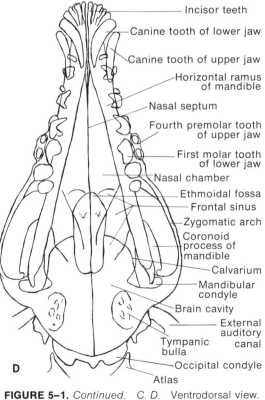

Incisor teeth

Canine tooth of lower jaw

Canine tooth of upper jaw

Horizontal ramus
of mandible

Nasal septum

Fourth premolar tooth
of upper jaw

First molar tooth
of lower jaw

Nasal chamber

Ethmoidal fossa

Frontal sinus

Zygomatic arch

Coronoid
process of
mandible

Calvarium

Mandibular
condyle

Brain cavity

External
auditory
canal

Tympanic
bulla

Occipital condyle

Atlas

D

FIGURE 5–1. *Continued. C. D.* Ventrodorsal view.

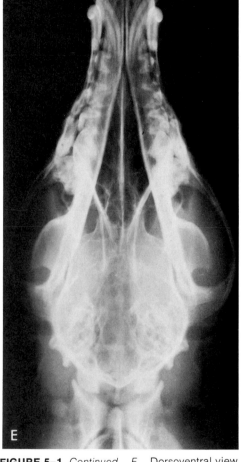

FIGURE 5–1. *Continued. E.* Dorsoventral view.
(Illustration continued on the following page.)

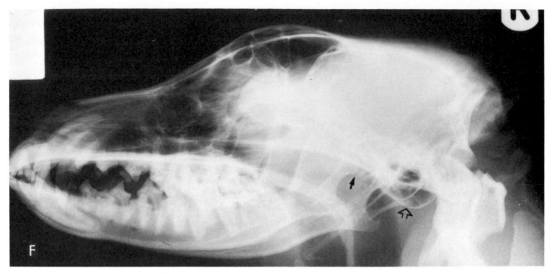

FIGURE 5–1. *Continued.   F.*   Oblique view. On this oblique view, made in right lateral recumbency, the right temporomandibular joint is demonstrated (black arrow). The osseous bullae (open arrow) are more clearly seen than on the true lateral view.

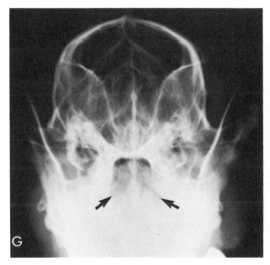

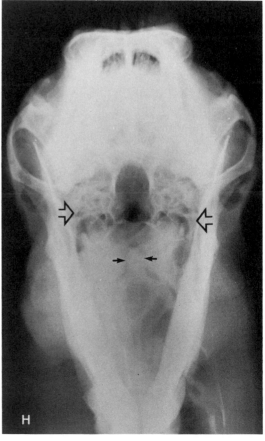

FIGURE 5–1. *Continued. G, H.* Frontal view. *G* is a frontal view showing the frontal sinuses and the nasal chambers (arrows). The calvarium is well outlined against the background of the air-filled sinuses. *H* is an open mouth view showing the osseous bullae (open arrows) and the foramen magnum. The dens (odontoid process) of the axis is also outlined (black arrows).

(Illustration continued on the opposite page.)

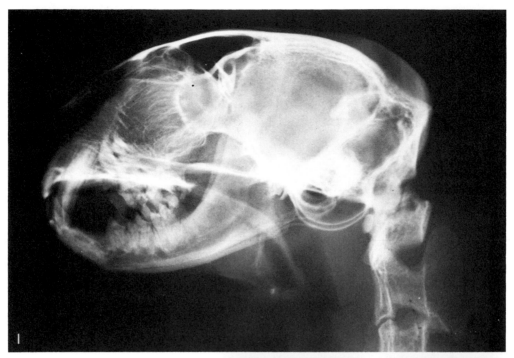

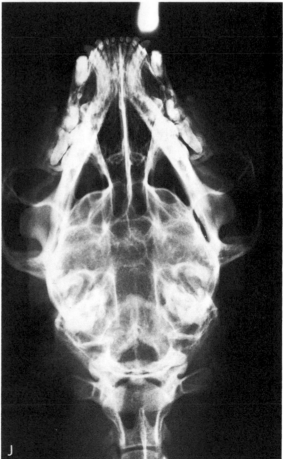

FIGURE 5–1. *Continued.   I, J.* Lateral and ventrodorsal views of the skull of a cat.

FRACTURES

Skull fractures in dogs are not very common except for fractures of the mandibles. The superimposition of bones makes fractures difficult to demonstrate. Lateral oblique views are useful in outlining the mandibular rami. Fractures involving the calvarium, the frontal bones or nasal bones are often depression fractures; skyline views of the area may be necessary to demonstrate them. Overriding of fracture fragments may cause a linear density. Fractures involving the nasal or frontal bones may be accompanied by hemorrhage into the frontal sinus or nasal cavity. This causes a soft tissue density within the air-filled cavity. (Fig. 5–2).

Suture lines should not be mistaken for fractures. In the dog and cat suture lines close within a few weeks after birth, although in some small breeds the suture lines may remain open permanently, as may the fontanelles. In such breeds no frontal sinus may be evident, for example in the Maltese terrier. Fontanelles are areas of unossified tissue found at the junction of several suture lines.

DISLOCATION OF THE TEMPOROMANDIBULAR JOINT

This is demonstrated in the ventrodorsal view when the mandibular condyle is seen to be displaced rostrally from the retroarticular (retroglenoid) process. A lateral oblique view may also show the displacement. If the dislocation is unilateral, comparison with the opposite side is helpful. Diagnosis of this dislocation can be difficult radiologically. (Fig. 5–3).

Text continued on page 387

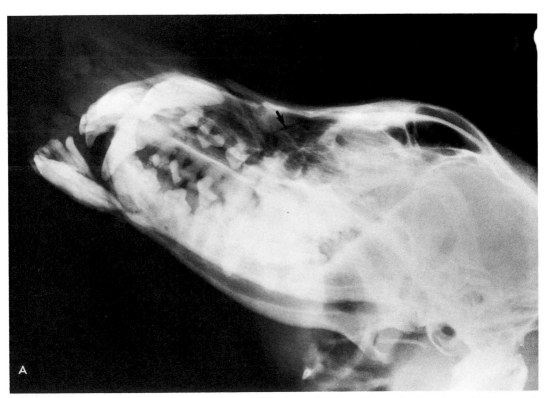

FIGURE 5–2. Fractures. *A.* Fracture of the mandible. There is also a fissure fracture (arrow) of the nasal bone.

(Illustration continued on the opposite page.)

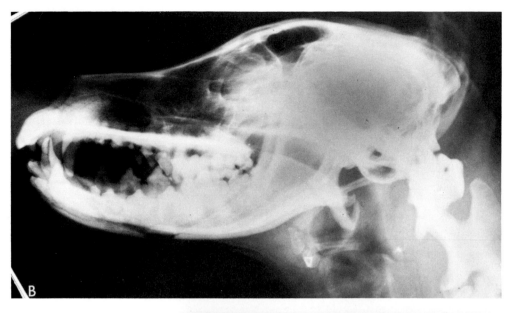

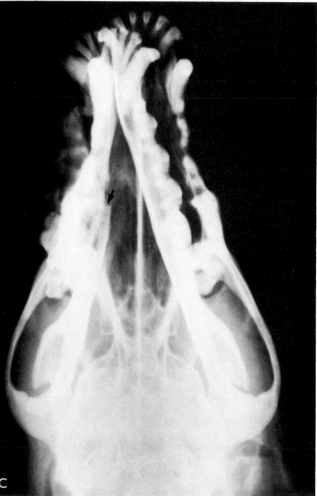

FIGURE 5-2. *Continued. B, C.* Fracture of the horizontal ramus of the mandible. The displacement in the lateral plane is demonstrated on the VD view (arrow). (*Illustration continued on the following page.*)

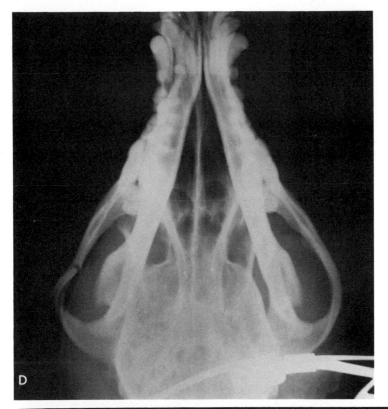

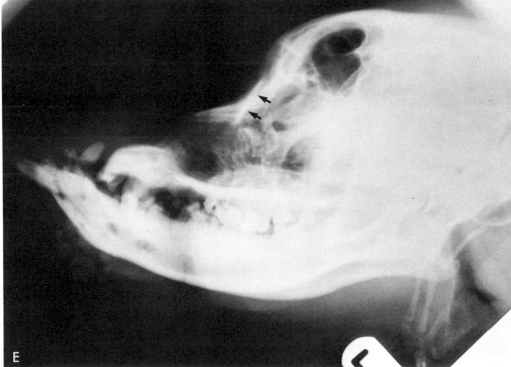

FIGURE 5–2. *Continued.* *D.* Fracture of the right zygomatic arch. The temporo-zygomatic suture, which is a late closing suture, should not be mistaken for a fracture line. *E.* A depressed fracture of the nasal bone (arrow). The mandible is also fractured.

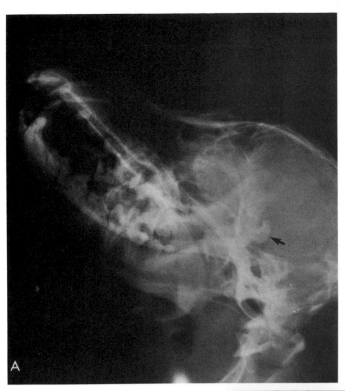

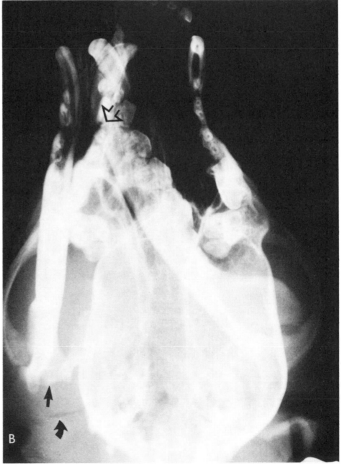

FIGURE 5–3. *A, B.* Dislocation of the right temporomandibular joint. The displaced mandibular condyle (straight arrows) can be seen both on the lateral and ventrodorsal views. There are also fractures of the right zygomatic arch and the left mandible (open arrow). The right external auditory canal is almost obliterated because of swelling in that area (curved arrow).

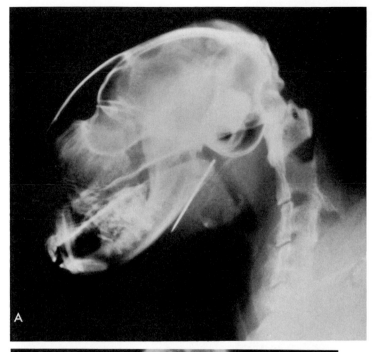

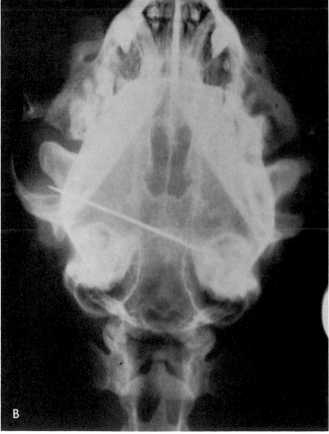

FIGURE 5–4. *A, B.* Foreign body. A needle in the pharyngeal region of a cat.

FOREIGN BODIES

Radiopaque foreign bodies are readily seen within the skull. They are usually located in the mouth, pharynx, or nasal chambers. Radiolucent bodies may require contrast medium to outline them. (Figs. 5–4 and 5–5).

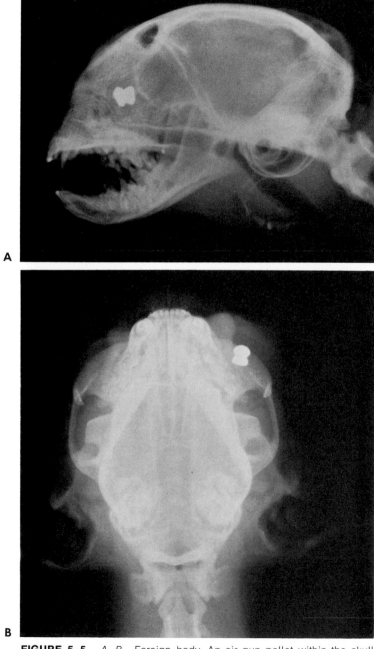

A

B

FIGURE 5–5. *A, B.* Foreign body. An air gun pellet within the skull shadow of a cat.

OSTEOMYELITIS

Osteomyelitis usually causes destruction of bone. There is usually a surrounding area of increased density (sclerosis) that sharply demarcates the affected area from the normal bone. Periosteal reaction is present. A sequestrum may form. Fungal osteomyelitis may simulate neoplastic changes. However, fungal lesions are usually multiple. While any of the bones of the skull may be affected with osteomyelitis, it is a rare condition except as an extension from infection in the nasal chambers or frontal sinuses.

NEOPLASIA

Neoplasia of the skull bones is not common. The dog is more commonly affected than the cat. Osteosarcoma may affect any of the bones of the skull. Its appearance is that of a destructive lesion with usually a profuse periosteal reaction. If the tumor is superficial there will be an associated large soft tissue swelling. Proliferative changes and sclerosis are more prominent than are destructive changes when the cranial vault is involved. Other neoplasms, such as fibrosarcoma and chondrosarcoma, are occasionally seen.

Differentiation of primary bone tumors is difficult. Osteomas are occasionally seen. They are dense, circumscribed, and provoke little, if any, reaction. Multiple myeloma has been reported in the dog, showing the typical punched-out lesions described in man.

Soft tissue tumors frequently invade and destroy adjacent skull bones, for example squamous cell carcinoma. (Fig. 5–6).

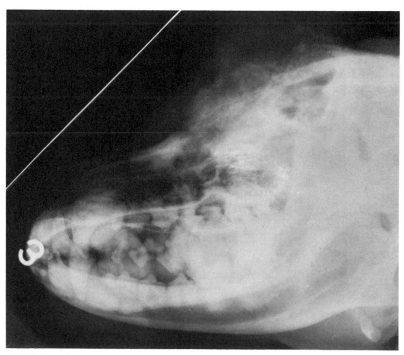

A

FIGURE 5–6. Neoplasia. *A.* Gross destruction of the frontal and nasal bones owing to invasion by a squamous cell carcinoma. The tumor originated in the caudal nares.

(Illustration continued on the opposite page.)

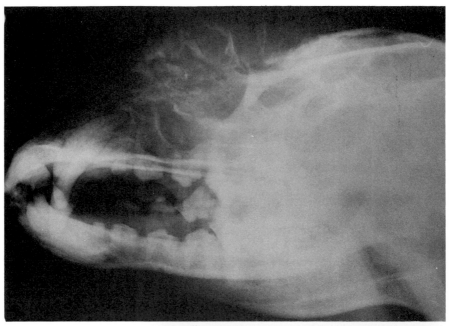

B

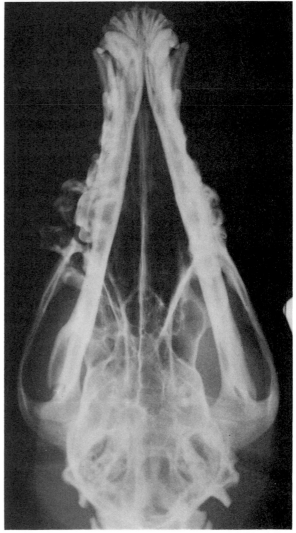

FIGURE 5–6. *Continued. B.* An osteosarcoma destroying the frontal, nasal, and maxillary bones. *C.* The right fourth premolar and the first molar tooth of the upper jaw are displaced owing to invasion of the maxilla by a carcinoma originating in the mouth.

C

OCCIPITAL DYSPLASIA

(Congenital Malformation of the Foramen Magnum; Arnold-Chiari Malformation.)

The term occipital dysplasia indicates a dysplasia associated with the occipital bone. The foramen magnum is completely surrounded by the occipital bone. A number of abnormalities are encountered in this area. The principal occurrence is in the small breeds of dogs. The foramen magnum may be abnormal in shape. The first cervical vertebra may be shortened and there may be hypoplasia and nonfusion of the odontoid process. There may be an associated hydrocephalus with open suture lines. Not all of the abnormalities may be present in any individual case. The symptoms are variable. Many cases are asymptomatic. Ataxia has been reported in about 25 per cent of cases with enlarged foramen magnum.

The foramen magnum is best demonstrated on a frontal view with the neck flexed so that the long axis of the head is 25° to 40° from the perpendicular. (Fig. 5–7).

METABOLIC DISEASES

Renal osteodystrophy (renal secondary hyperparathyroidism) causes demineralization of the skull bones, particularly of the mandibles and the maxillae. (See Fig. 4–33).

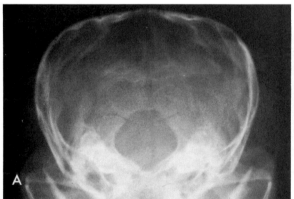

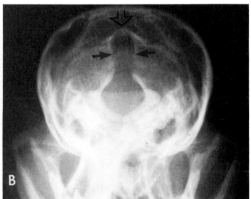

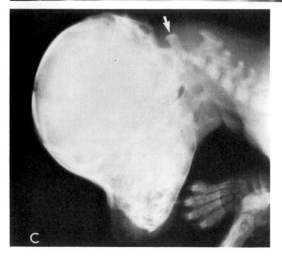

FIGURE 5–7. *A.* A normal foramen magnum. Suture lines can be seen in this young dog's skull. *B.* Malformation of the foramen magnum. The horizontal arrows indicate the dorsal limits of the foramen magnum. The area of radiolucency above the horizontal arrows, the dorsal limit of which is indicated by the open arrow, is the central sulcus of the caudal fossa. The bone of the central sulcus may be very thin and almost radiolucent in occipital dysplasia. As a result, the extent of the deformation of the foramen magnum may be overestimated. *C.* Shortening of the first cervical vertebra (arrow) associated with an occipital dysplasia. The space between the atlas and the axis, dorsally, is increased.

Juvenile osteodystrophy (nutritional secondary hyperparathyroidism) may cause changes similar to those seen with renal osteodystrophy.

Craniomandibular osteopathy causes proliferative changes particularly on the mandible and in the areas of the osseous bullae. The calvarium may be thickened. (Fig. 5–8). New bone formation at the distal radius and ulna has been reported in some cases. (See Chapter 4, page 331).

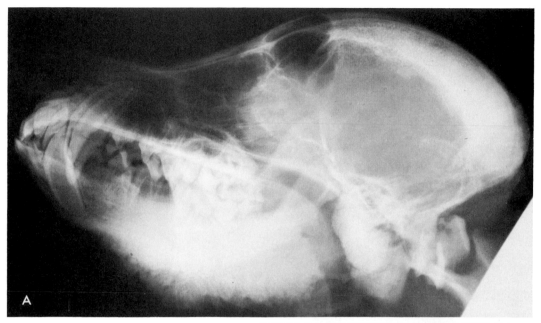

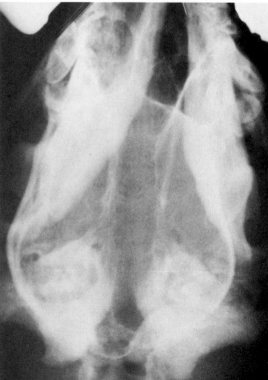

FIGURE 5–8. *A. B.* Thickening of the calvarium associated with craniomandibular osteopathy. There is extensive new bone formation on the mandibles and around the osseous bullae.

THE NASAL CHAMBERS

Anatomy

The nasal cavity is divided into right and left nasal chambers by the nasal septum. The septum is composed of the vomer bone rostrally and the septal processes of the frontal and nasal bones caudally. The nasal turbinate bones, covered by mucous membrane, fill the major portion of each nasal chamber.

Radiography

Most of the nasal chambers can be visualized on standard lateral and ventrodorsal views of the skull. A lighter technique than that used for the entire skull is required. The use of occlusal film in the dorsoventral view permits visualization of the nasal cavity without superimposition of the mandibles. An open-mouth view may also be used.

Normal Appearance

The nasal chambers normally project a fine bony trabecular pattern — the turbinate pattern. (Fig. 5–9).

Abnormalities

INFECTION. Infection in the turbinate bones causes an increased radiographic density on the affected side as compared with the normal side. The nasal septum provides a sharp demarcation line between the affected and the unaffected sides. If the condition is bilateral, there will be an increased density on both sides. The trabecular pattern of the turbinate bones is preserved, except in long-standing cases. It may be difficult to see, however, because of the increased density associated with exudation. (Fig. 5–10).

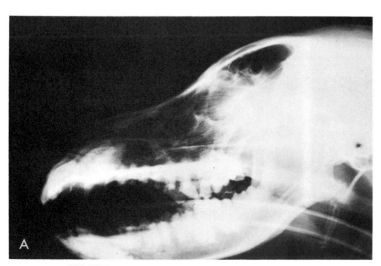

FIGURE 5–9. *See legend on the opposite page.*

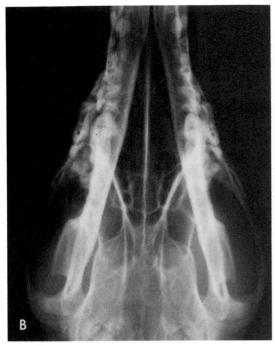 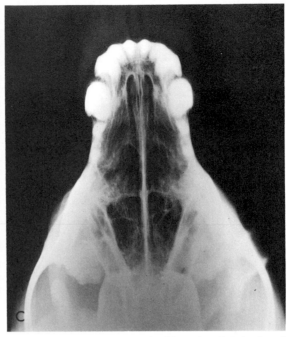

FIGURE 5–9. *Continued.* (*A*) and (*B*) show a normal turbinate pattern as seen on standard lateral and ventrodorsal views of the skull. (*C*) shows that the turbinate pattern is more obvious when demonstrated on an open mouth view.

FIGURE 5–10. Infection in the nasal chambers. *A.* Abnormal densities are seen in both nasal chambers. The nasal septum is intact. The turbinate pattern is partially obscured. This was a five year old dog with a history of bilateral nasal discharge for several months. *Candida* organisms were recovered from the discharge.

(*Illustration continued on the following page.*)

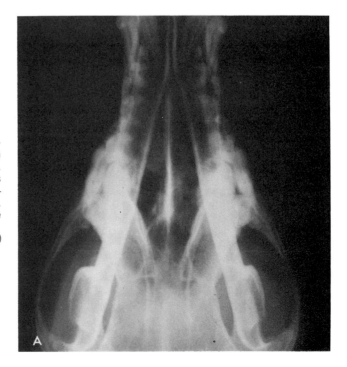

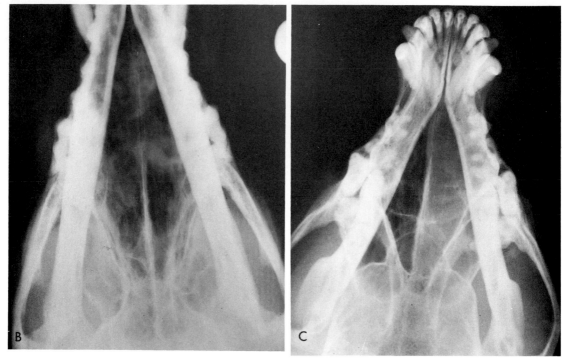

FIGURE 5–10. *Continued.   B.*   Diffuse densities are seen in both nasal chambers. The nasal septum cannot be identified rostrally. The turbinate pattern is obscured. The frontal sinuses have lost their normal air density. This was a seven year old German Shepherd that had a fight with a cat two years previously. The infection was of a mixed type. *C.* A unilateral nasal infection. An obvious loss of normal air density is seen on the left side as compared with the right (normal) side.

FOREIGN BODY.   Radiopaque foreign bodies are readily recognized on radiographs. Radiolucent foreign bodies are not seen. There may, however, be an increased density within the affected chamber due to exudation. The introduction of contrast material into the nasal chamber is not very informative except, perhaps, in the case of a large radiolucent foreign body. (Fig. 5–11).

NEOPLASIA.   Neoplasms may cause destruction of the turbinate bones, the nasal septum, and the walls of the nasal chambers.

RADIOLOGIC SIGNS

a. An increased density is seen in the affected chamber.

b. The turbinate bones are destroyed and the normal turbinate pattern is lost.

c. The nasal septum is frequently displaced by the growing tumor. It may be eroded as the neoplasm spreads into the adjacent chamber.

d. Loss of normal bone density in the surrounding bones and periosteal reaction become evident in advanced cases.

e. Soft tissue tumors often invade the nasal turbinates and the nasal septum. A soft tissue density is first noted within the nasal chamber. Later, invasion and destruction of the turbinate bone occurs with eventual involvement of the nasal septum and surrounding bones. Neoplasia may be difficult to distinguish from infection on radiographic studies alone. (Fig. 5–12).

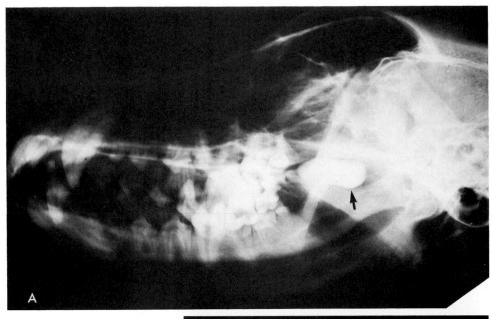

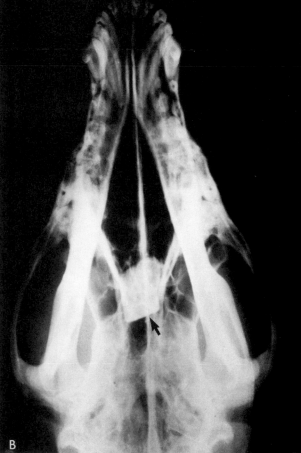

FIGURE 5–11. *A, B.* Foreign body. A mineral density (arrows) is seen in the caudal nares both on the lateral and ventrodorsal views. This was a stone. The dog had a bilateral nasal discharge for several weeks.

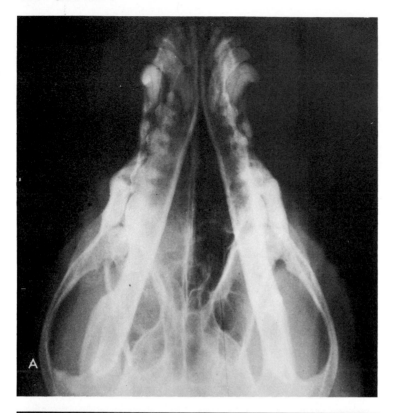

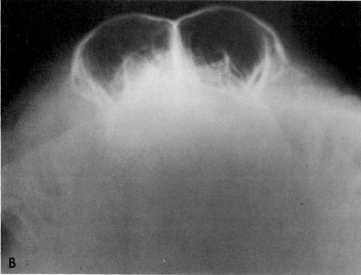

FIGURE 5–12. *A, B.* Neoplasia. The right nasal chamber shows a homogeneous density with loss of the normal turbinate pattern. The frontal sinus is also affected. Abnormal densities are seen in the left nasal chamber. The frontal view shows some loss of the normal air density in the right frontal sinus. This was a papillary cyst adenocarcinoma that totally occluded the right nasal chamber, encroached on the left nasal chamber, ethmoid bones, and frontal sinus. Radiographically, this is not distinguishable from changes due to infection.

THE SINUSES

Anatomy

Paranasal sinuses are located in the maxilla, frontal, and ethmoid bones. They are small at birth and enlarge as the animal grows. The frontal sinus is the largest and lies mainly between the lateral and medial tables of the frontal bone. The maxillary sinus is smaller and is a diverticulum of the nasal fossa. The ethmoid sinus is small.

Radiography

The frontal sinuses are most clearly seen on a lateral view. In the ventrodorsal or dorsoventral position the lateral extensions of the sinuses are superimposed on the mandibles. A frontal view shows the sinuses well.

Normal Appearance

On the lateral view the frontal sinuses are clearly seen above the orbit. Bony septa within them are visible. The sinuses are superimposed on one another in this view. On the ventrodorsal or dorsoventral view, a portion of the sinuses is seen rostral to the cranium. The maxillary or the ethmoid sinuses are not well seen on radiographs. (Fig. 5–13). See also Figure 5–1.

Abnormalities

INFECTION.   Infection in a frontal sinus causes loss of the normal air density within the affected sinus. A fluid density replaces the air density. Unless the condition is of very long standing there is usually no associated bone destruction. A thickened mucous membrane may be seen within the sinus. Infec-

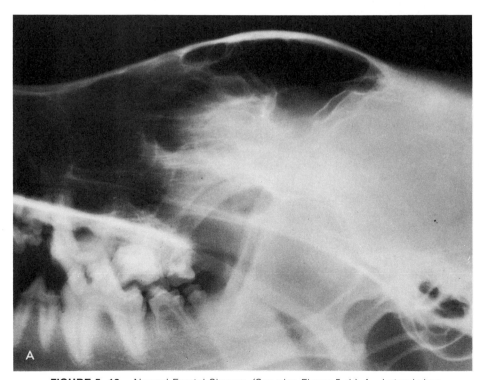

FIGURE 5–13.   Normal Frontal Sinuses. (See also Figure 5–1.) *A.* Lateral view.
(*Illustration continued on the following page.*)

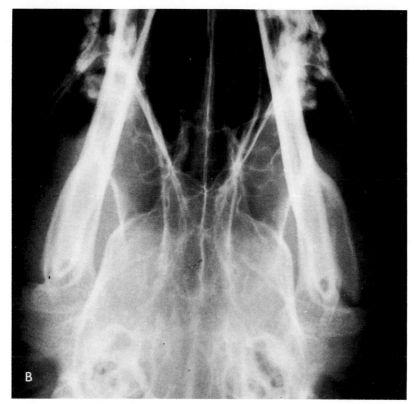

FIGURE 5–13. *Continued.*   *B.*   Ventrodorsal view.

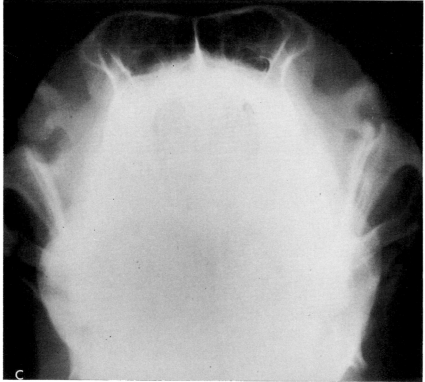

FIGURE 5–13. *Continued.*   *C.*   Frontal view.

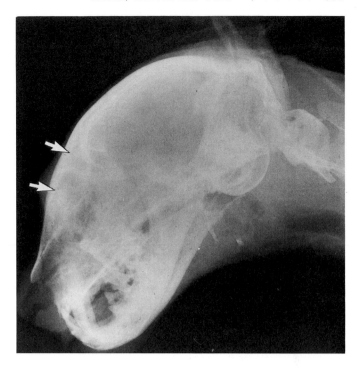

FIGURE 5–14. The normal air densities of the frontal sinuses (arrows) of this cat have been lost because of infection.

tion in the maxillary sinus associated with malar abscess is not readily demonstrable radiographically unless gross bone destruction is present. (Fig. 5–14).

NEOPLASIA. Neoplasms affecting the frontal sinus also cause loss of the normal air density within the sinus. Bone invasion and destruction with periosteal reaction are present in the later stages. Periosteal reaction is seen on the frontal bone. (Fig. 5–15).

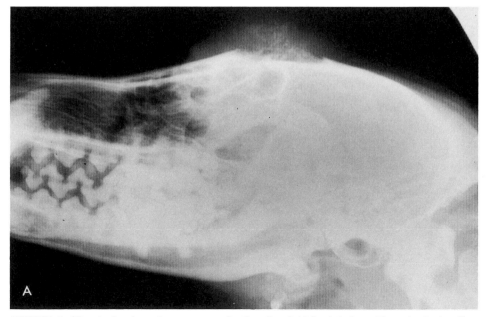

FIGURE 5–15. *A, B.* An osteosarcoma affecting the right frontal sinus. There is destruction of bone and invasion of the overlying soft tissues. The ventrodorsal view shows invasion of the cranium on the right side.

(*Illustration continued on the following page.*)

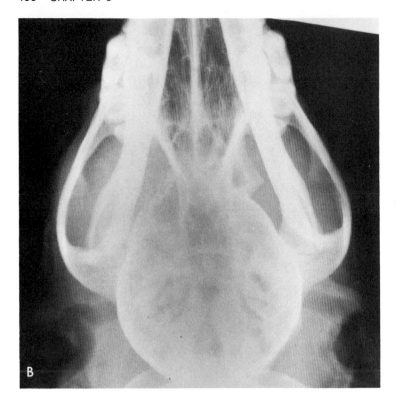

FIGURE 5–15. *Continued.*

THE TEETH

Radiography is of value in the assessment of periodontal and periapical disease, the demonstration of fractures, neoplasms, foreign bodies, malocclusion, and other tooth abnormalities.

Anatomy

The dental formula for the dog is as follows:

$$\text{Deciduous } 2 \times I\frac{3}{3} \, C\frac{1}{1} \, PM\frac{3}{3} \qquad = 28.$$

$$\text{Permanent } 2 \times I\frac{3}{3} \, C\frac{1}{1} \, PM\frac{4}{4} \, M\frac{2}{3} = 42.$$

The dental formula for the cat is as follows:

$$\text{Deciduous } 2 \times I\frac{3}{3} \, C\frac{1}{1} \, PM\frac{3}{2} \qquad = 26.$$

$$\text{Permanent } 2 \times I\frac{3}{3} \, C\frac{1}{1} \, PM\frac{3}{2} \, M\frac{1}{1} = 30.$$

The permanent teeth develop beneath or to one side of the deciduous teeth that they eventually displace. The first premolar tooth in the dog has no deciduous counterpart.

The exposed part of the tooth is covered by enamel. The tooth itself is composed of dentin, a bone-like structure that surrounds the pulp cavity and underlies the enamel. The tooth roots are covered by a thin layer of bone-like tissue called cementum, which cannot be distinguished, grossly or radiographically, from the underlying dentin. The pulp cavity, or hollow center of the tooth, contains nerves, arteries, veins, lymphatics, and connective tissue. At the tip of each root is the apical foramen, through which nerves and vessels enter the pulp cavity. The mandible has three mental foramina: the rostral foramen lies ventral to the alveolus of the central incisor tooth; the middle foramen lies ventral to the septum between the first two cheek teeth; the caudal foramen lies about 1 cm caudal to the middle mental foramen.

Radiography

Standard cassettes, using intensifying screens and screen film, can be used in lateral oblique open-mouth views to demonstrate the maxillary and mandibular dental arcades. The upper and lower canines, the premolars, and the molars are well seen. Greater detail and more accurate positioning can be achieved by the use of intraoral (occlusal), nonscreen film. Intraoral film is flexible and can be positioned to follow the contours of the mouth. A short focal-film distance, 16 inches, is recommended for intraoral film. Lateral and ventrodorsal or dorsoventral views of the skull result in superimposition of the dental arcades.

The incisors can be demonstrated by an oblique dorsoventral view for the upper incisors and an oblique ventrodorsal view for the lower incisors. The film is placed within the mouth and the x-ray beam is directed onto the teeth in a rostrocaudal direction at an angle of 20° to the vertical.

Normal Appearance

The pulp cavity can be seen as a relatively radiolucent canal surrounded by the more radiopaque dentin. A thin radiolucent line surrounds the tooth root. This represents the periodontal membrane. The bone lining the tooth socket is denser than the surrounding bone and appears as a dense radiopaque line called the *lamina dura*. The ridge of bone between adjacent teeth is called the alveolar crest. It forms a right angle with the lamina dura at the amelocemental junction, that is, the junction of enamel and cementum.

The mandibular canal appears radiolucent, as it lies parallel to the ventral border of the mandible. Occasionally, teeth roots project into the canal. (Fig. 5–16).

Abnormalities

VARIATION IN NUMBER. Anodontia, or complete absence of teeth, is rare. Oligodontia is a partial absence of teeth and is not infrequently seen in the brachycephalic type of skull. The first premolar and the lower third molar

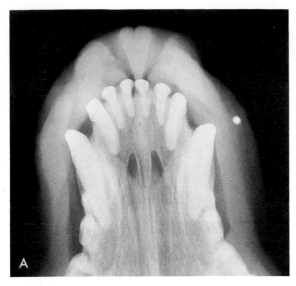

FIGURE 5–16. Normal teeth. *A.* Intraoral view of the upper incisors and canine teeth. There is a pellet in the lip.

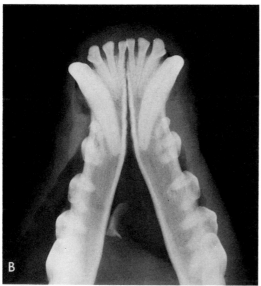

B. Intraoral view of the lower incisors, canine and molar teeth. A loose piece of tartar is seen.

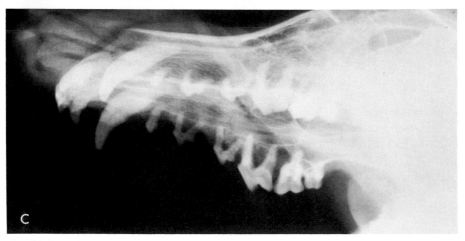

C. Oblique view to show the upper dental arcade. Superimposition of the dental arcades can be eliminated using oblique views. This is an old dog as evidenced by the narrow pulp cavities and the lack of sharp definition of the laminae durae.

  (Illustration continued on the opposite page.)

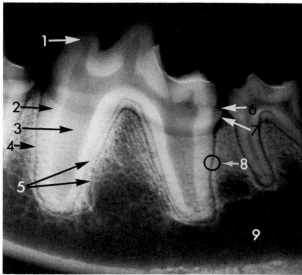

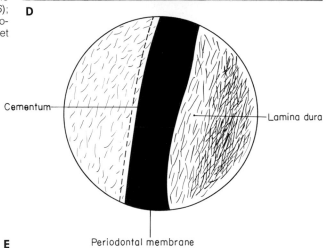

FIGURE 5–16. *Continued. D.* Normal teeth in a one year old Doberman pinscher. The anatomic landmarks are as follows: enamel (*1*); dentin (*2*); pulp cavity (*3*); lamina dura (*4*); both edges of the superimposed rostral root (*5*); tubercle (*6*); amelocemental junction (*7*); cementum, periodontal membrane, and lamina dura (*8*) [see inset *E;* and mandibular canal *(9)*.

(Courtesy of Dr. W. J. Zontine. Vet. Clinics of North America. Nov., 1974.)

are most commonly affected. Polydontia, or supernumerary teeth, may be seen in the area of the first two premolars, or less frequently there may be extra maxillary incisors or molars. Polydontia affects the permanent dentition. (Fig. 5–17).

PERIODONTAL DISEASE.   Periodontal disease is common in dogs and less common in cats. Oral infections involving the gingivae may spread to the periodontal membrane, the alveolar bone, the cementum, and dentin. In untreated cases there will be widespread infection, destruction of bone, and eventual loss of the affected tooth. Radiography helps to evaluate the spread of the disease in the periodontal space around the tooth root and in the surrounding bone.

RADIOLOGIC SIGNS

a. There is loss of the sharp angle at the junction of the alveolar crest and the lamina dura.

b. The periodontal space becomes wider.

c. The sharply defined radiopacity of the lamina dura is lost.

d. Rarefaction and, in more advanced cases, destruction of the alveolar bone occurs.

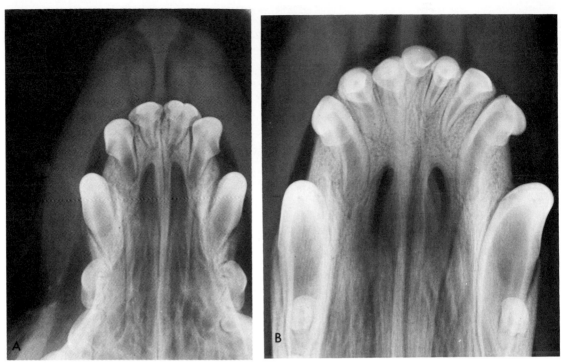

FIGURE 5–17. *A.* Oligodontia. Only four incisor teeth are present. The first incisor on the left side shows a cleft suggesting that there was partial development of two teeth in one alveolus. *B.* Polydontia. Seven incisor teeth are present. One has developed in the midline (mesiodens).

e. Resorption of the alveolar crest. Resorption of the alveolar crest may also be part of the normal aging process. (Fig. 5–18).

PERIAPICAL ABSCESS. Periapical abscess is an abscess surrounding the apex of one or more of the roots of a tooth. It may be the result of periodontal disease or it may result from trauma, cysts, or neoplasia.

RADIOLOGIC SIGNS

a. A zone of radiolucency surrounds the affected root apex. Overlying of a mental foramen may simulate this appearance.

b. The root may be partially resorbed.

c. A sclerotic margin often surrounds the radiolucent defect. (Fig. 5–18).

CARIES. Caries. Caries is rare in dogs and cats. If present, radiolucent defects may be seen in any part of the crown.

FRACTURES. While fractures are usually obvious on clinical examination, radiography may be helpful in demonstrating the degree of involvement of a tooth root.

THE AUDITORY SYSTEM

The external auditory canals are well seen on ventrodorsal or dorsoventral radiographs as radiolucent, tube-like structures. Exudates within them cause loss of the normal air density. Hemorrhage into the canals, such as may occur following a fracture at the base of the skull, will cause loss of their normal air density. (Fig. 5–1*C, D*). See also Fig. 5–3*B.*

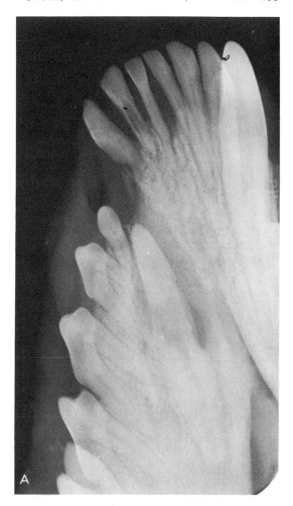

FIGURE 5–18. *A.* Periodontal and periapical disease. The right canine tooth has not erupted. A zone of radiolucency surrounds the tooth, and the adjacent alveolar bone is being destroyed. The dog presented with a mandibular sinus tract. *B.* Malocclusion. The mandibles project rostrally well beyond the level of the maxillae.

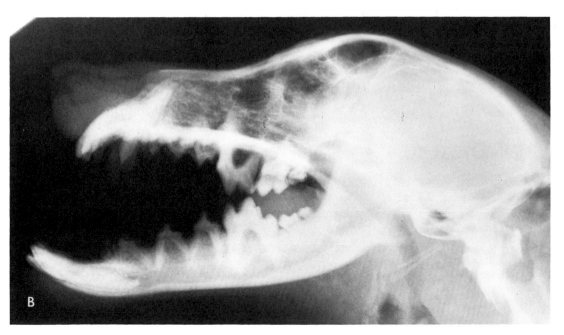

The middle ear and tympanic bullae also contain air. Infection in this region, accompanied by exudation, results in a loss of the normal air density. Usually only one ear is affected and comparison with the opposite side is helpful in detecting less obvious changes. Thickening of the tympanic bullae may be present.

THE SALIVARY GLANDS

The salivary glands and their associated ducts are not visible on plain radiographs. Sialography, that is the use of contrast medium to outline the ducts and glands, is sometimes employed. The principal indication for such studies is the presence of a so-called salivary cyst, or more correctly salivary mucocele. Sialography may outline rupture of a duct. The sublingual gland duct is the most commonly involved in salivary mucocele. In the case of a large mucocele, sialography helps to determine the side involved, that is whether left or right salivary gland complex. This is important if surgery is contemplated.

Anatomy

The parotid gland lies at the junction of the head and neck around the base of the auricular cartilage. Its duct opens in the mouth on a papilla on the mucosal ridge opposite the caudal margin of the fourth upper premolar (carnassial) tooth.

The zygomatic gland lies ventral to the zygomatic arch. Its duct opens about 1 cm caudal to the parotid papilla. Smaller ducts discharge individually into the mouth caudal to the opening of the main duct.

The mandibular gland lies just caudal to the angle of the jaw, between the external and internal maxillary veins. It is in a common capsule with the caudal portion of the sublingual gland. The mandibular duct opens on the lateral surface of the lingual caruncle at the frenum linguae.

The sublingual gland consists of several lobulated masses. The caudal portion is in a common capsule with the mandibular gland. The rostral portion of the gland lies along the line of the mandible. Its duct opens 1 to 2 mm caudal to the opening of the mandibular duct.

In about one-third of cases the sublingual and mandibular ducts join and have a common opening.

Radiography

Plain radiographs in the lateral and ventrodorsal positions are first made.

SIALOGRAPHY. Blunt cannulas made from fine gauge needles, 25 or 26 gauge, are necessary for cannulating the ducts. Oily (Dionosil Oily, Glaxo Laboratories) or water-soluble (Hypaque 50%, Winthrop Laboratories. Conray, Mallinckrodt.) contrast materials may be used. The dose depends on the size of the dog but may be from 0.1 to 0.3 ml of oily material or up to 2 ml of aqueous contrast medium.

The mandibular duct opening often appears as a small red spot on the lateral surface of the lingual caruncle. Gentle rubbing of the cannula tip in a rostrocaudal direction usually results in the cannula entering the duct. The sublingual duct, 1 to 2 mm caudally, is not so easy to find and enter; patience is required. The caruncle can be steadied by grasping with a fine forceps. However, it quickly becomes edematous if handled too much and unless care is exercised. Entry to the parotid duct is facilitated by grasping the oral mucosa with a forceps caudal to the duct papilla and pulling it gently rostromedially. Following injection of a duct lateral and ventrodorsal radiographs of the skull are made.

Normal Appearance

Following successful injection of a duct the duct and gland are outlined. A normal gland shows an arboreal type pattern, since branching ductules are outlined. The mandibular duct runs parallel to the ramus of the mandible and then dips ventrally into the gland. The sublingual duct parallels the mandibular duct and the several lobules of the gland are outlined. The parotid duct runs to the angle of the jaw, where it divides into several smaller ductules before entering the gland. The zygomatic duct is short and runs in a dorsocaudal direction to enter the gland. (Fig. 5–19).

Abnormalities

SALIVARY MUCOCELE. Salivary mucocele results from rupture of a salivary duct. The duct of the sublingual gland is most commonly affected. The cause remains obscure. If a duct is ruptured, sialography will show that the contrast medium leaks from the duct and into the fluid collected in the mucocele. This

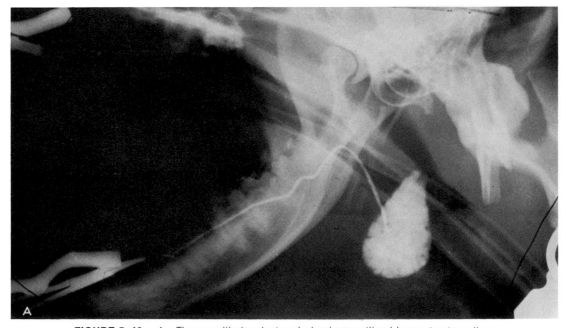

FIGURE 5–19. *A.* The mandibular duct and gland are outlined by contrast medium.

(*Illustration continued on the following page.*)

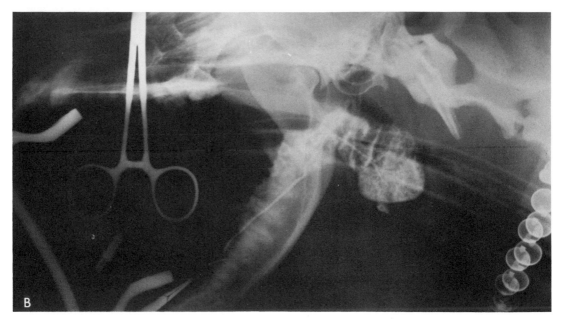

FIGURE 5–19. *Continued.*   B.   Less contrast medium outlines the glandular ductule system.

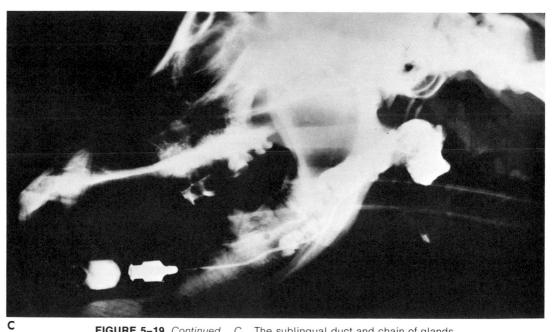

C

FIGURE 5–19. *Continued.*   C.   The sublingual duct and chain of glands.

(Illustration continued on the opposite page.)

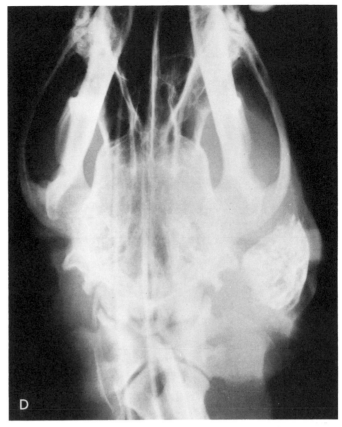

FIGURE 5–19. *Continued.* *D.* A normal parotid sialogram.

outlines the mucocele. If a duct is intact its integrity will be demonstrated on the contrast study and the corresponding gland will be outlined. (Fig. 5–20).

SIALOLITHS.   Sialoliths are rare in dogs and cats. When present they are seen as radiopaque densities along the course of a salivary duct. Air introduced into the duct during injection of positive contrast material may simulate sialoliths.

NEOPLASIA.   Adenocarcinoma of the mandibular or parotid glands is occasionally encountered in old dogs and cats. The condition is rare. While diagnosis is usually by methods other than radiographic, sialography may identify a salivary gland and distinguish it from an adjacent neoplastic mass.

THE NASOLACRIMAL DUCTS

The nasolacrimal ducts can be studied by dacryocystorhinography, that is, the introduction of contrast medium into the ducts. The medium is introduced by means of a cannula inserted into the superior puncta. Water-soluble (Hypaque 50%, Winthrop Laboratories; Renografin 60, Squibb & Sons) or oily (Dionosil Oily, Glaxo Laboratories, Ltd.) agents may be used. The information gained is limited. (Fig. 5–21).

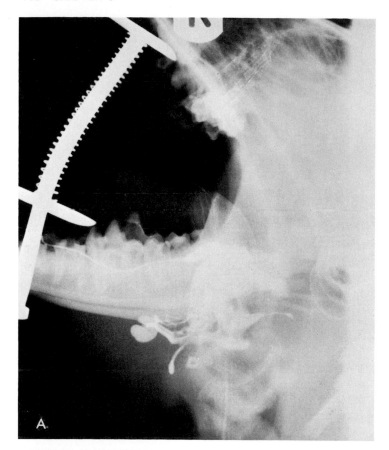

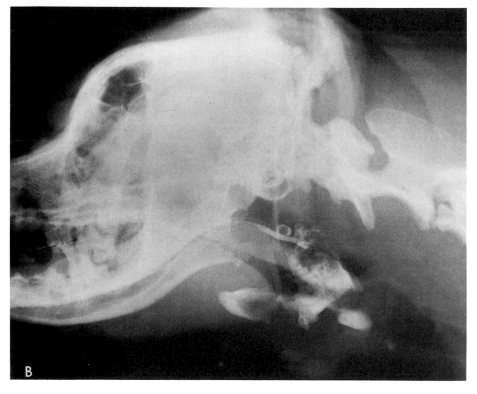

FIGURE 5–20. *A. B.* Leakage of contrast medium into salivary mucoceles following injections into ruptured ducts.

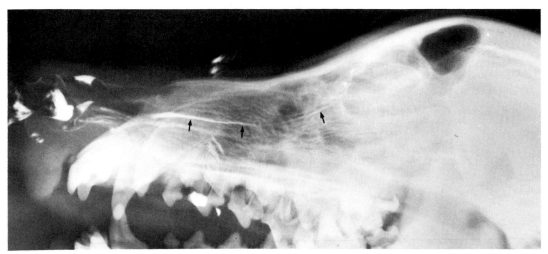

FIGURE 5–21. A nasolachrymal duct (arrows) outlined by contrast medium. The contrast material is leaking from the nose.

THE BRAIN

The brain lies within the bony cranium and is not visible on plain radiographs. Abnormalities within the brain are demonstrated by contrast studies. The usual methods of studying the brain are cerebral angiography, cranial sinus venography, and ventriculography.

Cerebral Arteriography

Cerebral arteriography is the outlining of the cerebral arteries by means of contrast medium.

ANATOMY

The left and right carotid arteries and the left and right vertebral arteries form the blood supply to the brain. These vessels are interconnected by several anastomotic branches.

The internal carotid artery, within the cranium, runs rostrodorsally, traversing the cavernous venous sinus that separates the dura mater into two layers. At the level of the optic chiasm it perforates the dura mater and reaches the subarachnoid space. Here it divides into rostral, middle, and caudal cerebral branches.

The vertebral arteries, branches of the subclavian arteries, anastomose within the cranium to form the basilar artery. The vertebral artery, having given off the caudal cerebellar, the acoustic, and the pontine arteries, bifurcates and contributes to the arterial circle at the base of the brain caudally, in common with the internal carotid artery rostrally and the caudal communicating artery laterally.

RADIOGRAPHY

Cerebral arteriography is the outlining of the cerebral arteries by contrast medium. It requires general anesthesia. Atropine is recommended 15 to 30 minutes before the induction of anesthesia. A rapid film changer is necessary for serial studies though much information can be gained from one or two films made three and six seconds after completion of the injection of contrast medium. Later films will show venous filling. A power syringe injector ensures complete filling of the cerebral vessels. The internal carotid and the vertebral arteries can be cannulated, the internal carotid directly in the neck and the vertebral via the femoral artery. The reader is referred to specialized works on the subject for technical details. Meglumine iothalamate 60 per cent (Conray, Mallinckrodt Lab.) is used at a dosage rate of 1 ml per 3 kg body weight. Sodium salts of iodine may cause severe reactions.

NORMAL APPEARANCE

The normal appearance of cerebral arteriograms is demonstrated in Figure 5–22.

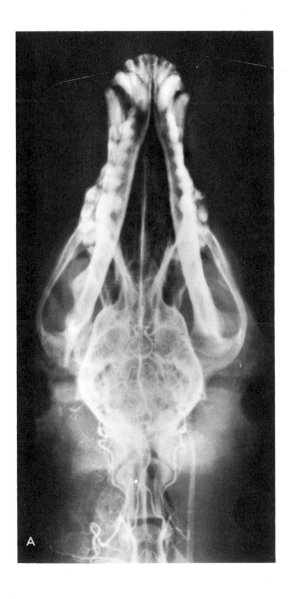

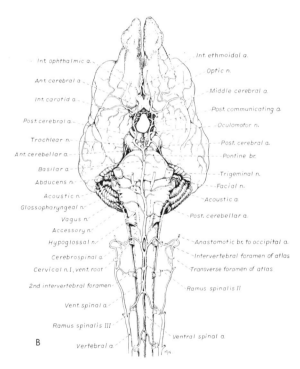

FIGURE 5–22. *A, B.* Cerebral arteriography. *A,* This normal arteriogram was taken 1.5 seconds after injection of contrast media into the vertebral artery at the C4 level. *B* identifies specific arteries. (*A* is from Ettinger. Textbook of Veterinary Internal Medicine. Phila. W. B. Saunders Co. *B* is from Miller, Christensen, and Evans. Anatomy of the Dog. Phila. W. B. Saunders Co.

(Illustration continued on the opposite page.)

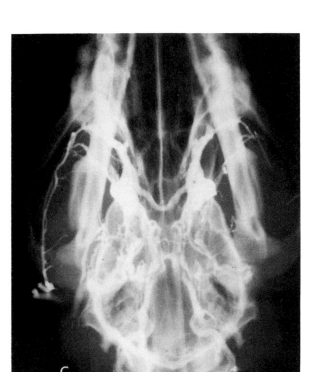

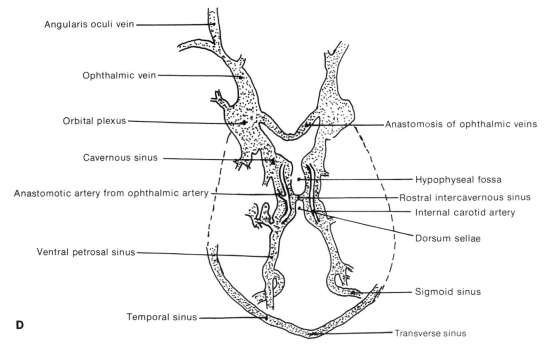

Angularis oculi vein

Ophthalmic vein

Orbital plexus

Cavernous sinus

Anastomotic artery from ophthalmic artery

Ventral petrosal sinus

Temporal sinus

Anastomosis of ophthalmic veins

Hypophyseal fossa

Rostral intercavernous sinus

Internal carotid artery

Dorsum sellae

Sigmoid sinus

Transverse sinus

D

FIGURE 5–22. *Continued. C.* A normal cranial sinus venogram following injection of contrast medium into the angularis oculi vein. *D.* A sketch of the vascular outlines. (After a drawing by Dr. R. Mitten.)

ABNORMALITIES

Internal carotid injection is recommended for the demonstration of abnormalities in the rostral portion of the brain; vertebral artery injection is recommended for midbrain and brain stem lesions. Diagnosis is based on the displacement of normal vessels or on the appearance of abnormal vessels in the case of tumors or aneurysms. (Fig. 5–23).

Cranial Sinus Venography

Cranial sinus venography is a relatively simple technique for outlining veins and sinuses at the base of the skull. It may demonstrate lesions on or near the floor of the cranium.

ANATOMY

Within the dura mater there are venous passages into which the veins of the brain and the surrounding bone drain. There are dorsal and ventral sinuses

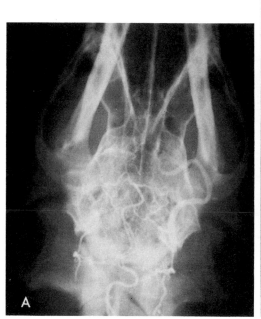
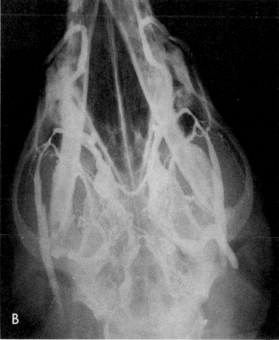

FIGURE 5–23. *A.* This arteriogram was performed via the right vertebral artery. There is good filling of the basilar artery and of the rostral cerebellar and caudal cerebral vessels. The right middle cerebral and rostral cerebral vessels also fill adequately. There is failure to fill the left rostral and middle cerebral vessels and an apparent deformity of the circle of Willis on the left side. The study suggests a space-occupying mass to the left of the midline compressing adjacent vessels. *B.* This study shows adequate filling of both angularis oculi veins, which were injected simultaneously. There is good filling of the orbital plexuses. However, within the cranium, there is normal filling of the right cavernous sinus but almost total absence of filling of the left cavernous sinus. The outline of the left internal carotid artery is lost. Caudally, both petrosal and sigmoid sinuses fill adequately. This study suggests an obstructing lesion on the left side. The two studies taken in combination suggest a left side lesion involving the hypothalamic region, causing pressure deformities in adjacent vessels. At autopsy there was a hypothalamic-hypophyseal tumor primarily on the left side. (Courtesy of Dr. R. Carithers).

that communicate with one another. Dorsally there is the dorsal sagittal sinus, straight sinuses, and the transverse sinus. Ventrally there is the intercavernous sinus and paired cavernous, sigmoid, occipital, dorsal, and ventral petrosal sinuses. The cavernous sinuses lie on the floor of the middle cranial fossa.

RADIOGRAPHY

General anesthesia is required. Contrast medium is injected into the angularis oculi vein. This outlines the intra- and extracranial venous systems. The injection can be made percutaneously into the vein just rostral to the orbit. Meglumine iothalamate 60 per cent (Conray, Mallinckrodt Lab.) is recommended at a dosage rate of 5 to 10 ml, depending on the size of the dog. Sodium diatrizoate 50 per cent (Hypaque, Winthrop Laboratories) is also suitable. The injection is made rapidly and radiographs are made as the injection is completed. The jugular veins should be compressed as the injection is made. Pressure on the facial vein during injection may reduce unwanted visualization of extracranial vessels. In many cases both right and left sides will be opacified following injection into either the right or left angularis oculi vein. If only one side is opacified the study can be repeated on the opposite side. Both veins may be injected simultaneously.

NORMAL APPEARANCE

The normal appearance of the sinuses is illustrated in Figure 5–22.

ABNORMALITIES

Abnormalities are manifested as displacement or obstruction of the normal vessels. (Fig. 5–23).

Orbital venography has been described as a means of demonstrating the veins around the orbit and retrobulbar space. Contrast medium is injected into the facial vein, the dorsal nasal vein, or the angularis oculi vein.

Ventriculography

Contrast medium, usually air, is injected into the ventricular system to outline the ventricles. Needles are passed through the cerebral cortex and into the lateral ventricles. The procedure is specialized and is used to demonstrate hydrocephalus, cerebral atrophy, or masses displacing the ventricles. In cases of hydrocephalus with open fontanelles, direct puncture of the ventricles is possible. (Fig. 5–24). Metrizamide may be used instead of air.

HYDROCEPHALUS

Hydrocephalus is an abnormal accumulation of fluid within the brain. It may be the result of increased production of cerebrospinal fluid or decreased resorption. It may be congenital or acquired. Obstruction to the normal flow of the cerebrospinal fluid may result in hydrocephalus.

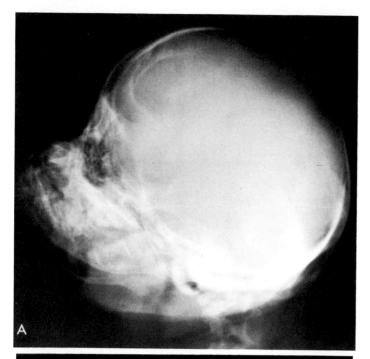

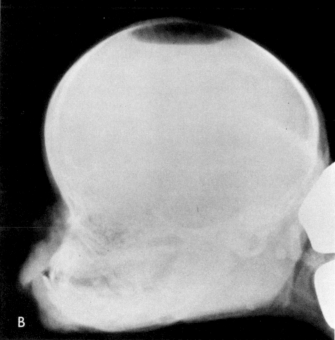

FIGURE 5-24. *A.* A grossly enlarged skull due to hydrocephalus. *B.* Air introduced into the ventricles shows a fluid level ventral to the calvarium. This indicates gross distention of the ventricles. (The hand, even when gloved, should not be in the x-ray beam).

In animals with congenital hydrocephalus the skull is often grossly enlarged and the fontanelles and suture lines remain open. No radiographic changes are seen on plain films in cases of acquired hydrocephalus because the skull bones are fused and fully formed. Ventriculography is used to outline the ventricular system. Varying degrees of hydrocephalus are encountered, from the gross, in which changes are obvious, to the mild, in which no radiographic evidence is visible on plain radiographs. (Fig. 5–24).

THE VERTEBRAL COLUMN

The vertebral column is frequently studied radiographically. Bone abnormalities are demonstrated on plain films. Associated soft tissue abnormalities can be demonstrated by the use of contrast media.

Anatomy

The vertebral column consists of approximately 50 vertebrae comprising cervical, thoracic, lumbar, sacral, and caudal (coccygeal) vertebrae. The dog and cat have seven cervical, thirteen thoracic, seven lumbar, three sacral, and a variable number of caudal vertebrae.

A typical vertebra consists of a body, an arch and a variable number of processes. Some vertebrae have modified shapes.

CERVICAL. There is a marked variation in the structure of the various cervical vertebrae.

The first cervical vertebra, or atlas, consists of a central arch and two wide horizontal wings. Each wing is penetrated by a foramen, which is visible radiographically.

The second cervical vertebra, or axis, carries a long, thin, dorsal spine. The transverse processes are directed caudally and each is perforated by a foramen — the foramen transversarius. The odontoid process, or dens, is a cranioventral eminence that is long and rounded and extends almost to the occiput.

From the third to the sixth cervical vertebrae, the transverse processes are bifid, and in the case of the fourth and fifth they take the form of a wide plate. The transverse process of the sixth has a small tubercle cranially and a broad plate caudally.

The body of the seventh vertebra is comparatively short.

The spinous processes become more prominent on each succeeding vertebra from the fourth caudally. (Fig. 5–25A–D).

THORACIC. The bodies of the thoracic vertebrae are shorter than those of the cervical vertebrae. The spinous processes are directed caudally as far as the anticlinal vertebra, which is usually the eleventh. Demifacets are present for rib articulations. Accessory processes are present on the last four or five vertebrae.

LUMBAR. The bodies of the lumbar vertebrae are longer than those of the thoracic. The spinous processes are directed cranially and the transverse processes cranially and laterally. Accessory processes are present on the first five vertebrae. They overlie the intervertebral foramina. The spinous processes increase in height from the first to the seventh. (Fig. 5–25E–H).

THE SACRUM. The sacrum is composed of three fused vertebrae and the spinous processes are fused to form a notched crest.

CAUDAL (COCCYGEAL). These vary in number from 6 to 23. Their shape is variable, being longer cranially and shorter caudally.

The intervertebral foramina are foramina that are formed from notches on the caudal aspects of the vertebrae that complement similar notches on the cranial aspects of succeeding vertebrae. They are present from the second cervical to the sacrum.

Text continued on page 422

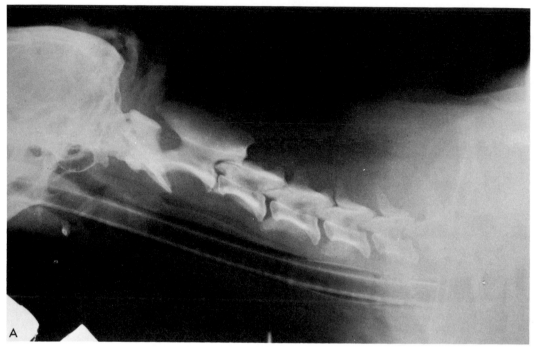

FIGURE 5–25. Normal vertebrae. *A–D.* Cervical vertebrae.

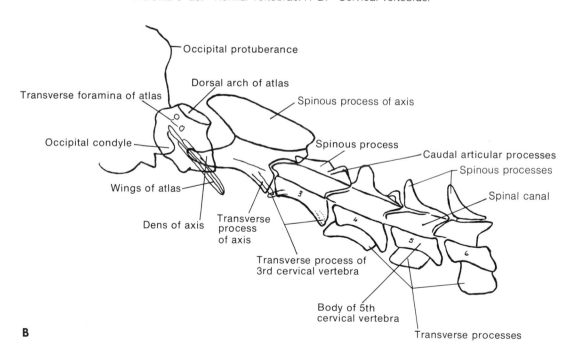

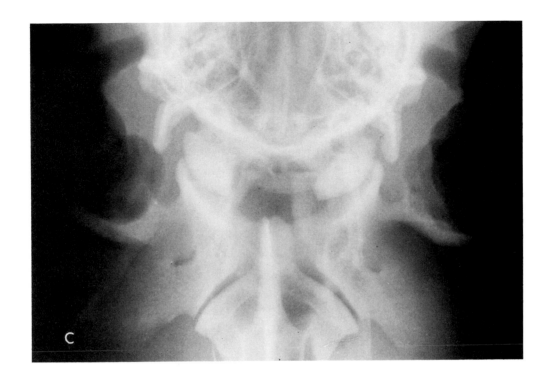

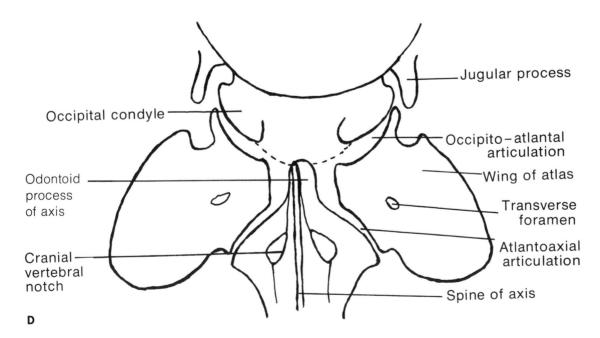

Jugular process

Occipital condyle

Occipito-atlantal articulation

Wing of atlas

Odontoid process of axis

Transverse foramen

Atlantoaxial articulation

Cranial vertebral notch

Spine of axis

D

(Illustration continued on the following page.)

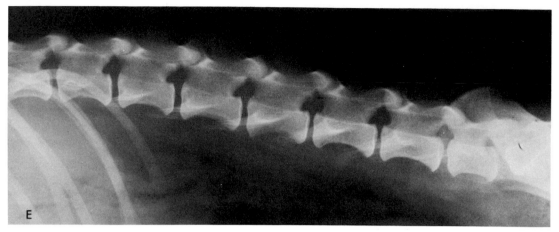

FIGURE 5–25. *Continued.* *E–H.* Lumbar vertebrae.

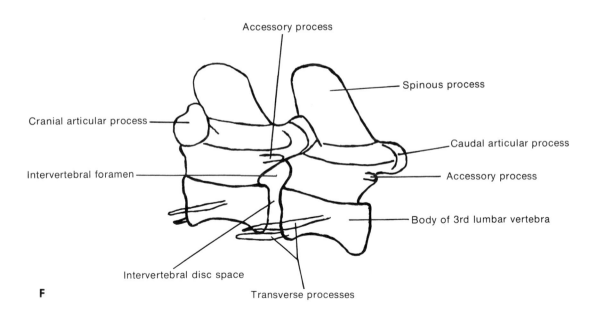

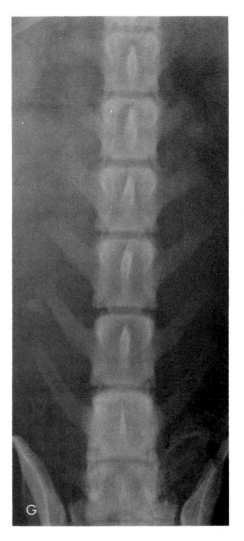

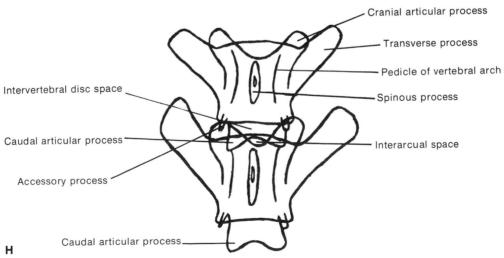

Cranial articular process

Transverse process

Pedicle of vertebral arch

Spinous process

Intervertebral disc space

Caudal articular process

Accessory process

Interarcual space

Caudal articular process

H

Radiography

The standard views for the study of the vertebral column are the lateral and the ventrodorsal. Sedation, or general anesthesia, greatly facilitates positioning and is a requirement for the proper study of the cervical region.

In the lateral view the spine should be parallel to the cassette and foam rubber cushions should be used under the cervical and lumbar vertebrae to achieve proper positioning. For cervical studies the forelimbs are drawn caudally over the thorax. Gentle traction, exerted between the forelimbs and the head, is useful. The head should be in a normal position relative to the neck. Slight stretching of the spine by drawing the forelimbs cranially and the hindlimbs caudally is also useful in making lateral exposures of the thoracic and lumbar vertebrae. In ventrodorsal views, the sternum should overlie the thoracic vertebrae.

MYELOGRAPHY

Myelography is the introduction of contrast material into the subarachnoid space. It is used to demonstrate pressure on the spinal cord from either intrinsic or extrinsic causes. Efforts to demonstrate spinal abnormalities using contrast medium in the epidural space or in the vertebral veins have not been wholly successful.

Myelography is indicated when it is required to demonstrate cord compression prior to surgery when other findings are inconclusive. Because of the associated hazards it should be employed only when absolutely necessary.

Myelography may be carried out using oily contrast medium or water-soluble contrast medium.

OILY CONTRAST MEDIUM.   The agent used is iophendylate (Pantopaque — General Electric, Keleket, Lafayette, Philips, Picker, Westinghouse; or Myodil — Glaxo Laboratories). This is given into the cisterna magna, which is a dilatation of the subarachnoid space. It lies at the junction of the occiput and the atlas. To enter the cisterna magna the anesthetized animal is placed in lateral recumbency and the atlanto-occipital articulation is flexed. A 1½ or 2 inch, 22 gauge needle is inserted on the midline, halfway between the occipital protuberances and the wings of the atlas. The needle is directed slightly caudad and slowly advanced into the cisterna magna. A good flow of cerebrospinal fluid results when the needle is correctly positioned. The dog often flinches as the needle penetrates the dura mater.

When the cisterna magna has been entered, about 3 ml of cerebrospinal fluid are withdrawn and a similar quantity of the contrast agent is injected. The animal is then placed on a tilt with the head higher than the tail.

While giving good contrast, oily preparations have not been found satisfactory in dogs. They tend to globulate when mixed with the cerebrospinal fluid. They may take a long time to gravitate down the subarachnoid space, particularly in smaller breeds. The contrast material is not readily recoverable from the subarachnoid space and it persists there for long periods of time, during which it can have irritant effects. (Fig. 5–26).

WATER-SOLUBLE CONTRAST MEDIUM.   Water-soluble contrast agents are irritant to the meninges. They do, however, mix readily with the cerebrospinal fluid and so give more consistent results than the oily preparations. Furthermore they are rapidly absorbed.

The agent most commonly used is methiodal sodium (Skiodan 40%, Winthrop Laboratories). It is used as a 20% solution being diluted with bacteriostatic water.

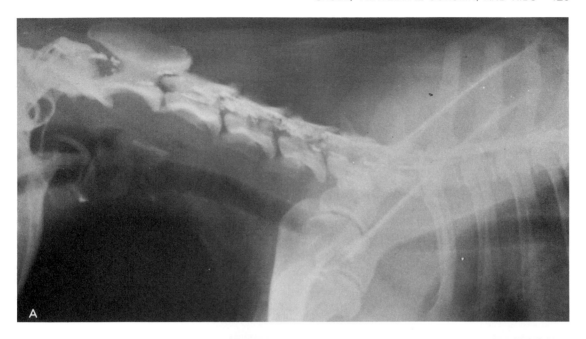

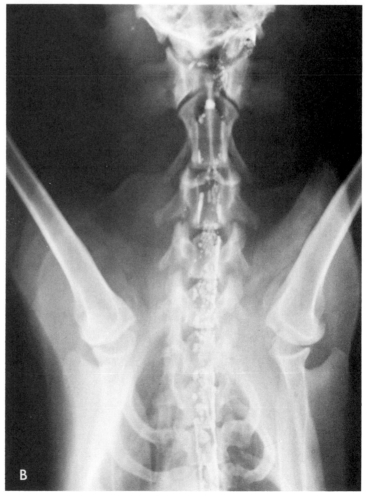

FIGURE 5–26. *A, B.* Oily contrast myelography. Marked globulation of the contrast medium has taken place in the cervical and cranial thoracic regions. Although the contrast is good, these are not diagnostic radiographs.

Five ml of Skiodan 40% are mixed with 4.5 ml of water and 0.5 ml of 2% Xylocaine (Xylocaine HCL 2%, Astra Pharmaceutical Products, Inc.). The dosage rate is 0.3 ml of the solution per kilogram body weight. If a cervical lesion is suspected, 3 ml of cerebrospinal fluid are withdrawn at the cisterna magna and the dosage rate is increased to 0.45 ml/kg. (Fig. 5–27).

The injection is made between the fifth and sixth lumbar vertebrae. Injection may also be made between the third and fourth or the fourth and fifth lumbar vertebrae. The more caudal site is preferred. Administration through the cisterna magna is not advisable because of the irritant nature of the contrast material. Adhesive arachnoiditis has been reported in man as a sequel to the use of water-soluble contrast media.

The dog is placed in lateral recumbency with the back arched. Alternatively, the dog may be placed in sternal recumbency with padding under the abdomen to arch the back. A 3 inch spinal needle is used. It is inserted just lateral to the sixth lumbar spinous process and directed medially and slightly cranial to enter the spinal canal through the dorsal intervertebral space. The needle is advanced to strike the floor of the canal. It is withdrawn slightly and the stylet removed. Leakage of spinal fluid from the needle confirms that it has been correctly placed. If no fluid is obtained, a small test injection is made and the position of the contrast medium is determined by making a radiograph. If fluoroscopy is available an attempt may be made to try to enter the subarachnoid space dorsally without transfixing the cord. This is not always successful. Fluoroscopy can also be used to monitor the test injection. Injection into the substance of the cord is disastrous. Injection into the epidural space results in a very irregular outline of the column of contrast medium. The spinal nerve roots may be outlined.

After the injection has been made the following radiographs are made immediately: lateral and ventrodorsal views of the thoracolumbar area; the animal is then rolled over onto the opposite side and a further lateral view is made of the thoracolumbar area; a coned-down view of the area of particular interest; a lateral view of the cervicothoracic region. The contrast solution is hypertonic and consequently is rapidly diluted and absorbed. If convulsions or muscular spasms ensue following the injection, they may be controlled by an injection of diazepam (Valium, Hoechst).

Metrizamide (Amipaque, Nyegaard & Co. Oslo, Norway) is a water-soluble contrast medium with a low osmolarity; it is, apparently, much less irritant than other water-soluble compounds. It may be given by cisternal puncture and it provides acceptable contrast. An isotonic solution is prepared by dissolving 3.75 g of metrizamide powder in 8.9 ml of the diluent provided (0.005% sodium bicarbonate). This gives an iodine concentration of 166 mg of iodine per ml. The dosage rate is 0.3 ml per kilogram body weight. Higher concentrations, up to 190 mg I/per ml., may be used. The contrast material is rather slowly absorbed and diagnostic films are still possible one hour after injection. The neck and forelimbs may be raised to facilitate caudal flow of the contrast medium. (Fig. 5–28).

Meglumine iocarmate (Dimer X, Andre Guerbert Laboratories, Paris, France) has also been used in dogs.

VENOGRAPHY

Venography has been described as a method of demonstrating cord compression. Depending on the size of the animal, 8 to 20 ml of a 60 per cent water-soluble contrast medium are injected into the saphenous vein. The caudal vena cava is compressed by compressing the abdomen. Films are made 15 and 20 seconds after

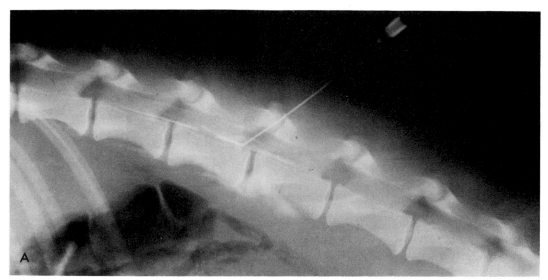

FIGURE 5–27. Myelography with methiodal sodium (Skiodan). *A.* A small test injection confirms accurate positioning of the needle. This is advisable if fluoroscopy is not available. The injection here is being made between the third and fourth lumbar vertebrae.

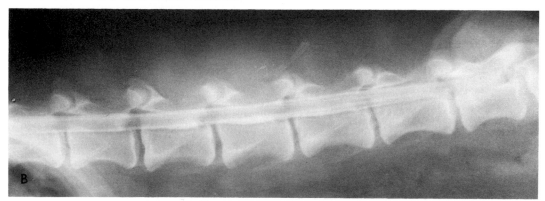

FIGURE 5–27. *Continued. B.* The lumbar subarachnoid space is outlined by the contrast medium.

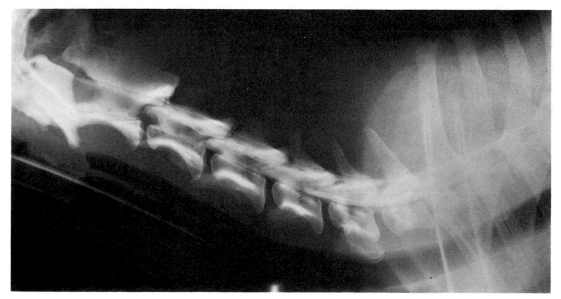

FIGURE 5–28. The cervical subarachnoid space is well outlined with metrizamide. The injection was made via the cisterna magna.

completing the injection. The vertebral veins are outlined. Compression is slowly released.

DISCOGRAPHY

Discography is the injection of contrast medium into the substance of a disc. Its use in the dog and cat has not gained general acceptance.

Normal Appearance

The normal appearance of the vertebral column is illustrated in Figure 5–25.

Abnormalities

DEVELOPMENTAL ANOMALIES

A congenitally malformed vertebral column may house a normal spinal cord. Most of the conditions seen have little clinical significance.

HEMIVERTEBRA.   This results from a failure of the vertebral body to develop fully. Various forms are seen. The vertebral body may show a midline cleft cranially and caudally giving the vertebra a "butterfly" appearance on the ventrodorsal view. Another form of hemivertebra appears wedge shaped on the lateral view, the apex of the wedge being ventrally located. Still another form appears wedge shaped on the ventrodorsal view. Compensatory changes in adjoining vertebrae are common. Hemivertebrae are most commonly seen in the thoracic vertebrae and are frequently associated with spondylosis in that area. They are most common in the bulldog and the Boston terrier. (Fig. 5–29).

BLOCK VERTEBRA.   Occasionally, two or more of the vertebral bodies are fused. This is a result of failure of the various segments to separate during development. The condition must be distinguished from inflammatory or degenerative conditions. There is usually no evidence of inflammatory reaction at the site. (Fig. 5–30).

TRANSITIONAL VERTEBRAE.   Sometimes vertebrae at the sacrolumbar junction or at the thoracolumbar junction may have some features that are common to both types of vertebrae. A transverse process may have the appearance of a rib. Clinically these anomalies are of no significance. They may be important from the point of view of accurately locating a surgical site. Similar anomalies may be seen in the sacrocaudal or cervicothoracic areas. (Fig. 5–31).

SPINA BIFIDA.   This is a rare condition that results from failure of the neural arch to close properly. There may be an associated hernia of the meninges. It is best seen on the ventrodorsal view by comparison with vertebrae that are normal cranial and caudal to the abnormality. Failure of fusion of the spinous processes can be seen so that the affected vertebra appears to have two spinous processes. Mild cases may show no clinical signs. (Fig. 5–32 A).

Because of the complex nature of spinal developmental processes other anomalies occur, but they are relatively rare.

Scoliosis is an abnomal curvature of the vertebral column in the lateral plane. It may be congenital or acquired due to an injury. (Fig. 5–32 B).

Kyphosis is an abnormal convex curvature of the spine as seen on the lateral view. (Fig. 5–29).

Text continued on page 430

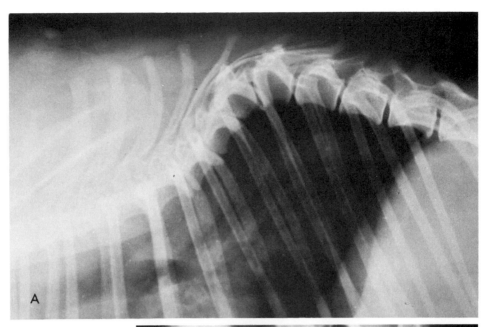

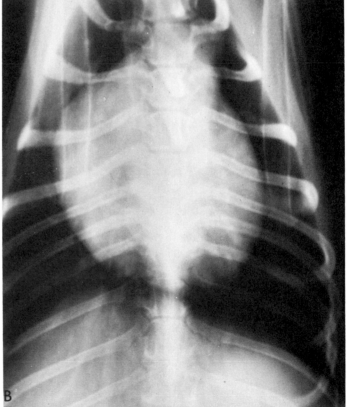

FIGURE 5-29. *A, B.* Hemivertebrae. The eighth and ninth thoracic vertebrae are wedge shaped, resulting in deformity of the spine with kyphosis. The ventrodorsal view shows crowding of the ribs in the area of the deformity.

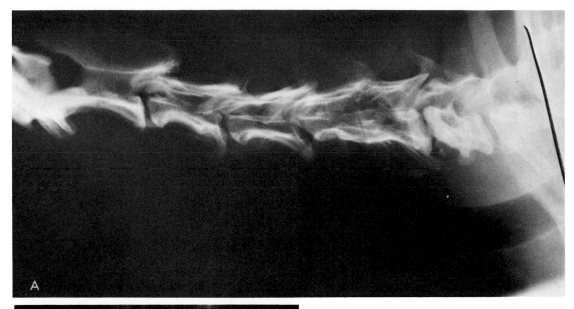

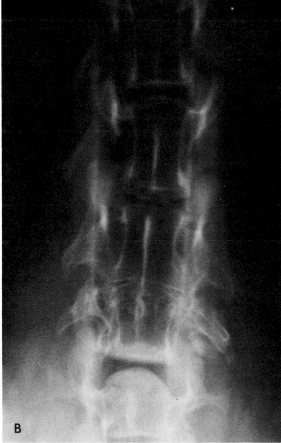

FIGURE 5–30. Block vertebra. The fifth and sixth cervical vertebrae are partially fused, a congenital anomaly. The vertebral bodies are also abnormal in shape.

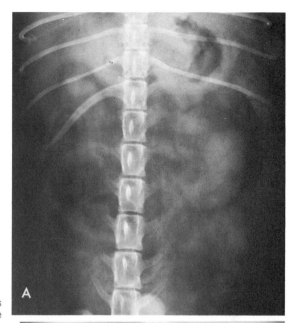

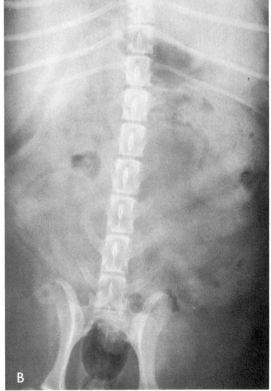

FIGURE 5–31. *A.* The thirteenth thoracic vertebra has only one rib. The rib that is present has some of the features of a lumbar transverse process. *B.* There are apparently only six lumbar vertebrae. The first lumbar vertebra has attached ribs.

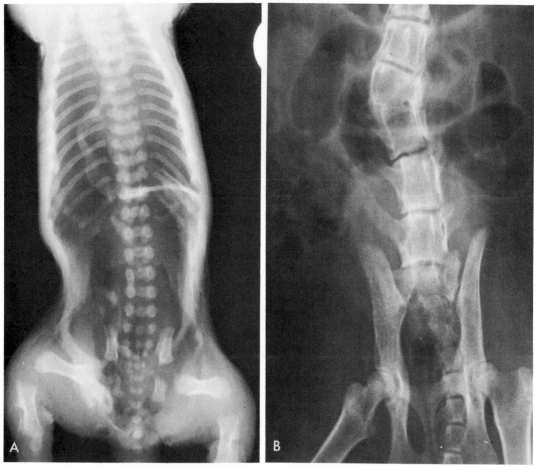

FIGURE 5–32. *A.* Spina bifida. This autopsy specimen shows failure of fusion of the spinous processes. *B.* Scoliosis in the spine of a cat due to deformities in the fourth and fifth lumbar vertebrae, which are almost entirely fused. The absence of inflammatory changes suggests that the deformity is congenital.

Deformity of the body of the third cervical vertebra has been reported as a cause of paralysis in young male Bassett hounds.

Dysgenesis and agenesis of the sacrum and other spinal anomalies have been described in the Manx cat.

DEGENERATIVE DISEASES

INTERVERTEBRAL DISC DISEASE.   Degeneration of the intervertebral discs is a common condition in dogs. It is less common in cats. Degeneration of the discs is a normal part of the aging process. Problems may arise, however, when the degenerative process proceeds more rapidly than usual. Degeneration of a disc may result in displacement of the pulpy nucleus, causing pressure on the spinal cord either directly or by causing the annulus fibrosus to bulge.

It is not unusual to detect degenerative changes in the intervertebral discs of animals that are showing no clinical signs of disease. Calcification of discs and narrowed intervertebral disc spaces, therefore, are not themselves indicative of cord pressure. For this reason correlation of radiologic and neurologic findings is essential in arriving at a diagnosis.

Anatomy

The intervertebral discs are spaced between the vertebral bodies from the junction of the second and third vertebrae caudally. Each disc has an outer laminated fibrous ring, called the annulus fibrosus, and a central nucleus, called the nucleus pulposus or pulpy nucleus, which is composed of a homogeneous gelatinous material. The ventral part of the annulus fibrosus is much thicker than the dorsal part.

Radiography

The intervertebral disc spaces are best evaluated on lateral radiographs of the spine. Short segments of the spine should be radiographed separately. There can be considerable distortion of the appearance of the intervertebral disc spaces cranial and caudad to the central beam. For this reason the use of a large film to give a survey view of a large segment of the vertebral column is not recommended.

Normal Appearance

On plain radiographs the intervertebral disc spaces are readily identified. The width of the spaces is about equal in any region of the vertebral column. Disc spaces appear to become narrower cranial and caudad to the level of the central ray of the x-ray beam. If the spine is not parallel to the film, pseudonarrowing of the disc spaces may be observed. Excessive stretching of the spine during radiography may mask small degrees of narrowing. The accessory processes on the caudal thoracic and cranial lumbar vertebrae may be mistaken for abnormal densities overlying the intervertebral foramina.

Radiologic Signs

Diagnosis of disc disease is based on finding one or more of the following signs:

a. Calcification of a disc or discs.

b. Narrowing of an intervertebral disc space.

c. Demonstration of nuclear material in the area of the intervertebral foramen. The disc material can sometimes be seen superimposed on the shadow of the foramen. The foramen provides a background contrast that is different from the bone density of the vertebrae. Hence, small amounts of nuclear material can sometimes be seen in that area when they would not be visualized were they overlying the vertebrae. (Fig. 5–33).

d. Myelography will demonstrate cord compression. (Fig. 5–34).

The fact that changes are seen radiographically does not necessarily imply that the changes seen are associated with clinical signs. It is necessary to demonstrate cord compression or to correlate the findings with the neurologic findings. An acute disc displacement may not be detected radiographically on plain films. Old lesions may be of no significance. The demonstration of cord compression is always significant.

Clinical signs associated with disc disease in cats are rare, though degeneration and protrusion of discs do occur.

SPONDYLOSIS (SPONDYLOSIS DEFORMANS). Spondylosis is a degenerative condition of the vertebrae that is seen in dogs and cats. It is characterized by new bone formation on the ventral aspects of the vertebral bodies at the intervertebral disc spaces. Bone spurs or bone bridges may form. The cause is unknown. The thoracic and lumbar vertebrae are most commonly affected. Spondylosis may cause no clinical signs.

Text continued on page 435

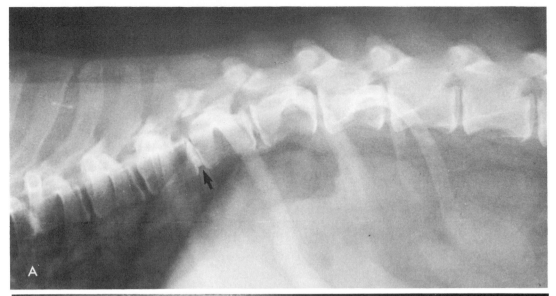

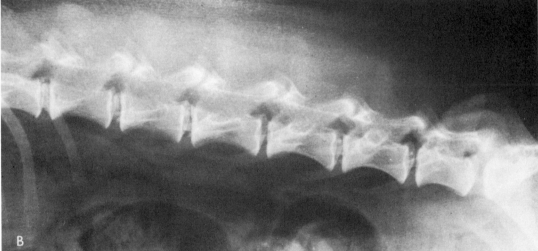

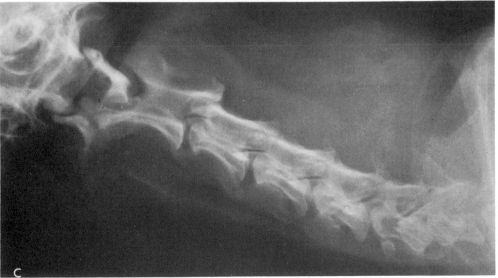

FIGURE 5–33.

432   (See legend on the opposite page.)

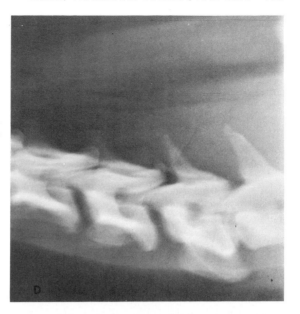

FIGURE 5–33. *A.* A calcified disc (arrow) is seen between the tenth and eleventh thoracic vertebrae. *B.* Several calcified discs are seen in the lumbar area. *C, D.* Evaluation of the disc spaces is frequently difficult in the caudal cervical region, particularly if muscle spasm is pronounced. Tomography is useful. In this case the plain radiograph is supplemented by a tomographic study. The tomogram shows a calcified disc between the sixth and seventh cervical vertebrae. *E.* A narrowed intervertebral disc space is present between the third and fourth lumbar vertebrae. The intervertebral foramen is different in shape from the foramina on either side. *F.* Calcified nuclear material (arrow) is seen within the spinal canal at the junction of the fourth and fifth lumbar vertebrae.

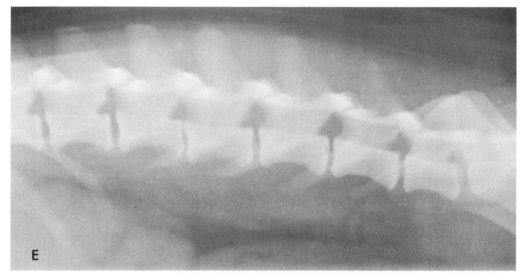

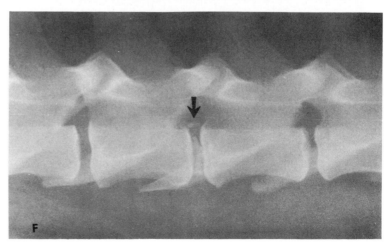

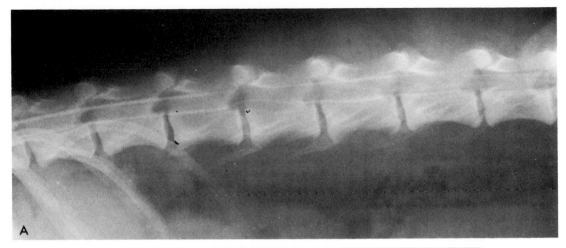

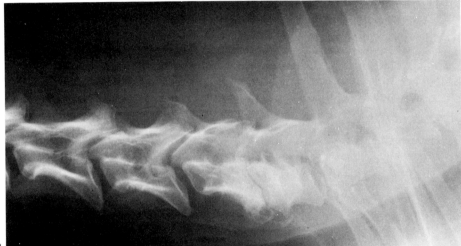

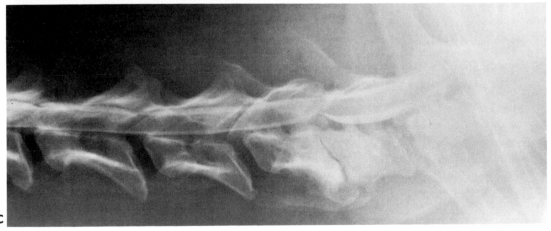

FIGURE 5–34. *A.* This contrast study shows narrowing of the subarachnoid space at the level of the disc be-tween the second and third lumbar vertebrae. This finding is consistent with displacement of the disc and cord pressure at this point. The contrast medium used was methiodal sodium. *B, C.* The plain film shows narrowing of the intervertebral disc space between the sixth and seventh cervical vertebrae. Both vertebrae show inflam-matory changes. This finding does not necessarily indicate that symptoms of cervical pain are referable to this area. The contrast study, however, shows pressure on the spinal cord at this point. The contrast medium used was metrizamide given via the cisterna magna.

Radiologic Signs

The lesions of spondylosis are best demonstrated on a lateral view.

a. In early cases small, hook-like projections develop on the ventral aspect of one or more vertebrae in the vicinity of the end-plate.

b. In more severely affected cases the new bone formation becomes more pronounced and large projections form on the ventral aspects of affected vertebrae. The projections on the caudal aspects of affected vertebrae appear to grow ventrocaudally toward the bodies of succeeding vertebrae, while those on the cranial aspects grow ventrocranially toward preceding vertebrae.

c. Complete bony bridges may develop, joining two or more of the vertebrae together. Care must be taken not to mistake two overlapping projections, seen on the lateral view, for union of the projections. In such cases the ventrodorsal view may be helpful. (Fig. 5–35).

SPONDYLOLISTHESIS (CERVICAL SPONDYLOPATHY; "WOBBLER" SYNDROME). This condition is most commonly seen in young Great Danes and Doberman pinschers. Other breeds may be affected and cases have been reported in the Bassett hound and the Rhodesian ridgeback. Clinically there is progressive incoordination of the hindlimbs. Affected animals are usually between 3 and 12 months of age. The cause would appear to be dorsal subluxation of the cervical vertebrae, particularly the fifth, sixth, and seventh. Less commonly the second, third, and fourth are involved. Other defects have also been described, such as deformity of vertebrae and osteochondrosis dissecans of the vertebral articulations.

Radiologic Signs

a. Flexed lateral views of the neck show the cranial end of affected vertebrae protruding dorsally into the spinal canal. Some dorsal movement is normally present at the cranial end of a vertebra when the neck is flexed; care should be exercised in evaluating this sign. The procedure should be carried out gently to avoid inflicting pressure damage on the cord.

b. Displacement of a vertebra may be seen on an extended view of the neck.

c. Myelography will demonstrate cord compression associated with flexion of the neck. (Fig. 5–36).

DURAL OSSIFICATION: (OSSIFYING PACHYMENINGITIS). This condition is characterized by the formation of bony plaques in the dura mater. The large breeds are more commonly affected. Radiographically, a fine linear bone density is seen running just above and parallel to the floor of the vertebral canal. This is best seen at the intervertebral foramina. Extensive plaque formation may be present in the absence of demonstrable radiographic changes. The condition would appear to have little clinical significance, though some authors believe otherwise. It has been reported to be associated with a degenerative myelopathy in old German Shepherd dogs. (Fig. 5–37).

HYPERVITAMINOSIS A. Excessive intake of vitamin A in cats, usually through being fed a liver-rich diet, may result in widespread confluent exostoses on the cervical and thoracic vertebrae. Presenting signs include rigidity of the neck and cervical sensitivity. Exostoses may spread to involve the entire spine. The limbs and ribs may also be affected. Joints may fuse. More advanced cases show ataxia, paralysis, or varying degrees of forelimb lameness. (See page 324.)

DEGENERATIVE JOINT DISEASE. Degenerative joint disease affecting the intervertebral joints is occasionally encountered. It is frequently not demonstrable radiographically. New bone formation about intervertebral joints may be seen. (Fig. 5–38).

Text continued on page 440

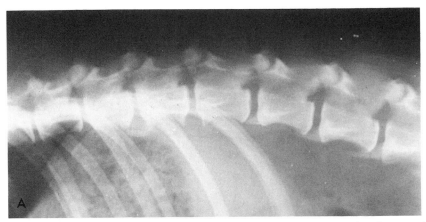

FIGURE 5–35. Spondylosis. *A.* Hook-like projections have developed on the ventral aspects of several vertebrae.

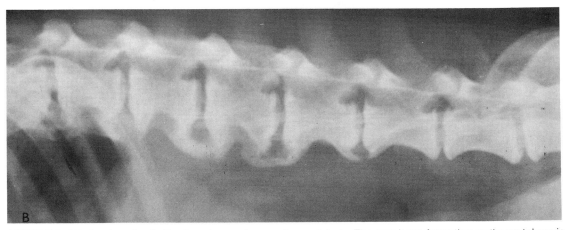

FIGURE 5–35. *Continued.* *B, C.* An advanced case of spondylosis. The new bone formation on the vertebrae is also evident on the ventrodorsal view.

(*Illustration continued on the opposite page.*)

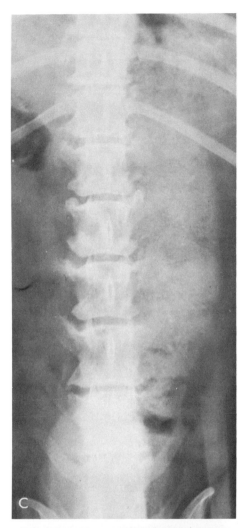

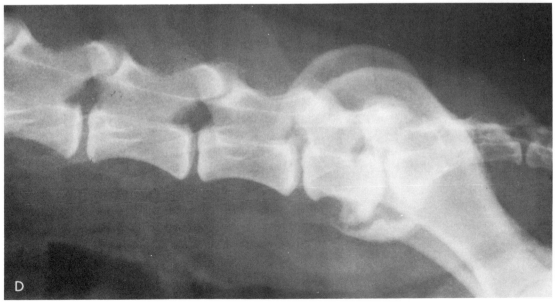

FIGURE 5–35. *Continued.* *D.* The lumbosacral junction is a common site of spondylosis.

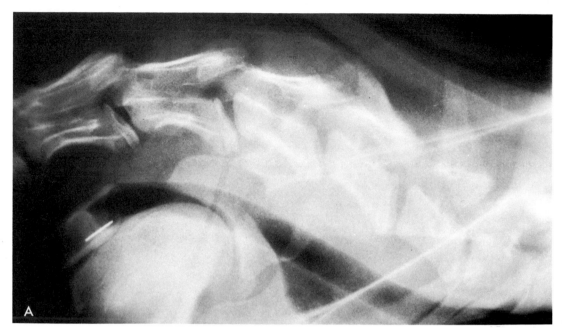

FIGURE 5–36. Spondylolisthesis. *A.* The flexed view of the neck shows dorsal displacement of the cranial aspect of the fifth cervical vertebra and, to a lesser extent, of the cranial aspect of the sixth.

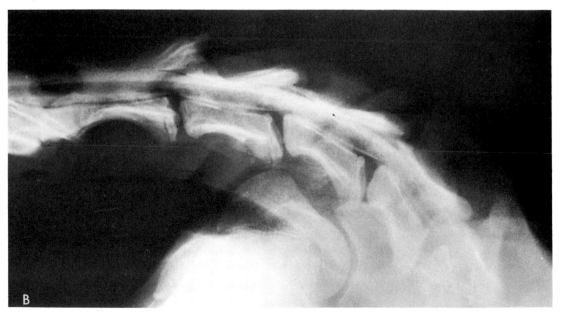

FIGURE 5–36. *Continued. B.* The myelogram shows marked pressure on the cord at the cranial aspect of the fifth cervical vertebra.

(*Illustration continued on the opposite page.*)

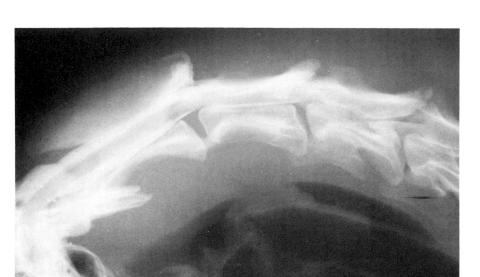

FIGURE 5–36. *Continued. C.* Care is required in assessing this sign. Some denting of the subarachnoid space is evident in normal dogs in the flexed position. Flexion of the neck may aggravate the clinical signs.

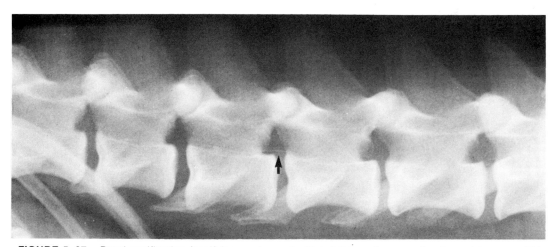

FIGURE 5–37. Dural ossification (ossifying pachymeningitis). A thin radiopaque line (arrow) is seen within the spinal canal above the intervertebral disc space between the third and fourth lumbar vertebrae. This represents ossification of the dura mater. A less evident line is seen between the first and second lumbar vertebrae. Ossification or calcification of the dorsal longitudinal ligament would show a line that is similar but more closely related to the floor of the canal.

INFECTIVE CONDITIONS

Infection involving the vertebral column is not very common. It may be the result of blood borne infection, the result of a wound, or it may be an extension from a nearby lesion.

OSTEOMYELITIS (SPONDYLITIS).   Osteomyelitis may affect the vertebrae just as it may affect other bones. The radiologic signs resemble those seen elsewhere with the condition. Bone destruction, periosteal reaction, and new bone formation with sclerosis of surrounding bone are usual features. Infection may spread to the spinal canal, causing meningitis and myelitis. The cranial lumbar vertebrae are most commonly affected. (The term "spondylitis" should be reserved to describe infection in a vertebra and the term "spondylosis" should be used to describe degenerative processes.) (Fig. 5–39).

DISCOSPONDYLITIS.   This is the term applied to a condition in which the disc and the vertebral end-plates are involved in an inflammatory process. The intervertebral disc space becomes narrow and changes in density are noted in the adjacent end-plates and vertebral bodies. The bodies become shorter as they undergo destruction. New reactive bone formation may simulate spondylosis deformans. *Brucella canis* and yeast-like organisms have been reported associated with discospondylitis. (Fig. 5–40).

TRAUMATIC CONDITIONS

FRACTURES.   Fractures are a common sequel to road traffic accidents. Pathologic fractures may affect the vertebrae.

Compression fractures cause the vertebral body to appear shorter than normal. Frequently, the affected vertebra assumes a wedge shape. Studies in both planes are necessary to evaluate the extent of the abnormality. Compression fractures may be associated with neoplasia, osteomyelitis, osteodystrophy, or trauma.

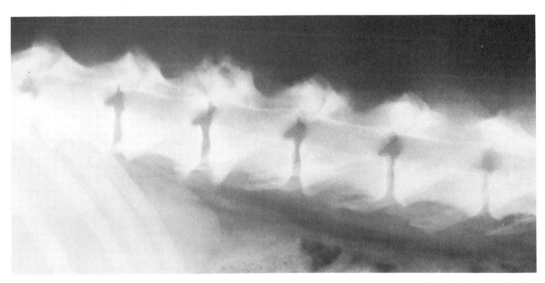

FIGURE 5–38. Degenerative joint disease. New bone formation is present around the lumbar articular facets. There is a concomitant spondylosis.

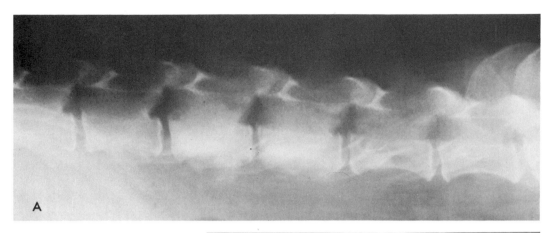

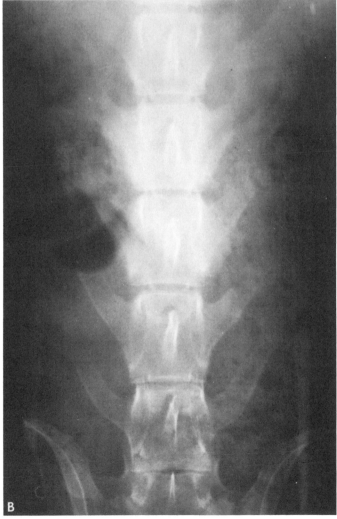

FIGURE 5–39. *A, B.* Osteomyelitis of the third and fourth lumbar vertebrae. Sclerosis is the primary radiologic sign in this case.

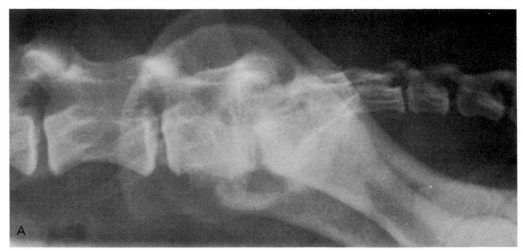

FIGURE 5-40. Discospondylitis. *A.* The inflammatory lesion at the lumbosacral junction has resulted in destruction of the vertebral end-plates. The disc space is narrowed and the lumbar vertebra and sacrum show sclerosis. Inflammatory new bone is visible ventrally.

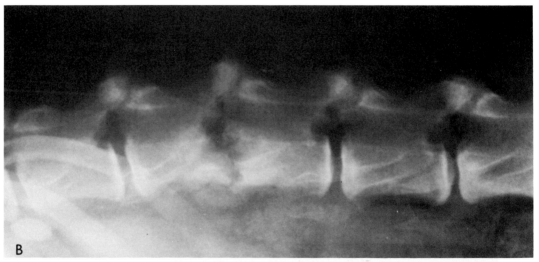

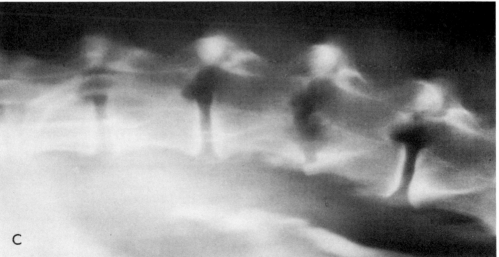

FIGURE 5-40. *Continued. B, C.* A destructive lesion affects the second and third lumbar vertebrae. The end-plates have been destroyed and the vertebral bodies invaded. Tomography shows the lesion in more detail. (Contrast medium is seen in a ureter).

Oblique fractures are often associated with considerable displacement of the fracture fragments. Separation of the vertebral end-plates is occasionally seen in young animals.

Fractures in the cranial cervical region are somewhat difficult to demonstrate. Fracture of the odontoid process is sometimes seen. Fractures with displacement cause a disruption of the normal line of the vertebra — a "step" effect is commonly seen along the lower border of the vertebra in the lateral view. A similar sign may be seen with dislocation. In all cases of suspected fracture, at least two views, made at right angles to one another, should be available for study. The spinous processes may be fractured but clinical signs are not always present. (Fig. 5–41).

DISLOCATIONS.   Complete dislocation of a vertebra is usually obvious radiographically. Subluxations are more difficult to evaluate. The intervertebral disc space may be narrowed and there will frequently be a slight disruption of the normal line of the vertebra relative to the preceding or succeeding vertebrae. Myelography will show cord compression at the site. In dislocation of the atlantoaxial articulation, the body of the axis is displaced dorsally and cranially and the distance between the arch of the atlas and the spine of the axis is greater than normal. (Fig. 5–42).

NEOPLASIA

Neoplasia of the vertebrae is relatively rare. Osteosarcoma and osteochondroma have been described, as have metastatic lesions. In most cases, malignancies associated with the vertebrae are destructive rather than proliferative in

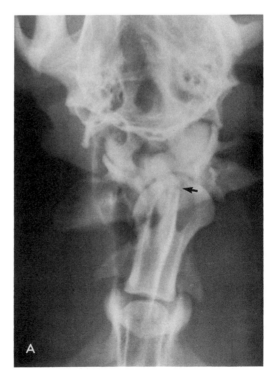

FIGURE 5–41. Vertebral fractures. *A.* The odontoid process of the axis is fractured. This is best seen on the ventrodorsal view (arrow).
(*Illustration continued on the following page.*)

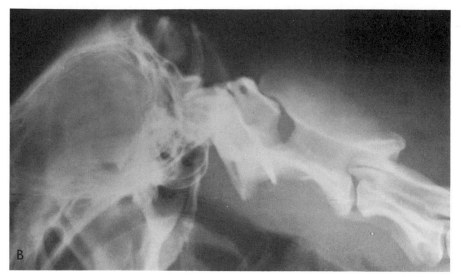

FIGURE 5–41. *Continued.* *B.* The lateral view shows that the normal space between the spinous process of the axis and the atlas has been narrowed.

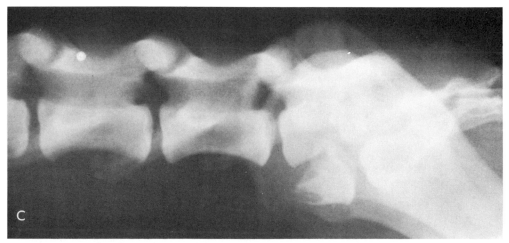

FIGURE 5–41. *Continued.* *C.* Fracture of the seventh lumbar vertebra.

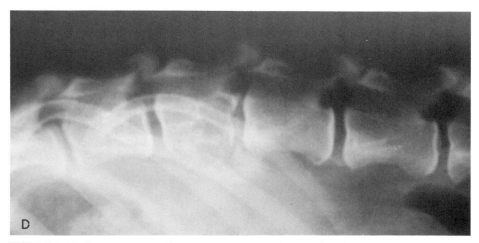

FIGURE 5–41. *Continued.* *D.* Collapse of the first lumbar vertebra due to an osteosarcoma.

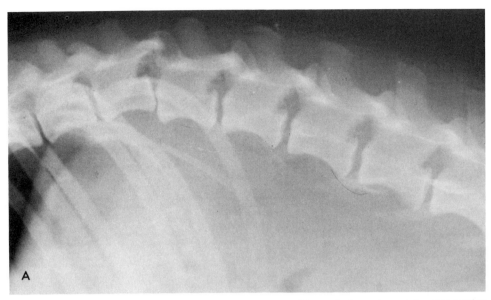

FIGURE 5–42.   *A.*   A subluxation is present between the thirteenth thoracic and the first lumbar vertebrae.

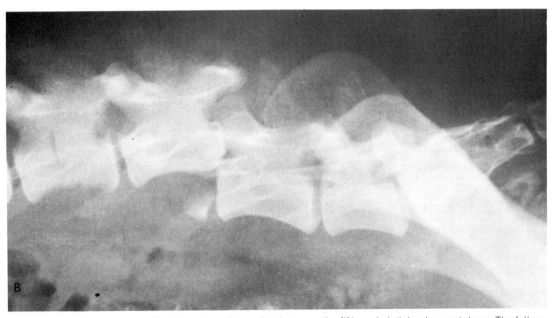

FIGURE 5–42. *Continued.*   *B, C.*   There is a dislocation between the fifth and sixth lumbar vertebrae. The full extent of the displacement is not evident on the ventrodorsal view. A small fracture fragment is seen cranial to the sixth vertebra.

(Illustration continued on the following page.)

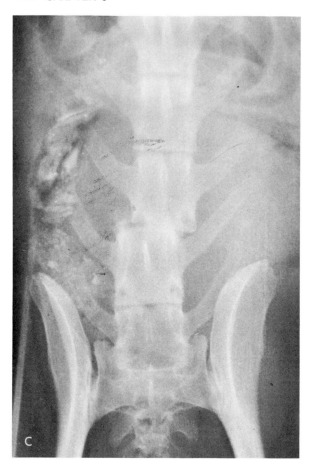

FIGURE 5–42. *Continued.*

nature. The vertebral end-plates and disc spaces are usually not involved in the destructive process. Compression fractures may occur. (Fig. 5–41*D*).

Neoplasms of the spinal cord may cause changes in the subarachnoid space that are demonstrable by myelography.

THE RIBS

Fracture of a rib or ribs is a common sequel to traffic accidents. Rib fractures may easily be missed radiographically if displacement is slight. Ventrodorsal and lateral views of the thorax should be made and a careful examination carried out of each rib for alteration in the normal rib line or for variation in density. Recent rib fractures usually have associated soft tissue damage. Rib fractures are often associated with other abnormalities, such as pulmonary hemorrhage, chylothorax, or pneumothorax.

Neoplasia of the ribs is not common but is occasionally seen. Chondrosarcoma is more common than osteosarcoma. Expansion of the rib and bone destruction are features. The ribs may be involved in an extension of an adjacent soft tissue tumor.

Ossification or calcification of the costochondral cartilages is common and is of no significance. (Fig. 5–43).

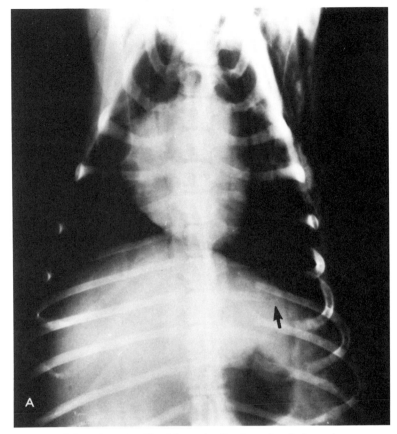

FIGURE 5–43.   The Ribs.   *A.*   Fracture of a rib (arrow).

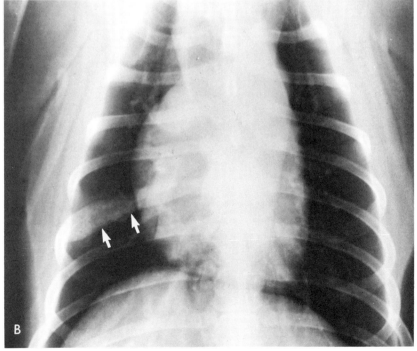

FIGURE 5–43. *Continued.*   *B.*   Coccidioidomycotic infection in a rib (arrows).
(*Illustration continued on the following page.*)

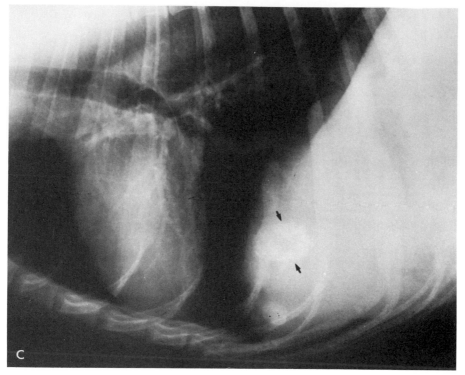

FIGURE 5–43. *Continued.*   *C.*   Osteocartilaginous exostosis on the rib cage (arrows).

THE STERNUM

Anatomy

The sternum is a series of eight bones. They form the floor of the thorax. The individual sternebrae are joined by cartilages, the intersternebral cartilages. The cranial sternebra is called the manubrium and the caudal sternebra the xiphoid process. The xiphoid cartilage prolongs the xiphoid process caudally. The first nine ribs articulate with the sternum through the costal cartilages. The first rib articulates with the manubrium and the others with the intersternebral cartilages. Ribs that have no sternal attachment are sometimes called "floating" ribs.

Radiography

The sternum is seen on lateral and ventrodorsal views of the thorax. It is best seen in the lateral view, since on the ventrodorsal view it overlies the thoracic vertebrae.

Abnormalities

FRACTURE.   The sternum is sometimes injured in traffic accidents or as the result of a blow or a kick. It usually heals well, though sometimes with a residual deformity. (Fig. 5–44).

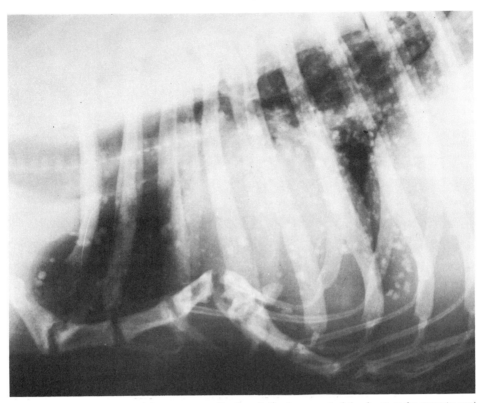

FIGURE 5–44. Fracture of the sternum with dorsal displacement of the fracture fragments and adjacent sternebrae. (The lungs show metastatic disease).

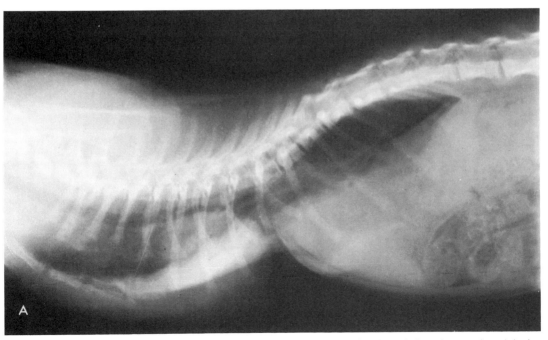

FIGURE 5–45. *A, B.* Pectus excavatum (chondrosternal depression). The lateral view shows a dorsal deviation of the caudal sternum. The heart is displaced dorsally. The ventrodorsal view, while slightly rotated, shows the heart displaced to the left side.

(*Illustration continued on the following page.*)

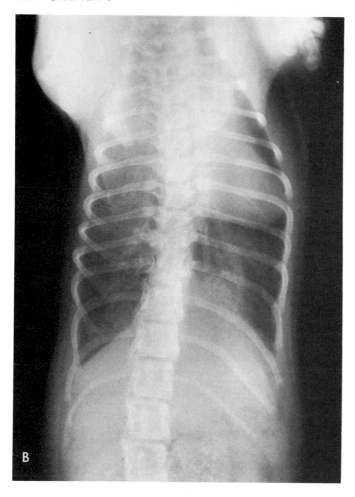

FIGURE 5–45. *Continued.*

PECTUS EXCAVATUM (CHONDROSTERNAL DEPRESSION). This is a congenital dorsal depression of the caudal portion of the sternum and the associated costal cartilages. Varying degrees of deformity are encountered in the costal cartilages and ribs. There may be some displacement of the heart. (Fig. 5–45).

NEOPLASIA. Neoplasia of the sternum is rare.

REFERENCES

Ackerman, N. and Corwin, L. A., Jr. (1975). Myelography with MP 2032–NMG meglumine iocarmate. J.A.V.R.S. XVI. 5. 174.

Bailey, C. S. and Holliday, T. A. (1975). Diseases of the spinal cord. In Textbook of Veterinary Internal Medicine. Diseases of the Dog and Cat. S. J. Ettinger, Editor. W. B. Saunders Co. Philadelphia.

Bardens, J. W. (1965). Congenital malformation of the foramen magnum in dogs. S. W. Vet. 18.

Brodey, R. S., Reid, C. F. and Sauer, R. M. (1966). Metastatic bone neoplasms in the dog. J.A.V.M.A. 148. 29.

Bullock, L. P. and Zook, B. C. (1967). Myelography in dogs using water soluble contrast medium. J.A.V.M.A. 151. 321.

Carlson, W. J. (1977). Veterinary Radiology. Gillette, E. L., Thrall, D. E. and Lebel, J. L., Editors. 3rd ed. Lea and Febiger. Philadelphia.

Conrad, C. R. (1975). Radiographic examination of the central nervous system. In Textbook of Veterinary Internal Medicine. Diseases of the Dog and Cat. W. B. Saunders Co. Philadelphia.

Dixon, R. T. and Carter, J. D. (1972). Canine orbital venography. J.A.V.R.S. XIII. 43.

Douglas, S. W. and Williamson, H. D. (1972). Principles of Veterinary Radiography. The Williams and Wilkins Co. Baltimore.

Douglas, S. W. and Williamson, H. D. (1970). Veterinary Radiological Interpretation. The Williams and Wilkins Co. Baltimore.

Ettinger, S. J. (1975) Editor. Textbook of Veterinary Internal Medicine. Diseases of the Dog and Cat. W. B. Saunders Co. Philadelphia.

Funkquist, B. (1962). Thoracolumbar myelography with water soluble contrast medium in dogs. Technique of myelography, side effects and complications. J. Sm. Anim. Pract. 3. 53.

Geary, J. C., Oliver, J. E. and Hoerlein, B. F. (1967). Atlantoaxial subluxation in the canine. J. Sm. Anim. Pract. 8. 557.

Gelatt, K. N., Cure, T. H., Guffy, M. M. and Jessen, C. (1972). Dacryocystorhinography in the dog and cat. J. Sm. Anim. Pract. 13. 381.

Glen, J. B. (1972). Canine salivary mucoceles. Results of sialographic examination and surgical treatment of 50 cases. J. Sm. Anim. Pract. 13. 515.

Hardy, W. D., Brodey, R. S. and Riser, W. H. (1967). Osteosarcoma of the canine skull. J.A.V.R.S. 8. 5.

Harvey, C. E. (1969). Sialography in the dog. J.A.V.R.S. X.18.

Henderson, R. A., Hoerlein, B. F., Kramer, T. T. and Meyer, M. E. (1974). Discospondylitis in three dogs affected with Brucella canis. J.A.V.M.A. 165. 451.

Hoerlein, B. F. Editor. (1971), Canine Neurology. 2nd ed. W. B. Saunders Co. Philadelphia.

James, C. C. M., Lassman, L. P. and Tomlinson, B. E. (1969). Congenital anomalies of the lower spine and spinal cord in Manx cats. J. Pathol. 97. 269.

Johnston, D. E. and Summers, B. A. (1971). Osteomyelitis of the lumbar vertebrae in dogs caused by grass seed foreign bodies. Aust. Vet. J. 47. 289.

King, A. S. and Smith, R. N. (1964). Degeneration of the intervertebral disc in the cat. Acta Orthop. Scand. 34. 139.

Koper, S. and Mucha, M. (1977). Visualization of the vertebral canal veins in the dog. A radiological method. J.A.V.R.S. XVIII. 4. 105.

Ladds, P., Guffy, M., Blauch, B. and Splitter, G. (1970). Congenital odontoid process separation in two dogs. J. Sm. Anim. Pract. 12. 46. 3.

Langham, R. F., Keahey, K. K., Mostosky, U. V. and Schirmer, R. G. (1965). Oral adamantinomas in the dog. J.A.V.M.A. 146. 474.

Larsen, J. S. (1977). Lumbosacral transitional vertebrae in the dog. J.A.V.R.S. XVIII. 3. 76.

Lee, R. and Griffiths, I. R. (1972). A comparison of cerebral arteriography and cavernous sinus venography in the dog. J. Sm. Anim. Pract. 13. 225.

Lindblad, G., Lunggren, G. and Olsson, S. E. (1962). On spinal cord compression in the dog. Adv. Sm. Anim. Pract. 3. 121.

Lord, P. F. and Olsson, S. E. (1976). Myelography with metrizamide in the dog. A clinical study on its use for the demonstration of spinal cord lesions other than those caused by intervertebral disc protrusions. J.A.V.R.S. XVII. 2. 42.

Miller, M. E., Christensen, G. C. and Evans, H. E. (1964). Anatomy of the Dog. W. B. Saunders Co. Philadelphia.

Morgan, J. P. (1967). Spondylosis deformans in the dog. A morphologic study with some clinical and experimental observations. Acta Orthop. Scand. (Suppl).

Morgan, J. P. (1969). Congenital anomalies of the vertebral column: a study of the incidence and significance based on a radiographic and morphologic study. J.A.V.R.S. 9. 21.

Morgan, J. P. (1969). Spinal dural ossification in the dog. Incidence and distribution based on a radiographic study. J.A.V.R.S. 10. 43.

Morgan, Joe P. (1972). Radiology in Veterinary Orthopedics. Lea and Febiger. Philadelphia.

Morgan, J. P., Suter, P. F., O'Brien, R. R. and Park, R. D. (1972). Tumors in the nasal cavity of the dog. A radiographic study. J.A.V.R.S. XIII. 18.

Morgan, J. P., Suter, P. F. and Holliday, T. A. (1972). Myelography with water soluble contrast medium: radiographic interpretation of disc herniation in dogs. Acta Radiol. (Suppl).

Morgan, J. P., Silverman, S. and Zontine, W. J. (1975). Techniques of Veterinary Radiography. The Printer. Davis, California.

Oliver, J. E. (1969). Cranial sinus venography in the dog. J.A.V.R.S. X. 66.

Oliver, J. E., Jr., Fletcher, O. J., Kneller, S. K. and Lewis, R. E. (1971). Pheochromocytoma metastases to the retrobulbar region of the canine skull. Demonstration by cavernous sinus venography. J.A.V.R.S. XII. 17.

Olsson, S. E. (1951). On disc protrusion in dogs (enchondrosis intervertebralis). Acta Orthop. Scand (Suppl. 8).

Palmer, A. C. and Wallace, M. E. (1967). Deformation of cervical vertebrae in Bassett hounds. Vet. Rec. 80. 430.

Parker, A. J. and Park, R. D. (1974). Occipital dysplasia in the dog. J. Amer. An. Hosp. Assoc. 10.5. 520.

Radberg, C. and Wennberg, E. (1973). Late sequelae following lumbar myelography with water soluble contrast media. Acta Radiol. 14.

Seawright, A. A., English, P. B. and Gartner, R. J. W. (1970). Hypervitaminosis A of the cat. Adv. Vet. Sci. Comp. Med. 14. 1.

Smallwood, J. E. and Beaver, B. V. (1977). Congenital chondrosternal depression (Pectus excavatum) in the cat. J.A.V.R.S. XVIII. 5. 141.

Stewart, W. C., Baker, G. J. and Lee, R. (1975). Temporomandibular subluxation in the dog. J. Sm. Anim. Pract. 16. 345.

Suter, P. F., Morgan, Joe P., Holliday, T. A. and O'Brien, R. R. (1971). Myelography in the dog. Diagnosis of tumors of the spinal cord and vertebrae. J.A.V.R.S. XII. 29.

Ticer, J. W. and Brown, S. G. (1974). Water soluble myelography in canine intervertebral disc protrusion. J.A.V.R.S. XV. 1. 3.

Ticer, J. W. (1975). Radiographic Technique in Small Animal Practice. W. B. Saunders Co. Philadelphia.

Wortman, J. A. (1974). Radiographic diagnosis of intervertebral disc disease in the dog. A comparison of noncontrast myelographic studies. Scientific Presentations and Seminar Synopses of the 41st Annual Meeting of the American Animal Hospital Association. 41. 698.

Wright, F., Rest, J. R. and Palmer, A. C. (1973). Ataxia of the Great Dane caused by stenosis of the cervical vertebral canal. Comparison with similar conditions in the Bassett hound, Doberman Pinscher, Ridgeback, and the thoroughbred horse. Vet. Rec. 92. 1.

Zontine, W. J. (1974). Dental radiographic technique and interpretation. in Vet. Clins. of North Amer. Nov., 1974. Radiology.

Zontine, W. J. (1975). Canine dental radiology. Radiographic technic, development and anatomy of the teeth. J.A.V.R.S. XVI. 3. 75.

MISCELLANEOUS

6

Calcification is a process by which calcium salts are deposited in tissue.

Dystrophic calcification is the deposition of calcium salts in abnormal tissue, that is in dead, degenerating, or damaged tissue.

Metastatic calcification is the deposition of calcium salts in tissue that is not the site of a disease process. It results from abnormalities in serum and in tissue calcium and phosphate levels. It is associated with metabolic disturbances such as hyperparathyroidism (hypercalcemia) or hypovitaminosis D.

The term ectopic calcification is used to denote the deposition of calcium salts in an organized fashion in soft tissue in radiographically visible amounts.

Examples of calcification in dogs are calcification of the external ear canals in old dogs, calcification of hematomas or bursae, or calcification in tumor tissue. Metastatic calcification is rare in dogs, but has been reported to affect the stomach wall.

Myositis ossificans is characterized by the deposition of bony plaques in muscle or the muscle itself may become ossified. Trabeculated bone densities may be seen.

Calcification cannot be distinguished from ossification unless a trabecular pattern can be identified. (Fig. 6–1).

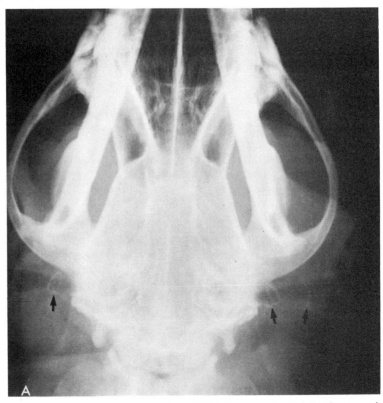

FIGURE 6–1. Calcification. *A.* Calcification (arrows) of the external ear canals in an old dog.

(*Illustration continued on the following page.*)

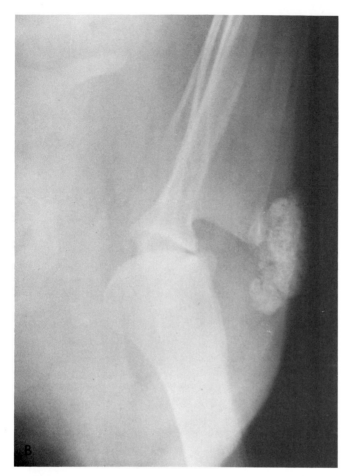

FIGURE 6–1. *Continued. B.* Calcification in a chronically inflamed infraspinatus bursa on the lateral aspect of a shoulder joint.

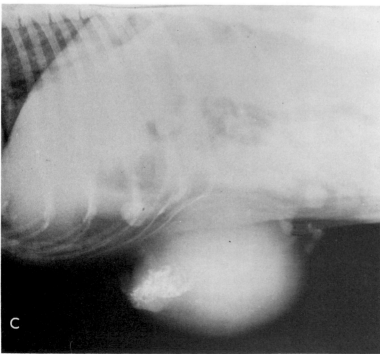

FIGURE 6–1. *Continued. C.* Calcification in a mammary tumor. The soft tissue swelling is well demonstrated.

Calcinosis Circumscripta

(Calcium Gout; Kalkgicht; Tumoral Calcinosis.)

In this condition, deposits of amorphous calcified material are laid down in the subcutaneous tissue and the skin. Lesions are usually found on the limbs, under the pads, or over bony prominences. Similar lesions have been described in the mouth. The etiology remains obscure. Chronic renal disease, hyperparathyroidism, and hypovitaminosis D have been suggested as possible causes. About half the cases seen occur in young German Shepherd dogs that are, otherwise, apparently normal. (Fig. 6–2).

Arteriovenous Fistula

An arteriovenous fistula is a direct communication between an artery and a vein without an interposed capillary bed. Such fistulas may be found centrally,

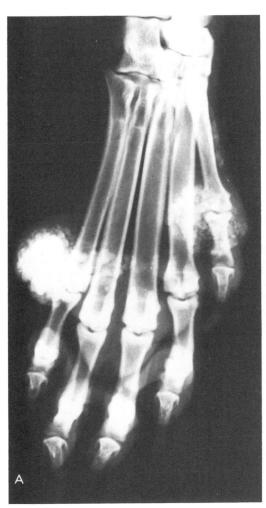
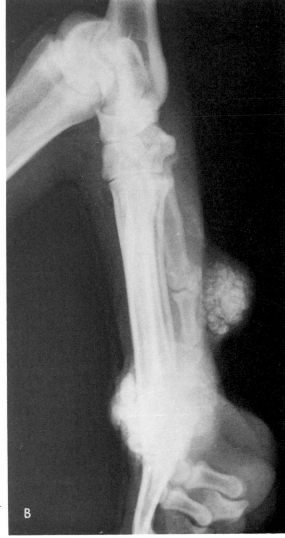

FIGURE 6–2. *A, B.* Lesions of calcinosis circumscripta.

as in patent ductus arteriosus or ventricular septal defect, or they may be peripheral. Peripheral fistulas may be congenital or acquired as the result of injury. While peripheral arteriovenous fistulas have been reported in dogs and cats, they are uncommon. Large fistulas may be painful and cause lameness if present on the limbs. Small fistulas may present as painless warm swellings. Pulsation is often a feature. Large fistulas in time produce compensatory cardiac changes.

Radiologically, arteriovenous fistulas on the limbs may cause alterations in the trabecular pattern of bones in the neighborhood. The changes seen are localized and nonspecific. The trabecular pattern becomes coarse. The vascular bed can be demonstrated by arteriography. (Fig. 6–3 and Fig. 4–43).

Fascial Planes

The fascial planes between muscles are frequently visible on radiographs because of the fat present in the connective tissue between the muscles. The use of a bright light assists in seeing them. If the fascial planes are of particular interest a soft tissue technique is used to demonstrate them. Air may be injected into the subcutaneous fascia from where it will spread to the intermuscular fascial planes and be visible radiographically.

Displacement of fascial planes is of diagnostic significance, for example displacement of the fascial plane usually visible caudal to the stifle joint indicates swelling of the joint capsule of the stifle joint. The infrapatellar fat pad may lose its radiolucency if intracapsular edema or hemorrhage is present. (Fig. 6–4).

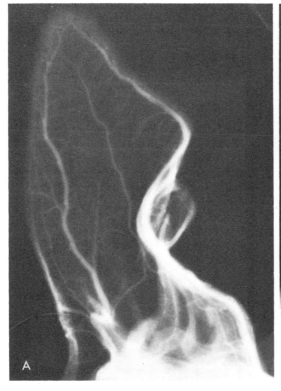

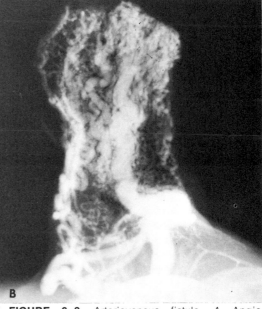

FIGURE 6–3. Arteriovenous fistula. *A.* Angiographic demonstration of the normal vascular pattern of the ear of a dog. *B.* Numerous abnormal vessels are present in the ear owing to an arteriovenous fistula. (Courtesy of the Editor of the Journal of the American Veterinary Radiology Society.)

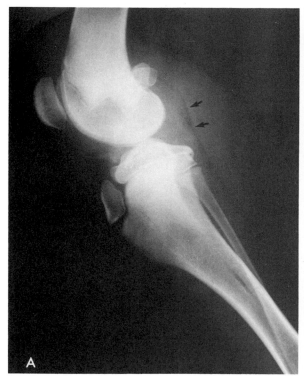

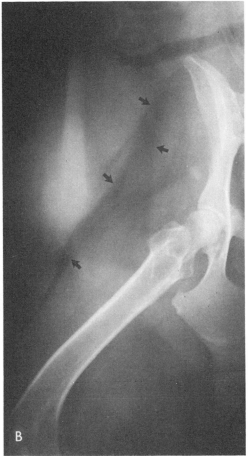

FIGURE 6–4. *A.* Displacement of the fascial plane (arrows) caudal to the stifle joint. This is indicative of swelling of the joint capsule and caudal displacement of the gastrocnemius muscle. *B.* Displacement of the fascial planes (arrows) in the thigh due to swelling of the vastus lateralis muscle. The cause was an undifferentiated sarcoma in the muscle.

Soft Tissue

Swelling of the soft tissue or soft tissue masses is frequently seen on radiographs. More detailed information is usually obtained by clinical examination. Emphysema is seen as gas shadows within the soft tissues or under the skin. Gas densities are seen within the soft tissues following puncture of the skin. Air shadows are seen within the soft tissues following surgery. Radiopaque foreign bodies in soft tissues are seen on radiographs.

Soft tissue masses may be recognized because they displace adjacent organs, for example a retropharyngeal mass will displace the larynx ventrally, a thyroid mass will displace the cervical trachea ventrally.

More specific details concerning soft tissue shadows are given in the earlier chapters. (Fig. 6–5).

Sinus and Fistula

A sinus tract is a blind purulent tract that shows no tendency to heal. The cause is often a foreign body. A fistulous tract is a communication between two

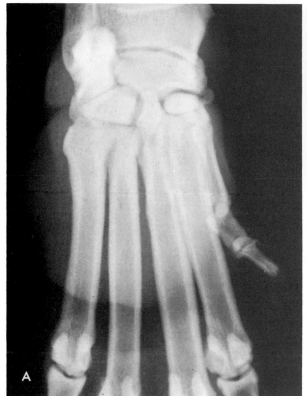

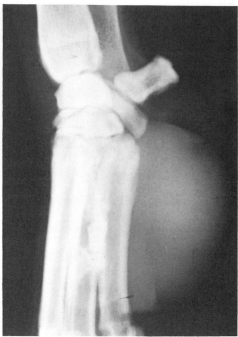

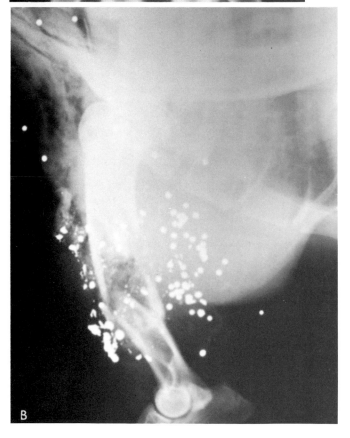

FIGURE 6–5. *A.* A large soft tissue mass is visible on both the lateral and dorso-volar views. The lesion was caused by a bite wound. *B.* Numerous shot grains are present in the shoulder region. Air has entered the soft tissues and is visible as dark shadows in the ventral neck and cranial to the shoulder.

body cavities or between a body cavity and the exterior. A fistulous tract is lined by epithelium. The terms sinus and fistula are often used interchangeably.

A tract may be visible on a radiograph because of gas (air) within it. A sinus tract may be outlined by injecting contrast medium into it. The procedure is frequently unsatisfactory in demonstrating the full extent of the tract. Such tracts regularly have many ramifications, not all of which are patent at any one time. Furthermore, it is difficult to inject the contrast medium under pressure to ensure that the entire tract is outlined. The contrast medium may outline a radiolucent foreign body.

A fistulous tract may be outlined by introducing contrast medium into an affected body cavity, for example barium in the esophagus will demonstrate an esophageal fistula.

Lymphography

Lymph nodes and ducts can be demonstrated radiographically following injection of contrast medium into the lymphatic system either through a lymph vessel or directly into a lymph node. Oily or water-soluble agents are used. The oily agents may persist in the lymphatic system for several months, while aqueous agents are absorbed within a few hours. Lymphography may be used to demonstrate chyloascites, chylothorax, and lymph node enlargement in lymphadenopathy or neoplasia. Its use is contraindicated in local infections near the site of the injection or inflammatory pulmonary disease because of the danger of embolization. Its use in veterinary practice is limited.

REFERENCES

Barrett, R. B. (1971). Radiography in trauma of the musculocutaneous soft tissues of dogs and cats. J.A.V.R.S. XII. 5.

Cotchin, E. (1960). Calcium gout (kalkgicht) and calcinosis circumscripta in dogs. Br. Vet. J. 116. 3.

Douglas, S. W. and Kelly, D. F. (1966). Calcinosis circumscripta of the tongue. J. Sm. Anim. Pract. 7. 441.

Ettinger, S., Campbell, L., Suter, P. F., DeAngelis, M. and Butler, H. (1968). Peripheral arteriovenous fistula in a dog. J.A.V.M.A. 153, 1055.

Kealy, J. K., Lucey, M. and Rhodes, W. H. (1970). Arteriovenous fistula in the ear of a dog. J.A.V.R.S. XI. 15.

Legendre, A. M. and Dade, A. W. (1974). Calcinosis circumscripta in a dog. J.A.V.M.A. 164. 12. 1192.

Meschan, I. (1966). Roentgen Signs in Clinical Practice. W. B. Saunders Co. Philadelphia.

Morgan, Joe P. (1972). Radiology in Veterinary Orthopedics. Lea and Febiger. Philadelphia.

Morgan, J. P., Silverman, S. and Zontine, W. J. (1977). Veterinary Radiography. 2nd ed. The Printer. Davis, California.

O'Brien, T. R. (1978). Radiographic Diagnosis of Abdominal Disorders in the Dog and Cat. W. B. Saunders Co. Philadelphia.

Rubin, L. F. and Patterson, D. F. (1965). Arteriovenous fistula of the orbit in a dog. Cornell Vet. 55. 471.

Slocum, B., Colgrove, D. J., Carrig, C. B. and Suter, P. F. (1973). Acquired arteriovenous fistula in two cats. J.A.V.M.A. 162, 271.

Suter, P. F., Gourley, I. M. and Rhode, E. A. (1971). Arteriovenous fistula of the temporal branches of the external carotid artery in a dog. J.A.V.M.A. 158. 349.

Suter, P. F. (1975). Diseases of the Peripheral Vessels. In Textbook of Veterinary Internal Medicine. Diseases of the Dog and Cat. S. J. Ettinger. Editor. W. B. Saunders Co. Philadelphia.

INDEX

Page numbers in *italics* refer to illustrations; (t) indicates tables.

S

T